WORKBOOK

Radiographic Image Analysis

second edition

Radiographic Image Analysis

Kathy McQuillen Martensen, MS, RT(R)

Director, Radiologic Technology Education
University of Iowa Hospitals and Clinics
Iowa City, Iowa

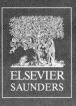

ELSEVIER
SAUNDERS

ELSEVIER
SAUNDERS

11830 Westline Industrial Drive
St. Louis, Missouri 63146

EXERCISES IN RADIOGRAPHIC IMAGE ANALYSIS

ISBN-13: 978-1-4160-2500-9
ISBN-10: 1-4160-2500-6

Publisher: Andrew Allen
Acquisitions Editor: Jeanne Wilke
Senior Developmental Editor: Linda Woodard
Publishing Services Manager: Patricia Tannian
Project Manager: Sarah Wunderly
Design Direction: Kathi Gosche

Printed in United States

Last digit is the print number: 9 8 7 6 5 4 3

This workbook has been designed to provide students with a means of testing his or her understanding of the information covered in *Radiographic Image Analysis*. It follows the same format as the textbook, which guides the student through the image-analysis process of each body structure in a systematic fashion. The text can be followed as written or the student may skip from chapter to chapter or procedure to procedure.

The workbook provides the following features for each chapter in the text

• **Learning objectives** that outline key issues within the chapter and indicate the knowledge the student should understand after the chapter is studied.

• **Study questions** that separately focus on each topic and procedure in the chapter. The questions first focus on how the patient should be positioned to obtain an accurately positioned image and what features are present when proper positioning has been obtained. The focus then shifts to questions that describe improperly positioned images. The student is asked to state how the patient was mispositioned to obtain such an image.

• **Poorly positioned images** that separately focus on each topic and procedure. Most of the images are different from those found in the text and present multiple positioning problems. Trauma scenarios and images are also presented.

• **Answer keys** to the study questions.

This workbook can be used with textbooks other than *Radiographic Image Analysis,* although the contents between these other textbooks and the workbook should be closely coordinated.

KMM

Prerequisite: It is suggested that a course in anatomy and basic medical terminology be taken prior to studying radiographic procedures and analysis. For best understanding, it is effective to study the radiographic procedure in conjunction with the analysis.

Guideline 1 Read the chapter learning objectives. These objectives outline key issues within the chapter and identify the knowledge you should understand after the chapter has been studied.

Guideline 2 Read the corresponding chapter in *Radiographic Image Analysis*, attend the procedure and analysis courses that focus on the subject matter.

Guideline 3 Fill in as many of the study question blanks as you can without referring to the textbook or the workbook answer key. The blanks you were unable to complete indicate the areas that require further study. Restudy the information that was covered in questions for which you left blank answers or were uncertain of the correct answer.

Guideline 4 Check your study question answers with the answers provided at the end of the chapter. Restudy the information covered in any questions you answered incorrectly.

Guideline 5 Consult with your instructor about taking a final examination.

CONTENTS

CHAPTER 1

Guidelines for Image Analysis

LEARNING OBJECTIVES

After completion of this chapter you should be able to:

_____ 1. Define the positioning, body plane, and general and technical terminology used in radiography.

_____ 2. State the characteristics of an optimal image.

_____ 3. Properly hang on the view box hard copy radiographs and present digital images on the cathode ray tube (CRT) monitor of any body structure.

_____ 4. State the information that is permanently imprinted onto the film's emulsion or displayed on the CRT monitor and why this information is required.

_____ 5. Describe how to determine the best place to position the identification plate on images of any body structure.

_____ 6. Discuss how to accurately mark images of any body structure.

_____ 7. Describe how to determine if an image is mismarked.

_____ 8. Explain the procedure to be followed if a radiograph has been mismarked or the marker is only faintly seen.

_____ 9. Identify differing degrees of patient obliquity when positioning a patient.

_____ 10. Identify differing degrees of patient flexion when positioning a patient and on images.

_____ 11. Explain how the centering of the central ray and x-ray beam divergence affect where structures are projected onto the image receptor (IR).

_____ 12. List the guidelines for performing mobile and trauma images.

_____ 13. State how technical factors should be adjusted to adapt for different mobile and trauma-related conditions.

_____ 14. List and define the different types of shape distortion that can be demonstrated on an image, and describe how they are obtained.

_____ 15. State how similarly appearing structures can be identified on an image.

_____ 16. Determine the amount of patient or central ray adjustment that is required when poorly positioned images are obtained.

_____ 17. Define size distortion and state how it is caused.

_____ 18. Explain the procedures taken to obtain sharply defined bony cortical outlines and soft-tissue structures on images.

_____ 19. Define voluntary and involuntary motion and discuss procedures that can be taken to avoid each on an image.

_____ 20. Identify images demonstrating motion, double exposure, and poor screen-film contact.

_____ 21. Discuss why good collimation practices are necessary, and list the guidelines to follow to assure good collimation.

_____ 22. State the situations in which gonadal shielding is recommended.

_____ 23. State the female and male gonadal structures that are shielded and describe their location.

_____ 24. Demonstrate how to properly position female and male gonadal shielding.

_____ 25. State and describe the three basic body types. Explain how the IR direction is adjusted to accommodate each type on chest and abdominal images and identify each on chest and abdominal images.

_____ 26. Discuss how to determine if an image is adequately exposed and penetrated.

_____ 27. Identify images that have been overexposed, underexposed, and underpenetrated. State what technical factor is adjusted and how much adjustment is required.

_____ 28. Describe how to accurately position the patient when using the automatic exposure controls.

_____ 29. Describe the digital radiography normalization process. Indicate when an image has been overexposed or underexposed.

_____ 30. State the guidelines to follow to obtain the most accurate digital image normalization.

_____ 31. Explain how an overexposed, underexposed, or underpenetrated image can result when the automatic exposure controls are used.

_____ 32. State the purpose of a compensating filter and describe how it should be positioned.

_____ 33. Describe the anode-heel effect, and state how it can be used to obtain uniform density on images that use a long 17-inch (43-cm) field size.

_____ 34. Identify images with high and low contrast. State how image contrast can be adjusted.

_____ 35. Explain why pediatric images demonstrate lower image contrast than adult images.

_____ 36. State how scatter radiation affects an image and how it can be controlled.

_____ 37. List and describe the different artifact categories. Give an example of an artifact that could be found under each category.

_____ 38. Discuss what items on the patient's requisition the technologist completes.

_____ 39. Define the difference between an optimal and an acceptable image.

STUDY QUESTIONS

1. An optimal image demonstrates what seven characteristics?

   A. _____

   B. _____

   C. _____

   D. _____

   E. _____

   F. _____

   G. _____

2. Use the lateral chest drawing in Figure 1-1 to complete the following statements.

Figure 1–1

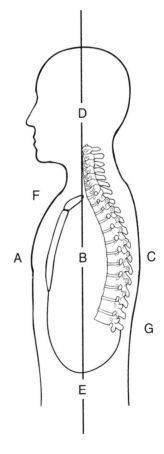

A. Letter B is situated on the _____ plane.

B. Letter A is placed _____ to letter B.

C. Letter C is placed _____ to letter B.

D. Letter D is placed _____ to letter B.

E. Letter E is placed _____ to letter B.

F. Letter F is placed _____ to letter B.

G. Letter G is placed _____ to letter B.

3. The inferior scapular angle moves toward the front and outer edge of the body when the humerus is abducted. What combination of the positioning terms is used to describe this movement? _____

4. When the humerus is brought from an abducted position to the patient's side, the inferior scapular angle moves toward the patient's back and closer to the midsagittal plane. What combination of the positioning terms is used to describe this movement?

_____

5. What combination of the positioning terms is used to describe the portion of the scapula that is positioned closest to the patient's front and head? _____

6. If the IR was placed against the lateral aspect of the patient's leg and the central ray was centered to the medial aspect, what projection of the leg was taken? _____

7. Use the abdominal drawing in Figure 1-2 to complete the following statements.

Figure 1–2

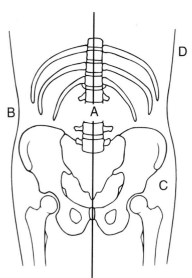

A. Letter A is situated on the _____ plane.

B. Letter B is placed _____ to letter A.

C. Letter A is placed _____ to letter B.

D. Letter C is placed _____ to letter A.

E. Letter D is placed _____ to letter A.

8. Use the drawing of the knee in Figure 1-3 to complete the following statements.

Figure 1–3

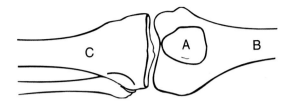

A. Letter B is placed _____ to letter A.

B. Letter C is placed _____ to letter A.

9. Circle the terms below that are projections.
anteroinferior
anteroposterior
posteroanterior
posteromedian
inferosuperior
anterolateral
anterosuperior
posteroinferior
posterosuperior
superoinferior
anteromedian
mediolateral
posterolateral
lateromedial

10. Use the positioning, body plane, and general and technical terminology or forms derived from these words, found in Chapter 1 of *Radiographic Critique*, to complete the crossword puzzle shown in Figure 1-4.

Figure 1–4

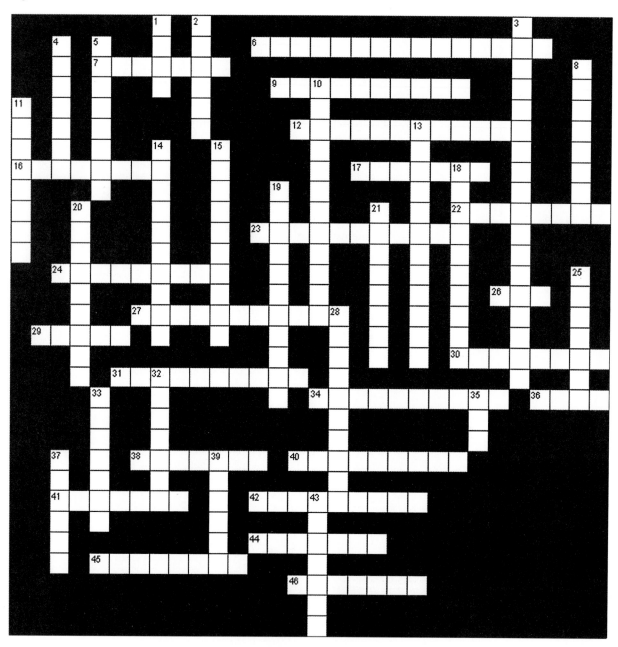

Across Clues:

6 Two structures on top of each other on an image.

7 Position where structure is rotated from a posteroanterior (PA) projection.

9 An object that prevents radiation from passing through it.

12 A joint.

16 Act of turning the plantar foot surface as far laterally as the ankle will allow.

17 Act of positioning the hand so the palm is turned down toward the IR.

22 Gown snap on an image.

23 To decrease the size of one axis of a structure.

24 Position in which patient lies on cart and a horizontal beam is used.
26 Acronym used to describe the distance from the source to the IR.
27 An object that allows radiation to pass through it.
29 To arrange the third metacarpal and forearm in a line.
30 Rotation used to describe the act of turning the anterior surface of a limb away from the torso.
31 Positioning the hand so the palm is turned up.
34 Ability to distinguish individual details from one another on an image.
36 Act of making a fist with the hand.
38 Backward movement of the jaw.
40 Act of locating a structure by feeling it through the skin.
41 Amount of darkness on an image.
42 Act of turning the plantar foot surface as far medially as the ankle will allow.
44 Position where the patient's side is placed adjacent to the IR.
45 To increase the size of one axis of a structure.
46 To equally increase the size of both axes of a structure.

Down Clues:
1 Device placed between the patient and IR to reduce scatter radiation reaching the IR.
2 Foot end of the patient.
3 An absorbing substance that removes photons from the beam to even out image density.
4 Shape of a structure that is rounded outward.
5 Number of gray shades that represent the structures on an image.
8 Head end of the patient.
10 The act of moving the toes and forefoot upward.
11 Rotation used to describe the act of turning the anterior surface of a limb toward the torso.
13 Axis that refers to the longest part of a structure.
14 Position that is the starting point from which image procedures are referenced.
15 To move the shoulders downward.
18 Axis that runs at a 90-degree angle to the longitudinal axis.
19 Forward movement of the jaw.
20 Act of unflexing the knee.
21 Outline of the medial femoral condyle on an image.
25 To move away from the normal or routine.
28 Pattern of cancellous bone's supporting material as seen on an image.
32 Movement of a structure that results from an angled central ray.
33 Plate used in computed radiography to receive the image.
35 Acronym used to describe the distance from the object to the IR.
37 Act of moving the arm laterally, away from the body.
39 Act of moving the arm toward the body.
43 To move the distal femur to a higher position.

11. State the distances indicated in Figure 1-5.

Figure 1–5

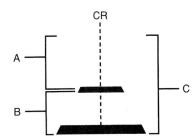

A. _____

B. _____

C. _____

12. Use the following (1 to 6) to define how hard copy radiographs of the listed body parts are accurately hung on the view box.

   1. Hanging as if the patient were standing upright
   2. Hanging from the fingertips
   3. Hanging from the shoulders
   4. Hanging from the toes
   5. Hanging from the hip
   6. Hanging from the anterior surface

A. _____ Chest

B. _____ Wrist

C. _____ Lumbar vertebrae

D. _____ Humerus

E. _____ Toes

F. _____ Oblique foot

G. _____ Lateral foot

H. _____ Ankle

I. _____ Lower leg

J. _____ AP hip

K. _____ Axiolateral shoulder

L. _____ Cervical vertebrae

M. _____ Abdomen

13. When an anteroposterior/posteroanterior (AP/PA) projection or oblique position of the torso is accurately hung on the view box, the patient's right side is on the viewer's _____ side.

14. If the image is accurately hung on the view box, will the marker appear correct or reversed for the following projections or positions of the torso?

A. PA projection: _____

B. AP projection: _____

C. Posterior oblique position: _____

D. Lateral position: _____

E. Anterior oblique position: _____

15. A. What marker is used for a patient that is placed in a right anterior oblique (RAO) position? _____

B. Where is the marker placed on the IR in reference to the patient? _____

16. A right lateral vertebral image is requested.

A. What marker is used for a patient in this position? _____

B. Where is the marker placed on the IR in reference to the patient? _____

17. Evaluate the following images for displaying (hanging) accuracy.

Figure 1–6

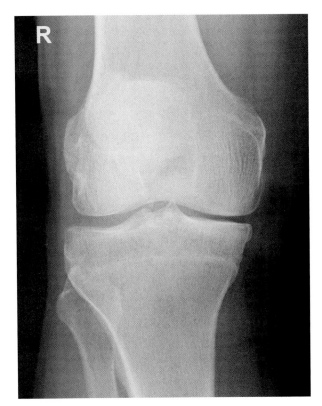

A. AP knee (Figure 1-6): _____

_____

Figure 1–7

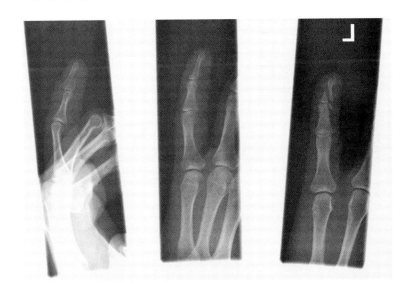

B. Left finger (Figure 1-7): _____

_____

C. Left lateral lumbar vertebrae (Figure 1-8): _____

Figure 1–8

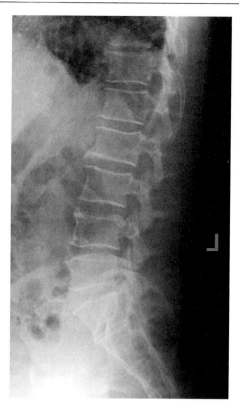

D. AP right forearm (Figure 1-9):_____

Figure 1–9

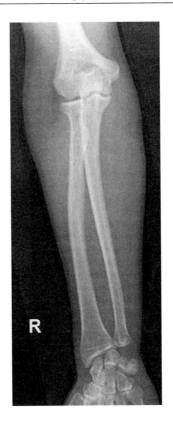

E. Mediolateral projection left foot (Figure 1-10): _____

Figure 1–10

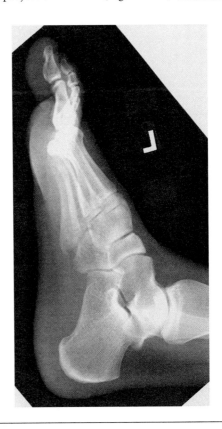

F. LPO lumbar vertebrae (Figure 1-11): _____

Figure 1–11

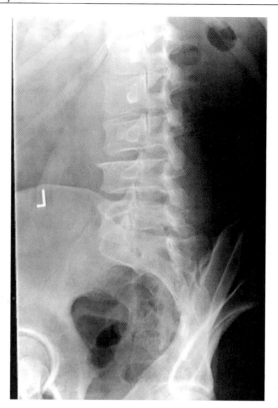

18. Evaluate the following images for marker placement accuracy.

A. AP lumbar vertebrae (Figure 1-12): _____

Figure 1–12

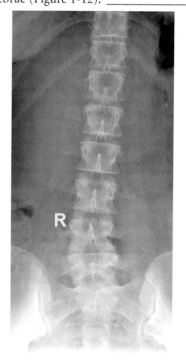

B. AP left hip (Figure 1-13): _____

Figure 1–13

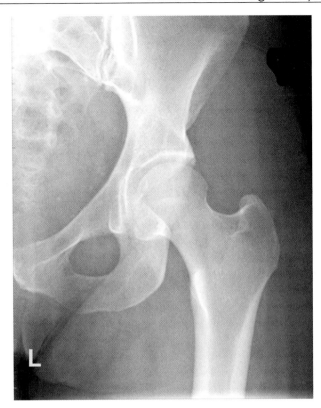

C. AP left shoulder (Figure 1-14): _____

Figure 1–14

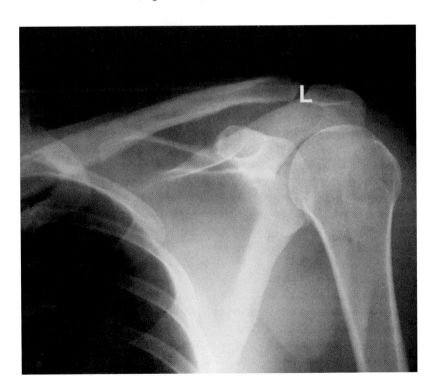

D. AP left lower ribs (Figure 1-15): _____

Figure 1–15

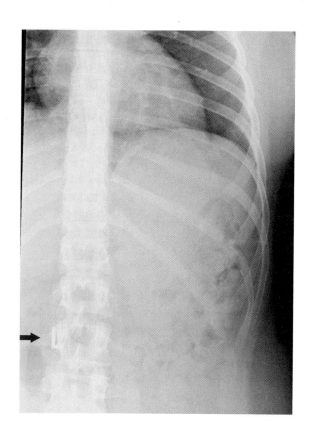

E. AP scapula (Figure 1-16): _____

Figure 1–16

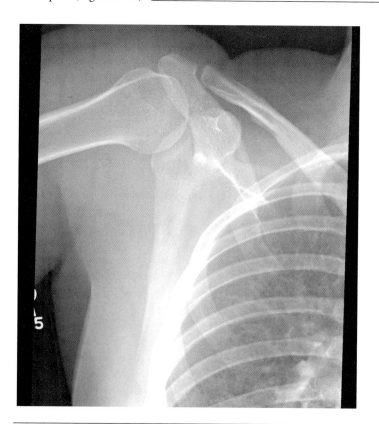

19. List the information that should be permanently photoflashed onto the ID plate or displayed on the CRT monitor.

A. _____

B. _____

C. _____

D. _____

E. _____

F. _____

20. State the guidelines that are followed when determining the best location to position the identification plate.

A. _____

B. _____

C. _____

21. The markers used in radiography are constructed of (A) _____ and are (B) _____ (radiolucent/radiopaque).

22. The marker placed on a lateral image of the torso or skull represents the side of the patient that is positioned _____ (closer to/farther from) the IR.

23. Place an R where the marker should be positioned on the hip diagram in Figure 1-17.

24. Place an L where the marker should be positioned on the lateral sacral diagram in Figure 1-18.

Figure 1-17

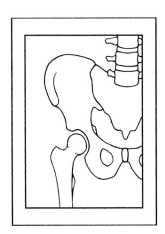

25. How is the image marked when a patient is placed in an oblique position (left posterior oblique [LPO], right posterior oblique

Figure 1–18

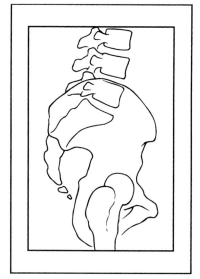

[RAO])? _____

_____

26. What procedure is followed if the marker has not been demonstrated within the collimated field but is faintly seen along its border?

_____

_____

_____

27. Estimate the degree of patient obliquity demonstrated in the diagrams in Figure 1-19.

   A. _____ degrees

   B. _____ degrees

   C. _____ degrees

   D. _____ degrees

   E. _____ degrees

28. Estimate the degree of elbow or knee flexion demonstrated on Figures 1-20 to 1-23.

Figure 1–19

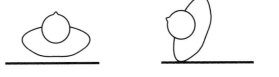

A. _____   B. _____   C. _____

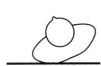

D. _____   E. _____

A. _____ degrees (Figure 1-20)

Figure 1–20

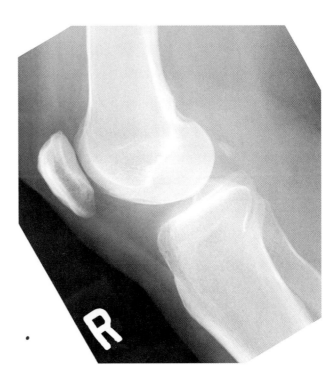

B. _____ degrees (Figure 1-21)

Figure 1–21

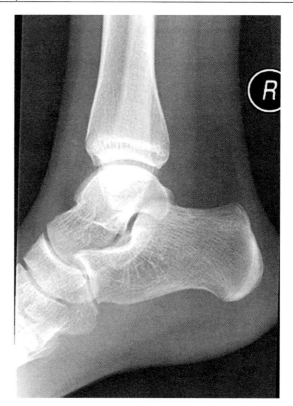

C. _____ degrees (Figure 1-22)

Figure 1–22

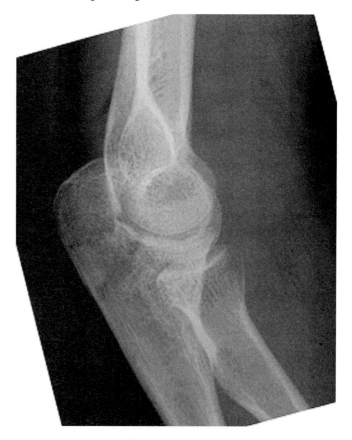

D. _____ degrees (Figure 1-23)

Figure 1–23

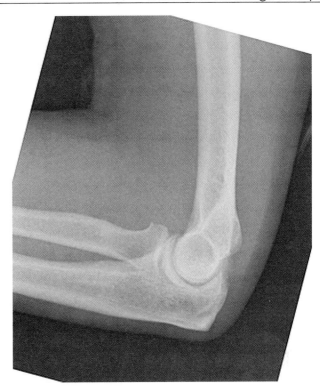

29. Use the lateral knee diagram in Figure 1-24 to answer the following questions.

Figure 1–24

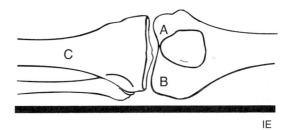

A. If a perpendicular central ray was centered to letter A on the knee diagram, where would letter A be positioned in reference to letter B on the resulting radiographic image?

_____

B. If a perpendicular central ray was centered to the letter C on the knee diagram, where would letter A be positioned in reference to letter B on the resulting image?

(1) _____

Will both letter A and letter B be projected the same distance?

(2) _____ (Yes/No)

Defend your answer.

(3) _____

_____

C. If the central ray was angled 15 degrees caudally and centered to letter A on the knee diagram, where would letter A be positioned in reference to letter B on the image?

(1) _____

How would the image change if the central ray angulation was increased to 45 degrees?

(2) _____

D. If the central ray was angled 15 degrees caudally and centered to letter C on the knee diagram, where would letter A be positioned in reference to letter B on the image?

_____

_____

30. State the goals for performing mobile and trauma imaging.

_____

_____

31. To obtain accurately positioned trauma and mobile images the central ray-part-IR must remain in the same alignment as if the image was taken under routine positioning situations. State what the part is for the following images.

A. Lateral hand: _____

B. AP elbow: _____

C. Lateral chest: _____

D. External oblique knee: _____

E. Towne cranium: _____

32. Complete the technical adjustments for the situations listed in Table 1-1.

TABLE 1-1 **Trauma Chart**		
Casts, Splints, Backboards or Patient Condition	**kVp Adjustment**	**mAs Adjustment**
Small to medium plaster cast		
Large plaster cast		
Fiberglass cast		
Inflated air splint		
Wood backboard		
Ascites (invasion of fluid into abdomen or swelled joint)		
Pleural effusion (fluid in pleural cavity)		
Pneumothorax (fluid within lungs)		
Postmortem imaging of head, thorax, and abdomen (resulting from pooling of blood and fluid)		
Soft tissue (used for foreign objects, such as slivers of wood, glass, or metal imbedded in the soft tissue, and to demonstrate the upper airway)		

33. To minimize shape distortion on an image, keep the part positioned (A) _____to the IR and the central ray (B) _____ to both the part and IR.

34. List the two types of shape distortion.

A. _____

B. _____

35. Which type of shape distortion will result in one axis of the part appearing disproportionately longer on the image than the opposite axis?

_____

36. For the central ray, part, and IR setups in Figure 1-25, state the type of shape distortion that will result.

Figure 1–25

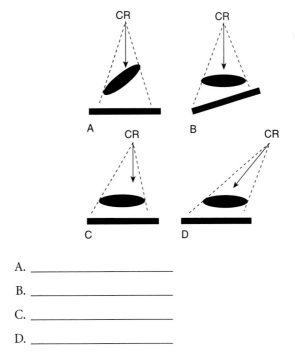

A. _____

B. _____

C. _____

D. _____

37. Figure 1-26 demonstrates a PA finger image with closed interphalangeal (IP) joints and foreshortened middle and distal phalanges. The patient was unable to fully extend the finger for the examination. Explain how the central ray and part should be positioned to obtain open IR joints and demonstrate the phalanges without foreshortening.

Figure 1–26

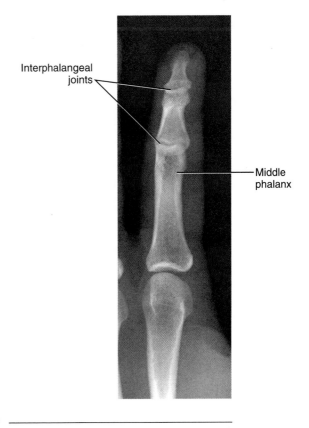

A. _____

Explain how the technologist would have to adjust the central ray to obtain open interphalangeal (IP) joints and nonforeshortened phalanges if the patient was unable to adjust the hand.

B. _____

_____

38. List three ways of identifying similarly appearing structures from one another on an image.

A. _____

B. _____

C. _____

39. If two structures are demonstrated without superimposition on a mispositioned image and they should be superimposed on an accurately positioned image of this projection or position, how does one determine how much to adjust the patient to obtain an optimal image, if both structures move in opposite directions when adjusted?

A. _____

_____

If only one structure moved when the patient was adjusted?

B. _____

_____

40. An angled central ray projects the structure situated (A) _____ (closer to/farther from) the IR farther than a structure situated (B) _____ (closer/farther) to/from the IR.

41. Figure 1-27 demonstrates an accurately and poorly positioned lateral hand image. On the poorly positioned image, the fifth metacarpal is situated 1 inch (2.5 cm) anterior to the second through fourth metacarpals. The second through fifth metacarpals should be superimposed on an optimal lateral hand image. The physical distance between the second and fifth metacarpals is 2½ inches (6.25 cm).

Figure 1–27

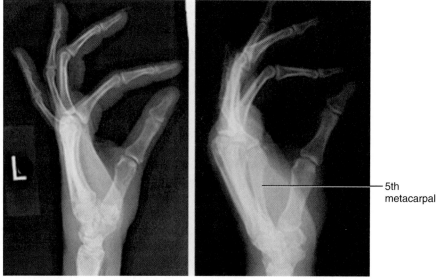

5th metacarpal

Accurate positioning

A. State how and by how much the patient's positioning could be adjusted to obtain an optimal image. The second and fifth metacarpals will move in opposite directions from each other when the hand is rotated.

_____

B. State how the central ray could be directed toward the hand and the amount of angulation needed to obtain an optimal image if the patient was unable to adjust positioning.

_____

_____

_____

42. Figure 1-28 demonstrates an accurately and a poorly positioned lateral knee image. On the poorly positioned image the lateral femoral condyle is situated 2 inches (5 cm) anterior to the medial femoral condyle. The condyles should be superimposed on an optimal lateral knee image. The physical distance between the femoral condyles is 2½ inches (6.25 cm).

Figure 1–28

Medial condyle

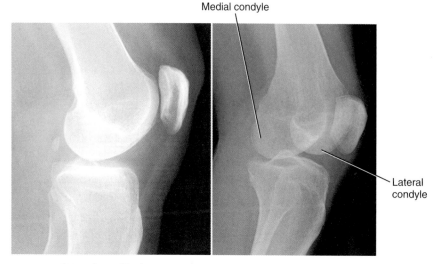

Lateral condyle

Accurate positioning

A. State how and by how much the patient's positioning could be adjusted to obtain an optimal image. The lateral and medial condyles will move in opposite directions from each other when the knee is rotated.

_____

B. State how the central ray could be directed toward the knee and the amount of angulation needed to obtain an optimal image if the patient was unable to adjust positioning.

_____

_____

_____

43. Figure 1-29 demonstrates an accurately and a poorly positioned lateral ankle image. On the poorly positioned image the lateral talar dome is situated ¼ inch (0.6 cm) posterior to the medial dome. The talar domes should be superimposed on an optimal lateral ankle image. The physical distance between the talar domes is 1 inch (2.5 cm).

Figure 1–29

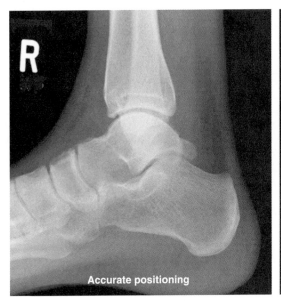
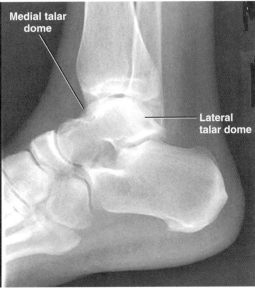

A. State how and by how much the patient's positioning could be adjusted to obtain an optimal image. The lateral and medial talar domes will move in opposite directions from each other when the ankle is rotated.

_____

B. State how the central ray could be directed toward the ankle and the amount of angulation needed to obtain an optimal image if the patient was unable to adjust positioning.

_____

_____

_____

44. Figure 1-30 demonstrates images of a humeral bone that has been size and shape distorted. Identify the type of distortion demonstrated on each image. If you identify elongation or foreshortening, state the aspect of the bone (proximal or distal humerus) that was positioned farther from the IR.

Figure 1–30

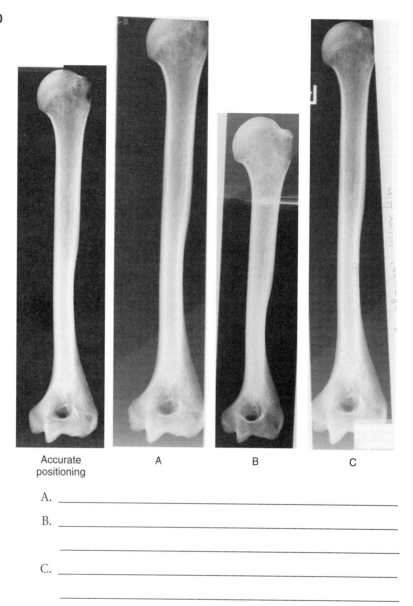

Accurate positioning   A   B   C

A. _____

B. _____

_____

C. _____

_____

45. The image of the lower leg diagrammed in Figure 1-31 will demonstrate what type of distortion?

Figure 1–31

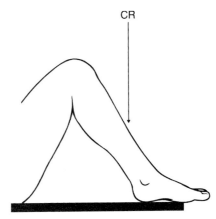

A. _____

Will the image be elongated or foreshortened?

B. _____

46. The image of the foot diagrammed in Figure 1-32 will demonstrate what type of distortion?

Figure 1–32

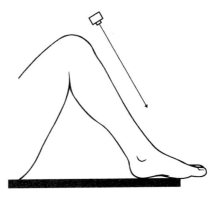

A. _____

Will the image be elongated or foreshortened?

B. _____

47. Which of the following images will have the greater image magnification? _____

Image 1 was exposed at a 72-inch source–image receptor distance (SID) and a 3-inch object–image receptor distance (OID).

Image 2 was exposed at a 72-inch SID and a 4-inch OID.

48. Which of the following images will have the greater image magnification? _____

Image 1 was exposed at a 72-inch SID and a 2-inch OID.

Image 2 was exposed at a 40-inch SID and a 2-inch OID.

49. A (A) _____ (large/small) focal spot size is used for fine detail demonstration because a detail that is (B) _____ (larger/smaller) than the focal spot size used to produce the image will not be demonstrated.

50. Define voluntary motion. _____

51. Define involuntary motion. _____

52. List four ways in which voluntary motion can be controlled.

    A. _____

    B. _____

    C. _____

    D. _____

53. When can normal voluntary motion be considered involuntary motion?

    _____

54. How can abdominal motion that is involuntary be controlled?

    _____

55. How can voluntary and involuntary motion be distinguished from each other on a supine abdominal image? _____

    _____

    _____

56. State whether the following situations are examples of voluntary or involuntary motions.

    A. The patient was extremely short of breath because of asthma and unable to hold it.

       _____

    B. After being in a car accident, the patient being imaged was unable to stop shaking.

       _____

57. How can a double-exposed film/screen image be distinguished from a film/screen image that has motion?

    _____

    _____

58. State whether the following images demonstrate motion or double-exposure.

Figure 1–33

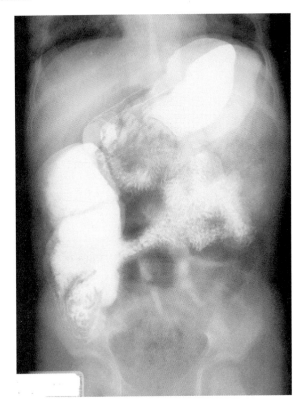

A. Figure 1-33: _____

Figure 1–34

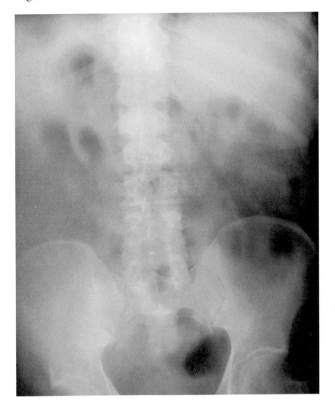

B. Figure 1-34: _____

Figure 1–35

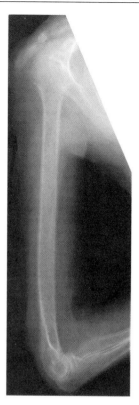

C. Figure 1-35: _____

59. How can one distinguish between poor screen-film contact and patient motion?

_____

_____

60. To prevent magnification on an image, the anatomical structure of interest is positioned as _____ (close to/far away from) the IR as possible.

61. List how an anatomical structure can be magnified.

    A. _____

    B. _____

62. Which of the following images will have the sharpest recorded details? _____

    Image 1 was exposed at a 40-inch SID and a 3-inch OID.

    Image 2 was exposed at a 72-inch SID and a 3-inch OID.

63. To obtain the greatest spatial resolution when using computed radiography, the _____ IR size should be selected.

64. How can the placement of the central ray be determined on an image?

_____

_____

65. Good collimation practices (A) _____ (increase/decrease) patient dosage and (B) _____ (increase/decrease) the visibility of recorded details and image contrast by reducing the amount of (C) _____ that reaches the IR.

66. The collimator's light field that is demonstrated on the patient's abdomen in Figure 1-36 measures 8 × 10 inches (18 × 24 cm). Does this mean that the IR placed in the Bucky needs to be only 8 × 10 inches, or should it be larger or smaller?

Figure 1–36

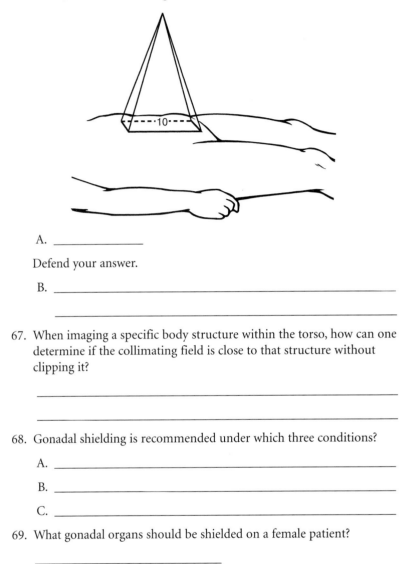

A. _____

Defend your answer.

B. _____

_____

67. When imaging a specific body structure within the torso, how can one determine if the collimating field is close to that structure without clipping it?

_____

_____

68. Gonadal shielding is recommended under which three conditions?

A. _____

B. _____

C. _____

69. What gonadal organs should be shielded on a female patient?

_____

70. Draw a shield on the female pelvic diagram in Figure 1-37 to indicate proper shield placement for the female patient.

Figure 1–37

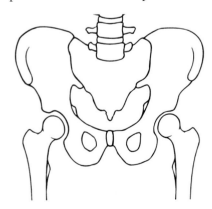

71. Describe how palpable pelvic structures are used to accurately position a flat contact shield on a female patient. _____

_____

72. Why should the size of the contact shield used for protecting the female patient be seriously considered? _____

_____

73. What gonadal organs are shielded on the male patient?

    A. _____

    Where are they located?

    B. _____

74. Approximately where is the top of the shield positioned when shielding the male gonadal organs?

    _____

75. Draw a shaded shield on the male pelvic diagram in Figure 1-38 to indicate proper shield placement for the male patient.

Figure 1–38

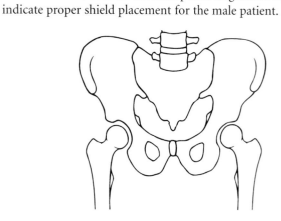

76. Evaluate the female gonadal shielding used on the pelvic image in Figure 1-39.

Figure 1–39

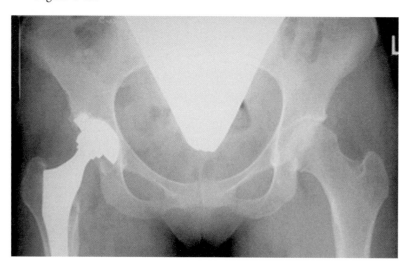

_____

_____

77. Evaluate the pediatric male gonadal shielding used on the femur image in Figure 1-40.

Figure 1–40

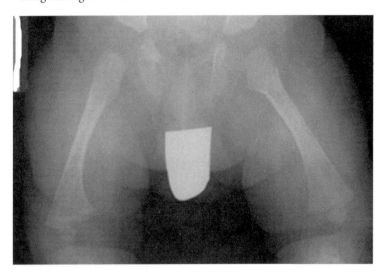

_____

_____

78. State how to shield a patient who is in a lateral position.

_____

_____

79. Radiosensitive cells such as the (A) _____,
    (B) _____, (C) _____, and
    (D) _____ should be shielded whenever they lie within
    (E) _____ inches of the primary beam.

80. The image in Figure 1-41 demonstrates poor radiation protection practices. What type of error is demonstrated?

Figure 1–41

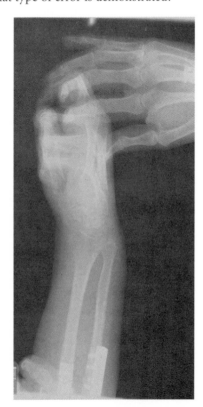

A. _____

How could this examination be taken without this error?

B. _____

_____

81. Describe the shape of the hypersthenic patient's thorax and peritoneal cavity.

A. Thorax: _____

B. Peritoneal cavity: _____

82. Describe the shape of the asthenic patient's thorax and peritoneal cavity.

A. Thorax: _____

B. Peritoneal cavity: _____

83. Identify what body habitus type is being demonstrated in each of the following images.

Figure 1–42

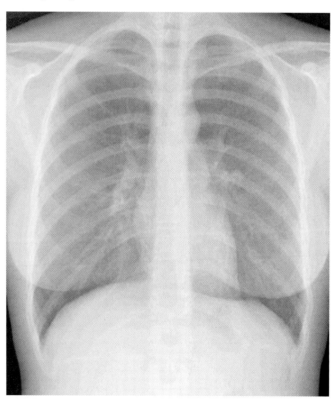

A. Figure 1-42: _____

Figure 1–43

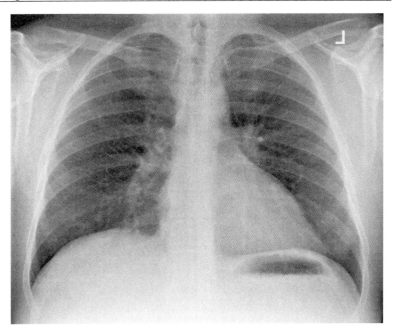

B. Figure 1-43: _____

Figure 1–44

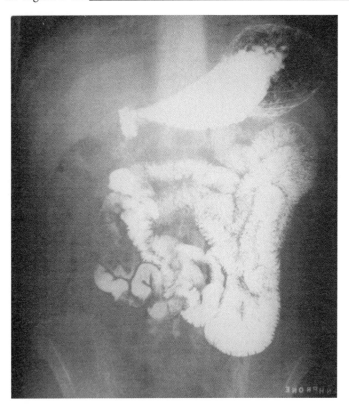

C. Figure 1-44: _____

Figure 1–45

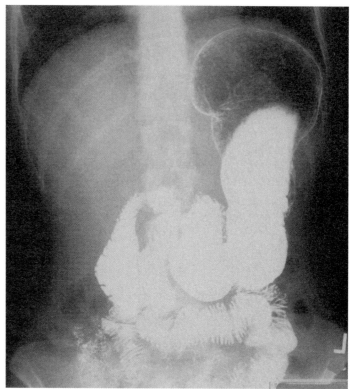

    D. Figure 1-45: _____

84. Is the IR placed crosswise or lengthwise for the following when producing a PA chest image?

    A. Hypersthenic body type: _____

    B. Asthenic body type: _____

85. What technical factor is primarily used to regulate image density?

    _____

86. How can one distinguish an underexposed image from an underpenetrated image? _____

    _____

87. How much mAs adjustment should be made if a conventional screen-film image requires repeating because of poor positioning and the image is slightly darker than optimal but not repeatable because of it?

    _____

88. How much mAs adjustment should be made if a conventional screen-film image definitely requires repeating because the image is too light?

    _____

89. What computed radiography error is demonstrated on the image in Figure 1-46?

Figure 1–46

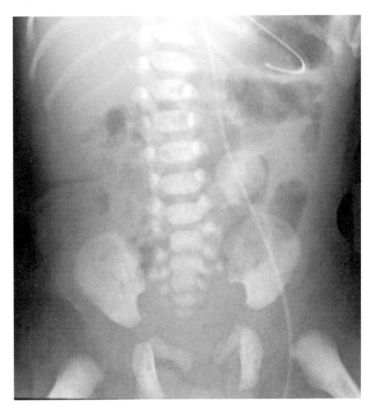

90. Evaluate the density, contrast, and penetration on the image in Figure 1-47. State a new manual technique that should be used to obtain an optimal image.

Figure 1-47: PA wrist; original technique: 60 kVp at 8 mAs

Figure 1–47

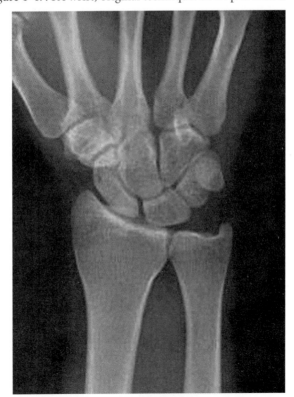

A. Density evaluation: _____

B. Contrast evaluation: _____

C. Penetration evaluation: _____

D. New technique: _____ kVP at _____ mAs

91. Evaluate the density, contrast, and penetration on the image in Figure 1-48. State a new manual technique that should be used to obtain an optimal image.

Figure 1-48: AP knee; original technique: 65 kVp at 5 mAs, nongrid

Figure 1–48

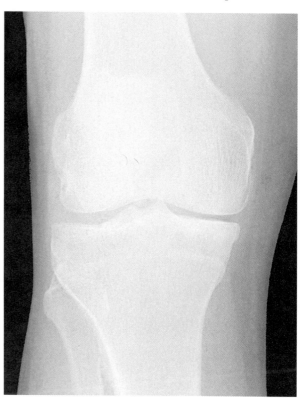

A. Density evaluation: _____

B. Contrast evaluation: _____

C. Penetration evaluation: _____

D. New technique: _____ kVP at _____ mAs

92. Evaluate the density, contrast, and penetration on the image in Figure 1-49. State a new manual technique that should be used to obtain an optimal image.

Figure 1-49: AP lumbar vertebrae; original technique: 85 kVp at 30 mAs, grid was used

Figure 1–49

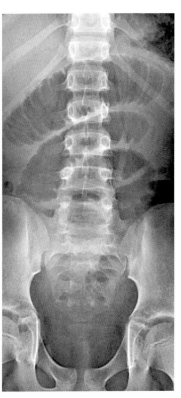

A. Density evaluation: _____

B. Contrast evaluation: _____

C. Penetration evaluation: _____

D. New technique: _____ kVp at _____ mAs

93. Will image contrast and density be adequate on an overexposed computed radiography image?

A. _____

Defend your answer.

B. _____

_____

94. Digital and computed radiography normalization corrections can be made without image degradation with (A) _____ as high as 120% and (B) _____ as low as 60% from the ideal range.

95. Why is it important to investigate the cause of exposure indicator numbers that specify that higher-than-ideal exposure values were used when an image was created with digital radiography?

_____

96. Digital radiography exposure values that result in exposure indicator numbers that specify lower-than-ideal exposure values would have required the normalization process to (A) _____ (increase/decrease) image density and may require repeating because of what image appearance? (B) _____

97. What is the most frequent cause of an underexposed or overexposed image when the automatic exposure controls are used? _____

_____

98. An overexposed image results when the ionization chamber is situated beneath a structure that has a (A) _____ (high/low) atomic number or is (B) _____ or (C) _____ than the structure of interest.

99. List five practices to follow to obtain correct normalization of a digital image.

A. _____

B. _____

C. _____

D. _____

E. _____

100. What technical factor is used to regulate penetration and image contrast?

_____

101. If an image had to be repeated because it was underpenetrated and the density was 100% too light, the kVp should be (A) _____ (increased/decreased) by (B) _____ % to obtain an optimal image.

102. Evaluate the compensating filter placement on the image in Figure 1-50.

Figure 1–50

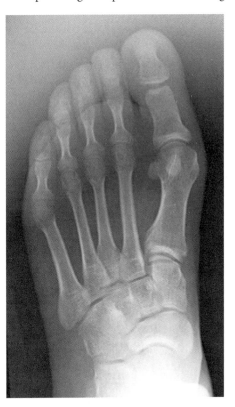

_____

_____

_____

103. Describe anode-heel effect. _____

_____

104. Complete Table 1-2.

TABLE 1-2 **Anode-Heel Positioning**		
Projection(s)	**Placement of Anode**	**Placement of Cathode**
AP and lateral forearm		
AP and lateral humerus		
AP and lateral lower leg		
AP and lateral femur		
AP thoracic vertebrae		
AP lumbar vertebrae		

105. What two factors affect the contrast an image demonstrates?

    A. _____

    B. _____

106. A low-contrast image will demonstrate (A) _____
    (little/great) difference between the shades of gray and results when
    the kVp level is too (B) _____ (high/low).

107. Explain why pediatric images demonstrate less image contrast. _____

_____

11. A. Source-object distance
     B. Object–image receptor distance
     C. Source–image receptor distance
12. A. 1 or 3
     B. 2
     C. 1
     D. 1 or 3
     E. 4
     F. 4
     G. 1 or 5
     H. 1 or 5
     I. 1 or 5
     J. 1 or 5
     K. 6
     L. 1
     M. 1
13. Left
14. A. Reversed
     B. Correct
     C. Correct
     D. Correct
     E. Reversed
15. A. Right
     B. Laterally, adjacent to the patient's right side
16. A. Right
     B. Anteriorly
17. A. The knee image is accurately displayed.
        Marker is correct, and it is accurately displayed
        as if hanging from the patient's hip.
     B. The marker is reversed, indicating that the
        image needs to be flipped horizontally.
        The image is accurately displayed by the
        fingertip.
     C. The marker is reversed, indicating that the
        image needs to be flipped horizontally. The
        image is accurately displayed as if the patient
        were in an upright position.
     D. Forearm images should be displayed as if
        hanging by the fingertips and not the elbow.
        The image is horizontally displayed correctly, as
        indicated by the correctness of the marker.
     E. Lateral feet images should be displayed as if
        hanging from the patient's hip. The image
        should be moved 90 degrees counterclockwise.
        The marker is also reversed and should be cor-
        rect for a lateral foot image. Flip the image hor-
        izontally.
     F. The marker is reversed and should be correct
        for posterior oblique positions. The image
        should be flipped horizontally, with the left
        marker positioned on the viewer's right side.

The image is accurately displayed as if the
patient were in an upright position.
18. A. The marker is situated too medially, superim-
        posing anatomical structures of interest. It
        should remain within the collimated field but
        be moved as far laterally as possible.
     B. The marker is situated at the midsagittal plane.
        It should be placed on the left side of the verte-
        bral column as far laterally as possible, while
        staying within the collimated field.
     C. The marker is superimposed on the shoulder
        anatomy of interest. Move the marker as far
        laterally as possible, while staying within the
        collimated field.
     D. The marker is placed to the right of the verte-
        bral column. It should be placed on the left
        side of the vertebral column as far laterally as
        possible, while staying within the collimated
        field.
     E. The marker is only partially demonstrated.
        Move the marker completely within the colli-
        mated field.
19. A. Facility's name
     B. Patient's name
     C. Patient's age or birth date
     D. Hospital identification number
     E. Date of examination
     F. Time of examination
20. A. Place it outside the collimated field whenever
        possible.
     B. Position it away from the direction in which
        the central ray is angled.
     C. Position it next to the narrowest anatomical
        structure.
21. A. Lead
     B. Radiopaque
22. Closer to
23.

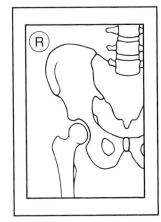

24.

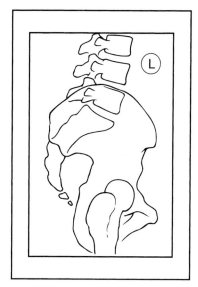

25. Mark the side that is positioned closer to the IR, and place a face-up marker laterally, adjacent to that side.
26. Circle the marker and restate the information it displays next to it for hard copy images, or add a marker next to the original during postprocessing for digital systems.
27. A. 0
    B. 68
    C. 45
    D. 23
    E. 90
28. A. 45
    B. 45
    C. 30
    D. 105
29. A. It would superimpose it.
    B. (1) Proximal
       (2) No
       (3) Because letter A is farther from the IR it will be projected further proximally than letter B.
    C. (1) Distally
       (2) Letter A would be projected even more distally.
    D. Possibly superimposed over it or positioned only slightly distal or proximal to it depending on the SID used. The placement would vary depending on the SID, because the angle used to record A and B could be perpendicular or proximal if a short SID was used and caudal if a long SIS was used.
30. The goal of mobile and trauma imaging is to demonstrate accurate relationships between the anatomical structures for the projection or position imaged, without further patient injury and with minimal discomfort.
31. A. Line connecting the metacarpals
    B. Line connecting the humeral epicondyles

C. Midsagittal plane
D. Line connecting the femoral epicondyles
E. Orbitomeatal line (OML)

32.

Casts, Splints, Backboards or Patient Condition	kVp Adjustment	mAs Adjustment
Small to medium plaster cast	+5-7 kVp	+50%-60%
Large plaster cast	+8-10 kVp	+100%
Fiberglass cast	+3-4 kVp	+25%-30%
Inflated air splint	No adjustment	No adjustment
Wood backboard	+5 kVp	+25%-30%
Ascites (invasion of fluid in abdomen or swelled joint)		+50%-75%
Pleural effusion (fluid in pleural cavity)		+35%
Pneumothorax (fluid within lungs)	−8% kVp	
Postmortem imaging of head, thorax, and abdomen (resulting from pooling of blood and fluid)		+35%-50%
Soft tissue (used for foreign objects, such as slivers of wood, glass, or metal imbedded in the soft tissue, and to demonstrate the upper airway)	−15%-20% kVp	

33. A. Parallel
    B. Perpendicular
34. A. Elongation
    B. Foreshortening
35. Elongation
36. A. Foreshortening
    B. Elongation
    C. Elongation
    D. Elongation
37. A. Fully extend the patient's finger.
    B. Align the central ray parallel with the IP joint or perpendicular to the phalange of interest. For this examination the central ray would have needed to be angled proximally until it was parallel with the joint of interest.
38. A. Use identifiable structures that surround the identical structures.
    B. Use surrounding bony projections.
    C. Identify expected magnification.
39. A. Adjust the patient half the distance demonstrated between the two structures that should be superimposed.
    B. Adjust the patient the entire distance between the structures that should be superimposed.
40. A. Farther from
    B. Closer to

41. A. Internally rotate the hand ½ inch (1.25 cm).
    B. Direct the central ray anteriorly to move the second metacarpal toward the fifth metacarpal. Because the physical distance between the second and fifth metacarpals is 2½ inches (0.6 cm) and a 5-degree angle will move the second metacarpal ½ inch (1.25 cm) for this amount of physical separation, and the amount of mispositioning is off by 1 inch (2.5 cm), a 10-degree angle should be placed on the central ray.

42. A. Externally rotate the leg 1 inch (2.5 cm).
    B. Direct the central ray anteriorly to move the medial condyle toward the lateral condyle. Because the physical distance between the condyles is approximately 2 inches (5 cm), a 5-degree angle will move the medial condyle ¼ inch (0.6 cm) for this amount of physical separation, and the condyles are mispositioned by 2 inches (5 cm), a 40-degree angle should be placed on the central ray.

43. A. Internally rotate the leg ¼ inch (0.6 cm).
    B. Direct the central ray posteriorly to move the medial talar dome toward the lateral dome. Because the physical distance between the talar domes is 1 inch (2.5 cm), a 5-degree angle will move the medial condyle ¼ inch (0.6 cm) for this amount of physical separation, and the domes are mispositioned by ¼ inch (0.6 cm), a 5-degree angle should be placed on the central ray.

44. A. Magnification. Proportional magnification of proximal, distal, and midshaft of humerus.
    B. Foreshortening. The proximal humerus was placed farther from the IR as demonstrated by the increased magnification of the proximal humerus when compared with the distal humerus.
    C. Elongation. The distal humerus was placed farther from the IR as demonstrated by the increased magnification of the distal humerus when compared with the proximal humerus.

45. A. Shape
    B. Foreshortened

46. A. Shape
    B. Elongated

47. Image 2

48. Image 2

49. A. Small
    B. Smaller

50. Motion the patient is capable of controlling

51. Motion the patient is incapable of controlling

52. A. Explain examination to patient.
    B. Make patient comfortable.
    C. Keep exposure time short.
    D. Use positioning devices.

53. When patient is unable to control the motion

54. Use a short exposure time.

55. Voluntary motion demonstrates blurred gastric patterns and bony cortical outlines, whereas involuntary motion demonstrates blurred gastric patterns and sharp cortical outlines.

56. A. Involuntary
    B. Involuntary

57. A double-exposed image will demonstrate two cortical outlines of each anatomical structure and unexplainable overexposure.

58. A. Double-exposure
    B. Motion
    C. Double-exposure (noticeable at the proximal forearm)

59. Motion will demonstrate blur throughout radiograph, whereas poor screen-film contact will demonstrate blur only where the film and screen are not in direct contact.

60. Close to

61. A. Increase the OID.
    B. Decrease the SOD or SID.

62. Image 2

63. Smallest

64. Make an imaginary X diagonally connecting the corners of the collimated field. The center of the X indicates where the central ray was centered.

65. A. Decrease
    B. Increase
    C. Scatter radiation

66. A. Larger
    B. The x-ray beams continue to diverge as they move through the patient to the IR.

67. Use palpable anatomical structures located around the area of interest.

68. A. When gonads are within 3 inches (5 cm) of the primary x-ray beam
    B. If the patient is of reproductive age
    C. If the gonadal shield does not cover information of interest

69. Ovaries, uterine tubes, and uterus

70.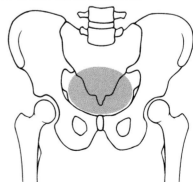

71. Place the narrow end of the shield superior to the palpable symphysis pubis and determine side-to-side centering by placing the shield at equal distances from the anterior superior iliac spines.

72. The shield is placed at a large OID and will greatly magnify, possibly covering needed information.
73. A. Testes within scrotal pouch
    B. Along midsagittal plane, inferior to the symphysis pubis
74. 1 to 1½ inches (2.5 to 4 cm) inferior to the symphysis pubis
75.

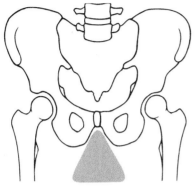

76. This is a male shield used on a female patient. It covers too much of the sacrum and does not cover the required gonadal organs. The shield is situated too superiorly and is not the correct shape.
77. The shield is poorly shaped for a male and does not cover the gonadal organs. The shield should be moved superiorly.
78. Palpate the patient's coccyx and elevated anterior superior iliac spine (ASIS). Draw an imaginary line connecting the coccyx with a point 1 inch (2.5 cm) posterior to the ASIS. Position the flat contact shield against this imaginary line.
79. A. Breasts
    B. Eyes
    C. Thyroid
    D. Gonads
    E. 2½ inches (6.25 cm)
80. A. Anatomical artifact
    B. Use positioning devices such as sponges and sandbags to aid patient in holding position.
81. A. Wide and short
    B. Wide
82. A. Long and narrow
    B. Narrow
83. A. Asthenic
    B. Hypersthenic
    C. Hypersthenic
    D. Asthenic
84. A. Crosswise
    B. Lengthwise
85. Milliamperage/second
86. The cortical outlines will still be visible on an underexposed image but not on an underpenetrated image.
87. 30%
88. 300% to 400%
89. Quantum mottle
90. A. Image density is too high by 100%. Soft-tissue structures are not visible.

B. Contrast is acceptable.
C. Penetration is acceptable.
D. 60 kVp at 4 mAs.
91. A. Image density is too light by 400%. Bony trabeculae are not well demonstrated.
    B. Contrast is low because of low density.
    C. Penetration is acceptable. The cortical outlines are light but can be visualized. The fibular head is visible through the tibia, and the patella can be seen.
    D. 65 kVp at 20 mAs.
92. A. Density is acceptable.
    B. Contrast is too low. Vertebral images should have high contrast to best visualize the bony structures.
    C. Penetration is acceptable.
    D. kVp needs to be lowered to obtain high contrast, and mAs needs to be increased to offset the density change that would occur because of the kVp adjustment. A 15% change in kVp was chosen because more than this would take the kVp level below optimal for the part and below the 70 kVp required when a grid is used. 72 kVp at 60 mAs.
93. A. Yes
    B. The reader acquisition system will adjust (normalize) the image.
94. A. Overexposures
    B. Underexposures
95. The patient would have received more radiation than needed to create the image.
96. A. Increase
    B. Noisy, quantum mottle
97. Poor patient and ionizing chamber alignment
98. A. High
    B. Thicker
    C. Denser
99. A. Choose the correct diagnostic specifier for the anatomical structure and position or projection imaged.
    B. For nonroutine positioning situations, pathological conditions, internal artifacts, and missing or added anatomy, follow the manufacturer's guidelines for choosing the most appropriate diagnostic specifier or processing mode to meet the situation.
    C. Center the structure being imaged to the center of the IR.
    D. Do not overlap collimation edges when more than one image is placed on the IR.
    E. Collimate tightly.
100. Kilovoltage
101. A. Increased
    B. 15
102. The density is not even from toes to the metacarpals demonstrating increased density at distal metacarpals. The filter needs to be

moved approximately 1 inch (2.5 cm) proximally.

103. A density variation that is present on images that require a long (17-inch) field size. It is a result of greater photon absorption that occurs at the thicker "heel" portion of the anode compared with the thinner "toe" portion.

104.

Projection(s)	Placement of Anode	Placement of Cathode
AP and lateral forearm	Wrist	Elbow
AP and lateral humerus	Elbow	Shoulder
AP and lateral lower leg	Ankle	Knee
AP and lateral femur	Knee	Hip
AP thoracic vertebrae	Cephalic	Caudal
AP lumbar vertebrae	Cephalic	Caudal

105. A. Kilovoltage level
     B. Amount of scatter radiation that reaches the IR
106. A. Little
     B. High
107. The bones of infants and children are less dense and more porous than adult bones.
108. A. Use a grid.
     B. Use tight collimation.
     C. Place a flat contact shield or edge of an apron along the appropriate collimated border.
109. A. An anatomical structure within collimated field that could have been removed
     B. Two exposures are taken on the same IR without processing being done between them
     C. Patient and hospital belongings that are found outside the patient's body that could have been removed but were not and are demonstrated on an image
     D. Objects located within the patient's body that cannot be removed and are demonstrated on the image

E. Artifacts that are caused by the imaging equipment
F. Artifacts that are caused by the processor or the way the IR was handled or stored
110. A. External artifact
     B. Anatomical artifact
     C. Internal artifact
     D. Equipment-related artifact
     E. Improper film handling or processor artifact
111. A. Inverted or off-focused
     B. Off-center
112. A. Toward
     B. Increase
     C. Higher
113. Normalization
114. A stationary grid is used and the image plate is placed in the plate reader so that the grid lines are aligned parallel with the scanning direction
115. A. When the IR plate is not adequately erased
     B. When the IR is exposed to scatter radiation when the IR is left in room during other exposures or has been used for 24 hours and has collected sufficient exposure from background radiation
116. They produce small white dots or curved white lines.
117. When the artifact can be eliminated and is obscuring a portion of the area of interest
118. A. Number of images taken for examination
     B. Sizes of films used for examination
     C. Technical factors used for examination
     D. Technologist's name
     E. Date of procedure
     F. Time of procedure
     G. Imaging room number
     H. Pertinent patient history
119. An optimal image is perfect in all aspects, whereas an acceptable image does not have to be repeated but has aspects that could be improved.

Image Analysis of the Chest and Abdomen

LEARNING OBJECTIVES

After completion of this chapter you should be able to:

_____ 1. Identify the required anatomy on all chest and abdominal images.

_____ 2. Describe how to properly position the patient, image receptor (IR), and central ray for adult and pediatric chest and abdominal images.

_____ 3. State the technical data used in chest and abdominal images.

_____ 4. State how to properly mark and display chest and abdominal images.

_____ 5. List typical artifacts that are found on chest and abdominal images.

_____ 6. List the image analysis requirements for accurately positioned adult and pediatric chest and abdominal images.

_____ 7. State how to properly reposition the patient when chest and abdominal images with poor positioning are produced.

_____ 8. Discuss how to determine the amount of patient or central ray adjustment that is required to improve poor positioning on chest and abdominal images.

_____ 9. State the kilovoltage routinely used for adult and pediatric chest and abdominal images and describe what anatomical structures are visible when the correct technical factors are used.

_____ 10. Discuss when the IR is placed crosswise and when it is placed lengthwise for posteroanterior/anteroposterior (PA/AP) projection chest images.

_____ 11. Explain why a 72-inch (183-cm) source–image-receptor distance (SID) is routinely used for chest images.

_____ 12. List the chest dimensions that expand and contract when the patient exhales and inhales and how much they expand and contract.

_____ 13. Discuss how to determine if full lung expansion is obtained on chest images.

_____ 14. State when an expiration PA chest image is required.

_____ 15. Describe scoliosis, and identify a chest image of a patient with this condition.

_____ 16. Describe methods of identifying the right and left hemidiaphragms on lateral chest images.

_____ 17. Explain the location of the liver and discuss how its location affects the height of the right hemidiaphragm and the location of the right kidney.

_____ 18. State the differences that are found when comparing a left and a right lateral chest image.

_____ 19. Discuss how to identify the eleventh thoracic vertebra on a lateral chest image.

_____ 20. State why the kilovolt peak (kVp) level used for mobile chest images is lower than that for routine chest images. Discuss why a different kVp level is used when an image is taken to evaluate the patient's lung field versus the mediastinal region.

_____ 21. State the purpose and proper location of the internal tubes and lines demonstrated on AP chest images.

_____ 22. Describe how and why the level at which the diaphragm is located on full inspiration is different when the patient is upright versus supine.

_____ 23. State when to expose chest images when the patient is unconscious or on a ventilator to obtain a fully aerated lung.

_____ 24. Discuss how the patient is positioned for a lateral decubitus chest image to rule out pneumothorax and pleural effusion.

_____ 25. State how the patient and central ray are positioned to best demonstrate air and fluid levels within the pleural cavity. Explain how this detection is affected on an AP/PA chest image if the patient is placed in a supine or partial upright position.

_____ 26. State an indication for taking an AP lordotic chest image.

_____ 27. Explain the difference in the degree of patient obliquity needed to see the heart shadow without spinal column superimposition for right anterior oblique (RAO) and left anterior oblique (LAO) chest images.

_____ 28. Describe the location of the psoas muscles and the kidneys.

_____ 29. Discuss how technique is adjusted for imaging of the abdomen of patients with large amounts of bowel gas, ascites, or bowel obstructions. Explain why this adjustment is required.

_____ 30. State the difference between voluntary motion and involuntary motion. Describe how they can be identified on an abdominal image and ways motion can be reduced.

_____ 31. Explain why a patient is positioned in the upright or lateral decubitus position for at least 10 to 20 minutes before the abdominal image is taken.

_____ 32. Describe why it is necessary to center differently for female and male patients when positioning for an AP abdominal image.

_____ 33. State why it is necessary for the diaphragm to be included in all upright and lateral decubitus abdominal images.

_____ 34. Discuss why abdominal images are taken on expiration.

_____ 35. State why the long SID used for adult chest images is not needed for pediatric chest images.

_____ 36. Explain how neonates' lungs develop and change as they grow.

_____ 37. Describe the purpose and location of the internal lines and tubes found in pediatric chest images.

_____ 38. State why cross-table lateral chest images are preferred to overhead images on neonates.

_____ 39. Explain why the abdominal organs are not well defined on pediatric abdominal images.

STUDY QUESTIONS
Chest

1. Describe how the following chest images should be hung on a view box or displayed on a cathode ray tube (CRT) monitor.

   A. PA: _____

   B. Left lateral: _____

   C. AP lordotic: _____

   D. RAO: _____

   E. Right lateral decubitus (AP projection): _____

   _____

2. State why chest images are taken at a 72-inch (183-cm) SID.

   _____

   _____

3. List how to obtain sharply defined recorded details on chest images.

   A. _____

   B. _____

   C. _____

   D. _____

4. Adequate contrast and density are present on chest images when what lung structures are clearly demonstrated?

   _____

5. Sufficient penetration has been obtained on chest images when the

   _____

   are demonstrated.

6. Complete Table 2-1.

TABLE 2-1   Abdominal Technical Data

Position or Projection	kVp	Grid	AEC Chamber(s)	SID
PA projection				
Lateral position				
AP projection		Grid		
AP projection		Nongrid		
Lateral decubitus position				
AP axial (lordotic) projection				
Oblique position				

AEC, Automatic exposure control; AP, anteroposterior; kVp, kilovolt peak; SID, source–image receptor distance.

7. Complete Table 2-2.

TABLE 2-2   IR Size, Placement, and Direction

Position or Projection	IR Size	Placement and Direction
PA projection		
Lateral position		
AP projection		
Lateral decubitus position		
AP axial (lordotic) projection		
Oblique position		

AP, Anteroposterior; IR, image receptor; PA, posteroanterior.

PA Projection

8. Identify the labeled anatomy in Figure 2-1.

Figure 2–1

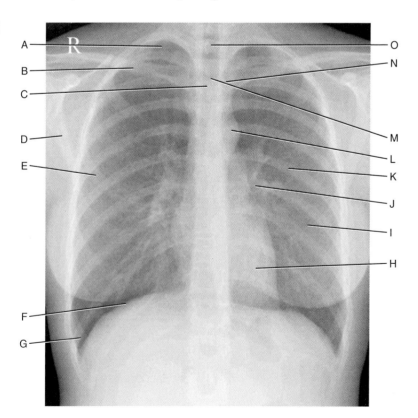

A. _____

B. _____

C. _____

D. _____

E. _____

F. _____

G. _____

H. _____

I. _____

J. _____

K. _____

L. _____

M. _____

N. _____

O. _____

9. Define the terms in the following list.

A. Pleural cavity: _____

B. Pneumothorax: _____

C. Pneumectomy: _____

D. Intraperitoneal: _____

E. Vertebra prominens: _____

F. Apex (apical): _____

G. Air-fluid line: _____

H. Anterior rotation: _____

10. How must the patient and central ray be positioned for a PA chest image to obtain the most accurate assessment of air-fluid levels in the thorax?

A. Patient: _____

B. Central ray: _____

11. Identify the pathological condition demonstrated in the following images (Figures 2-2 to 2-4).

Figure 2–2

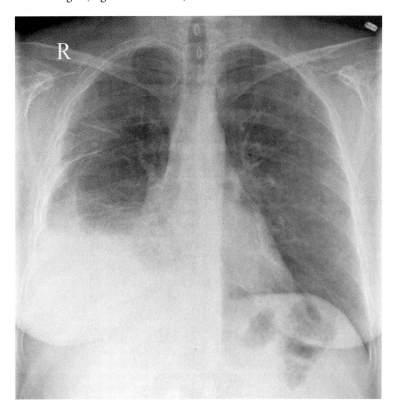

Right inferior lung (Figure 2-2):
A. _____

Figure 2–3

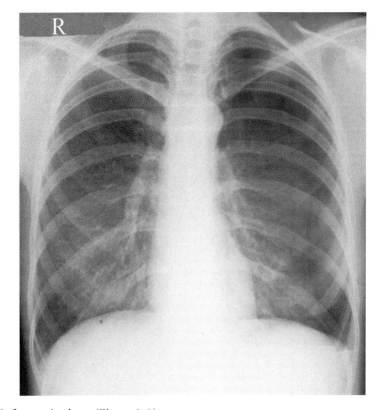

Left superior lung (Figure 2-3):
B. _____

Figure 2–4

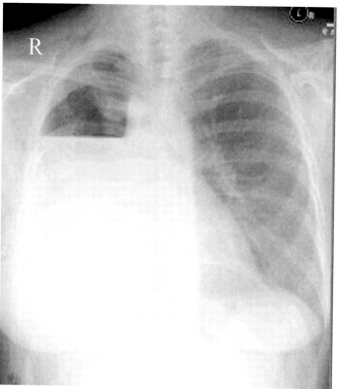

Right inferior lung (Figure 2-4):

    A. _____

12. List the three dimensions in which the lungs expand and contract during inspiration and expiration.

    A. _____

    B. _____

    C. _____

13. The _____ dimension of the thorax expands the most during inspiration.

14. List two situations that could prevent full lung expansion during the taking of chest images.

    A. _____

    B. _____

15. What body type requires the IR to be placed crosswise when a PA chest image is taken?

    A. _____

    Describe the lung shape of such a patient.

    B. _____

16. What body types will require the IR to be placed lengthwise when a PA chest image is taken?

    A. _____, _____

    Describe the lung shapes of such patients.

    B. _____

17. When it is difficult to decide whether the IR should be placed crosswise or lengthwise for a PA chest image, what method can be used to determine if the transverse IR dimension is sufficient?

_____

_____

18. Where is the best place to position the identification nameplate and marker for a screen-film PA chest image? _____

19. State how the patient is positioned to prevent rotation on a PA chest image.

_____

_____

20. A nonrotated PA chest image is demonstrated when the distance from the vertebral column to the (A) _____ and the lengths of the (B) _____ are equal.

21. A. What spinal condition may result in a rotated appearance on a PA chest image? _____

B. Can patient positioning be adjusted to offset this rotated appearance on such a patient? _____

C. How can this condition be distinguished from rotation on a PA chest image?

_____

_____

_____

22. How is the patient positioned to place the clavicles on the same horizontal plane on a PA chest image?

_____

23. How is the patient positioned for a PA chest image to place the scapulae outside the lung field?

_____

24. The level at which the manubrium is visible on the vertebral column and the amount of apical lung field demonstrated above the clavicles are determined by the tilt of the patient's (A) _____ plane. When this plane is vertical, the manubrium will be at the level of the (B) _____ thoracic vertebra and approximately (C) _____ inch(es) of the apices will be demonstrated above the clavicles.

25. On an accurately positioned PA chest image, the clavicles should be horizontal. What two aspects of the setup procedure can be mispositioned to result in somewhat vertically running clavicles?

A. _____

B. _____

26. Why will an increase in lung aeration be obtained when a chest image is taken with the patient in an upright position versus a supine or seated position?

_____

_____

27. What two positioning procedures will provide a PA chest image with the greatest amount of vertical lung field?

   A. _____

   B. _____

28. Why are chest images exposed after the patient has taken the second full inspiration?

   _____

29. When the lungs have been fully aerated for an upright PA chest image, _____ posterior ribs will be demonstrated above the diaphragm.

30. List two patient conditions that may indicate the need for an expiration chest image to be taken.

   A. _____

   B. _____

31. On an expiration PA chest image, the diaphragm will be positioned (A) _____ (higher/lower), (B) _____ posterior ribs will be demonstrated above the diaphragm, the heart shadow will appear (C) _____ and (D) _____, and the image density will be (E) _____ (lighter/darker).

32. On an accurately positioned PA chest image, the (A) _____ will be centered within the collimated field. This is accomplished by centering a (B) _____ central ray to the (C) _____ plane at a level approximately 7.5 inches (18 cm) inferior to the (D) _____.

33. What anatomical structures are included on an accurately positioned PA chest image?

   _____

For the following descriptions of PA chest images with poor positioning, state how the patient would have been mispositioned for such an image to result.

34. The vertebral column is superimposed over the right sternoclavicular (SC) joint, whereas the left SC joint is demonstrated without vertebral superimposition.

   _____

35. The clavicles are not positioned on the same horizontal plane. The lateral clavicular ends are elevated. The manubrium is at the same level as the fourth thoracic vertebra.

   _____

36. The right scapula is demonstrated within the superolateral lung field.

   _____

37. The clavicles are horizontal, the manubrium is situated at the level of the fifth thoracic vertebra, and more than 1 inch (2.5 cm) of the chest apex is demonstrated superior to the clavicles.

   _____

38. The manubrium is situated at the level of the first thoracic vertebra, and less than 1 inch (2.5 cm) of the chest apex is demonstrated superior to the clavicles.

_____

39. The image demonstrates the first through eighth posterior ribs above the diaphragm.

_____

For the following PA chest images with poor positioning, state what anatomical structures are misaligned and how the patient should be repositioned for an optimal image to be obtained.

Figure 2–5

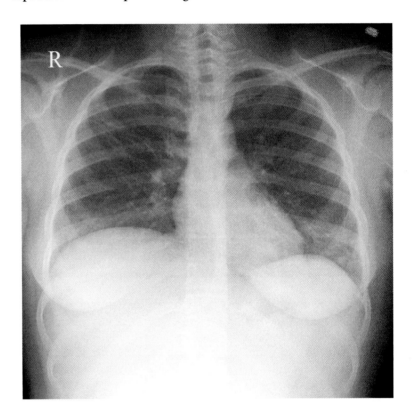

40. (Figure 2-5): _____

_____

_____

_____

Figure 2–6

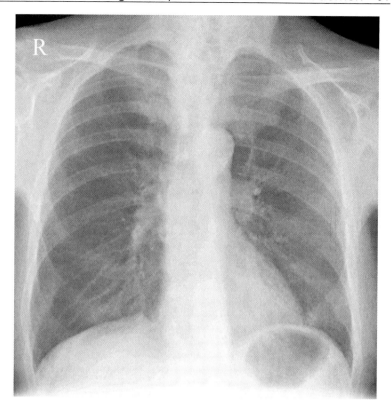

41. (Figure 2-6): _____

_____

_____

_____

Figure 2–7

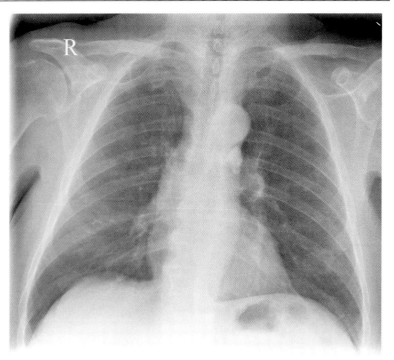

42. (Figure 2-7): _____

    _____

    _____

    _____

Figure 2–8

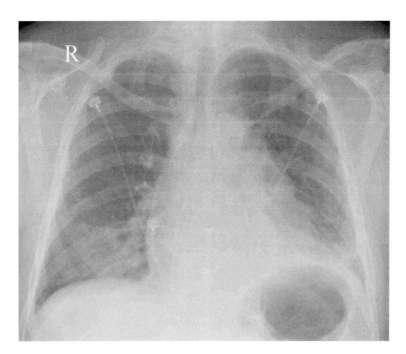

43. (Figure 2-8): _____

    _____

    _____

    _____

Left Lateral Position

1. Identify the labeled anatomy in Figure 2-9.

Figure 2–9

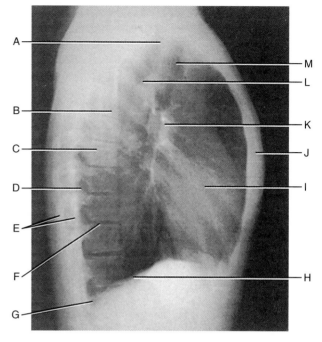

A. _____

B. _____

C. _____

D. _____

E. _____

F. _____

G. _____

H. _____

I. _____

J. _____

K. _____

L. _____

M. _____

2. Define the following terms.

A. Spinal scoliosis: _____

B. Hemidiaphragm: _____

C. Deviation: _____

D. Kyphotic: _____

E. Lordotic: _____

3. A nonrotated lateral chest image will demonstrate approximately
(A) _____ inch(es) of space between the (B) _____ or
(C) _____ ribs.

4. How is the patient positioned to prevent rotation on a lateral chest image?

_____

_____

5. Which side of the thorax will demonstrate the greatest magnification when a left lateral chest image is taken?

A. _____

Defend your answer.

B. _____

_____

6. How is rotation identified on a lateral chest image?

_____

_____

7. List two methods that can be used to identify the right and left hemidiaphragms on a lateral chest image with poor positioning.

A. _____

B. _____

8. Where is the gastric air bubble located on an upright lateral chest image?

_____

9. Which side of the chest cavity contains most of the heart? _____

10. A rotated lateral chest image demonstrates the left lung posteriorly, with 2½ inches (6.25 cm) of space between the posterior ribs. How should the patient be adjusted, and how much movement from the original position should be made?

_____

_____

11. State a method of distinguishing scoliosis from rotation on a lateral chest image.

_____

_____

12. How is the patient positioned with respect to the IR for a lateral chest image to prevent lung foreshortening? _____

_____

13. Which lung and diaphragm are situated higher on the average patient?

_____

14. List two expected differences that would be demonstrated between a right and a left lateral chest image.

A. _____

_____

B. _____

_____

15. State whether it is best to take a right or left lateral chest image for the following.

    A. To evaluate right lung details: _____

    B. To evaluate the heart: _____

    C. To evaluate left lung details: _____

16. How is the patient positioned for a lateral chest image to prevent the humeral soft tissue from being superimposed over the anterior lung apices?

    _____

17. It is best to take a lateral chest image of an obese patient with the patient in a standing position to better demonstrate the _____ aspect of the lung and heart.

18. How can one determine if full lung aeration has occurred for a lateral chest image? _____

    _____

19. What two positioning procedures will provide a lateral chest image with the greatest amount of vertical lung field?

    A. _____

    B. _____

20. Which thoracic vertebra has the last rib attached to it? _____

21. On an accurately positioned lateral chest image, the
    (A) _____ plane located at the level of the
    (B) _____ thoracic vertebra is centered within the collimated field. This is accomplished by centering the central ray to the (C) _____ plane at a level 8.5 inches (21.25 cm)
    (D) _____ to the vertebral prominens.

22. What anatomical structures are included in a lateral chest image for which the subject was accurately positioned?

    _____

    _____

For the following descriptions of left lateral chest images with poor positioning, state how the patient would have been mispositioned for such an image to result.

23. The humeri soft-tissue shadows are superimposed over the anterior lung apices.

    _____

    _____

24. The posterior ribs are separated by more than ½ inch (1.25 cm), and the superior heart shadow is seen extending beyond the sternum into the anteriorly situated lung. _____

    _____

25. One hemidiaphragm is demonstrated superior to the other, and the gastric bubble is situated beneath the superior hemidiaphragm.

    _____

    _____

For the following lateral chest images with poor positioning, state what anatomical structures are misaligned and how the patient should be repositioned for an optimal image to be obtained.

Figure 2–10A

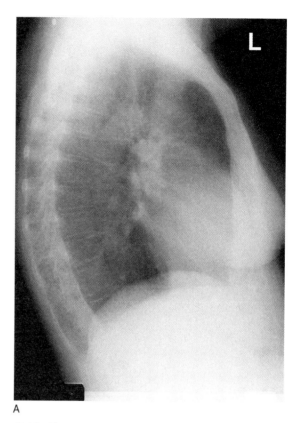

A

26. (Figure 2-10, *A*): _____

   _____

   _____

Figure 2–10B

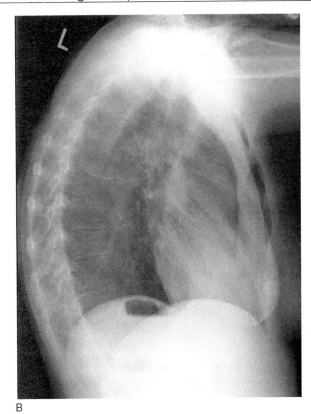

B

(Figure 2-10, *B*): _____

_____

_____

Figure 2–11

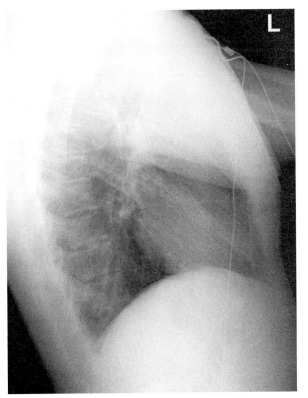

27. (Figure 2-11): _____

_____

_____

_____

_____

The following chest case study includes PA and lateral chest images from the same patient. Evaluate the images for accurate positioning.

Figure 2–12

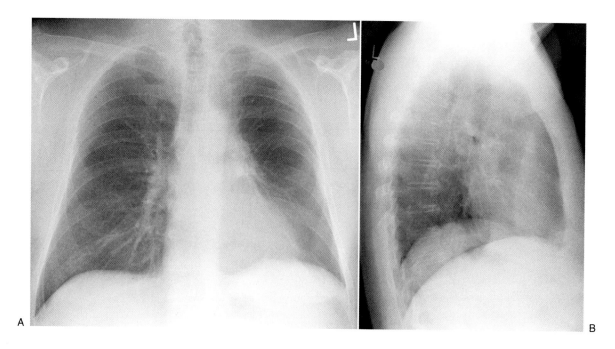

A   B

28. (Figure 2-12):

A. _____

_____

_____

B. _____

_____

_____

AP Projection (Supine or with Mobile X-Ray Unit)

1. Identify the labeled anatomy in Figure 2-13.

Figure 2–13

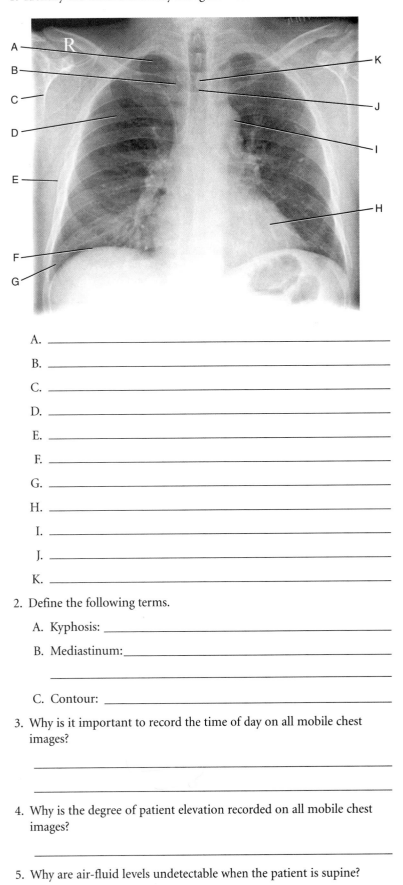

A. _____

B. _____

C. _____

D. _____

E. _____

F. _____

G. _____

H. _____

I. _____

J. _____

K. _____

2. Define the following terms.

A. Kyphosis: _____

B. Mediastinum: _____

_____

C. Contour: _____

3. Why is it important to record the time of day on all mobile chest images?

_____

_____

4. Why is the degree of patient elevation recorded on all mobile chest images?

_____

5. Why are air-fluid levels undetectable when the patient is supine?

_____

6. The thoracic vertebral column may not be visible through the heart shadow on an AP mobile chest image because the _____ used is too low.

7. Describe the function of each of the following lines and tubes, and state the area of the thorax that should be best demonstrated to show the apparatus.

    A. Endotracheal tube: _____

    _____

    B. Chest tube: _____

    _____

    C. Central venous line: _____

    _____

    D. Pulmonary arterial line: _____

    _____

8. Identify the internal tube or line demonstrated in Figures 2-14 to 2-16.

Figure 2–14

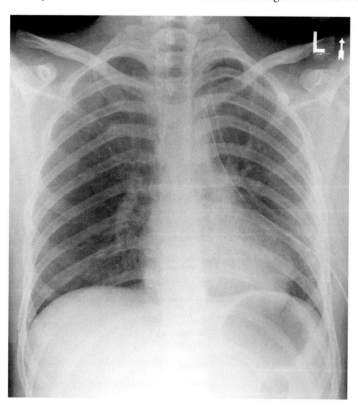

    A. (Figure 2-14): _____

Figure 2–15

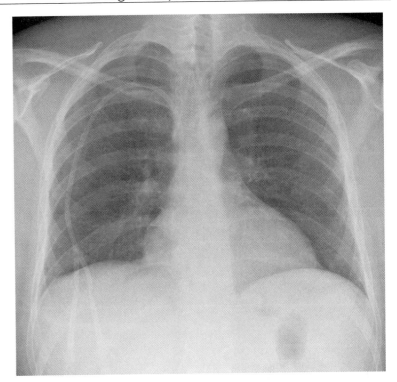

B. (Figure 2-15): _____

Figure 2–16

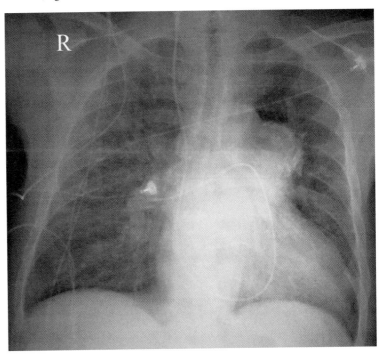

C. (Figure 2-16): _____

9. A. Why is it safe to position the IR crosswise for all mobile AP chest images on most body types?

_____

_____

B. Why is it more likely for the lateral edges of the lung field to be clipped if the IR is placed lengthwise for mobile AP chest images?

_____

_____

10. State how the patient is positioned to prevent rotation on an AP chest image.

_____

_____

11. A nonrotated PA chest image is demonstrated when the distance from the vertebral column to the (A) _____ and the length of the (B) _____ are equal.

12. How can rotation be identified on an AP chest image?

_____

_____

13. When the patient's condition allows, the shoulders should be depressed for an AP chest image. How can this movement be identified on the image?

_____

14. When an AP chest image is obtained that demonstrates somewhat vertically appearing clavicles, how can one determine if this appearance is a result of poor central ray alignment or poor shoulder positioning?

_____

_____

_____

15. When the patient's condition allows, how can the scapulae be drawn from the lung field on an AP supine chest image?

_____

_____

16. Accurate central ray, IR, and patient positioning on an AP chest image have been obtained when the manubrium is superimposed over the (A) _____ thoracic vertebra, approximately (B) _____ inch of the apices is present above the clavicles, and the posterior ribs demonstrate a gentle (C) _____ contour.

17. Poor central ray alignment on a mobile chest image will affect the amount of apical lung field demonstrated superior to the clavicles and the contour of the posterior ribs. For each of the following situations, describe the expected change in apical lung visualization and posterior rib contour.

A. The central ray was angled too caudally.

_____

_____

_____

B. The central ray was angled too cephalically.

_____

_____

_____

18. How can the central ray be adjusted to improve the posterior rib contour and eliminate superimposition of the chin on the apices when imaging a kyphotic patient for an AP chest image?

_____

19. A. How is the central ray angled for a supine AP chest image?

_____

B. Why is this angle needed?

_____

20. A fully aerated supine AP chest image will demonstrate_____ posterior ribs above the diaphragm.

21. Why are fewer posterior ribs demonstrated above the diaphragm on a supine AP chest image than on an upright PA chest image?

_____

_____

22. How is the patient instructed to breathe to obtain maximum lung aeration?

_____

23. Why is it unnecessary to watch an unconscious patient on a high-frequency ventilator?

_____

24. On an accurately positioned AP chest image, the (A) _____ vertebra will be centered within the collimated field. This is accomplished by centering the central ray to the (B) _____ plane at a level (C) _____ inches inferior to the (D) _____.

25. What anatomical structures are included on an accurately positioned AP chest image? _____

_____

For the following descriptions of AP chest images with poor positioning, state how the patient would have been mispositioned or the central ray misaligned for such an image to result.

26. The left SC joint is visible away from the vertebral column, whereas the right SC joint is superimposed over the vertebral column (list both patient and central ray mispositioning that could cause this image).

_____

_____

_____

27. The manubrium is shown superimposed over the fifth thoracic vertebra with more than 1 inch (2.5 cm) of the apical lung field visible above the clavicles, and the posterior ribs demonstrate a vertical contour. _____

_____

28. The manubrium is shown superimposed over the third vertebra with less than 1 inch (2.5 cm) of apical lung field visible above the clavicles, and the posterior ribs demonstrate a horizontal contour.

_____

29. An image of a patient with severe kyphosis demonstrates the chin superimposed over the apical region, and the posterior ribs demonstrate a vertical contour. _____

_____

_____

For the following AP chest images with poor positioning, state what anatomical structures are misaligned and how the patient should be repositioned for an optimal image to be obtained.

Figure 2–17

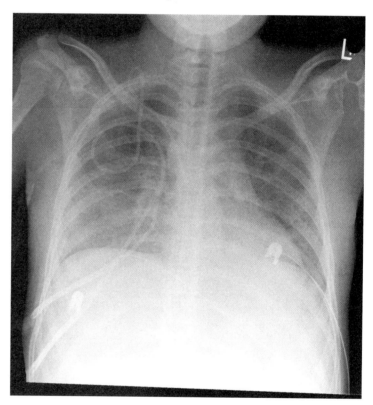

30. (Figure 2-17): _____

_____

_____

_____

Figure 2–18

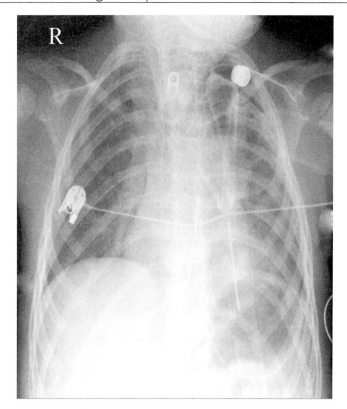

31. (Figure 2-18): _____

_____

_____

_____

Figure 2–19

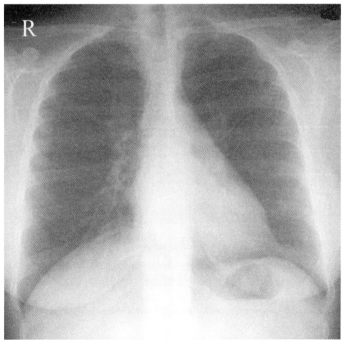

32. (Figure 2-19): _____

_____

_____

_____

_____

_____

Lateral Decubitus Position

1. Identify the labeled anatomy in Figure 2-20.

Figure 2–20

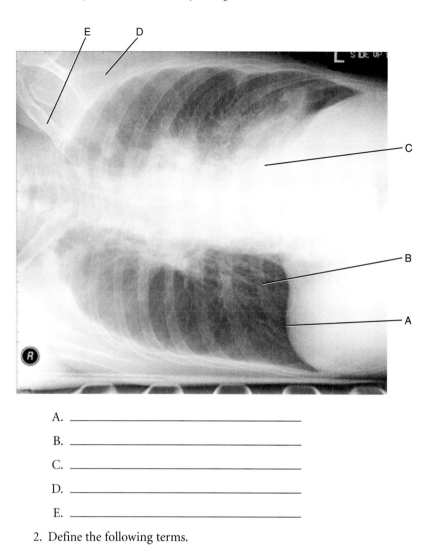

A. _____

B. _____

C. _____

D. _____

E. _____

2. Define the following terms.

A. Aerate: _____

B. Pleural effusion: _____

C. Radiolucent: _____

3. How is a left lateral decubitus chest image accurately marked and displayed on the view box or CAT monitor?

A. Marked: _____

_____

B. Displayed: _____

4. Adequate density is present on a decubitus chest image when what lung structures are clearly visible?

_____

5. The lateral decubitus position is primarily performed to confirm the presence of (A) _____ or (B) _____ levels within the pleural cavity.

6. If fluid is present within the pleural cavity on a decubitus chest image, where will it be located? _____

   _____

7. How are the technique factors used for a decubitus chest image adjusted for a patient with the following conditions?

   A. Pneumothorax: _____

   B. Pleural effusion: _____

8. For each situation below, state whether a right or left decubitus chest image should be taken.

   A. Right pneumothorax: _____

   B. Left pleural effusion: _____

9. A nonrotated PA chest image is demonstrated when the distance from the vertebral column to the (A) _____ and the length of the (B) _____ are equal.

10. To avoid rotation on decubitus chest images, align the patient's (A) _____, (B) _____, and (C) _____ perpendicular to the cart.

11. Will an AP or PA projection chest image demonstrate the sixth and seventh cervical vertebrae without distortion and open intervertebral disk space? _____

12. The lateral scapular borders are situated outside the lung field when the arms are positioned _____ for a decubitus chest image.

13. The manubrium and the _____ thoracic vertebra are superimposed on an accurately positioned decubitus chest image.

14. Chest foreshortening can be avoided on a decubitus chest image by positioning the (A) _____ plane (B) _____ (perpendicular/parallel) to the IR.

15. If the lungs are fully aerated for a decubitus chest image, _____ posterior ribs will be demonstrated above the diaphragm.

16. How can the patient be positioned for a decubitus chest image to prevent the cart pad from creating an artifact line along the lung field positioned against it?

   _____

For the following descriptions of decubitus chest images with poor positioning, state how the patient would have been positioned for such an image to be obtained.

17. A PA decubitus chest image demonstrates the vertebral column superimposed over the right SC joint, whereas the left SC joint is demonstrated without vertebral superimposition.

   _____

18. An AP decubitus chest image demonstrates the right SC joint superimposed over the vertebral column, whereas the left SC joint does not demonstrate vertebral superimposition.

_____

19. An AP decubitus chest image demonstrates the manubrium at the level of the second thoracic vertebra.

_____

For the following decubitus chest images with poor positioning, state what anatomical structures are misaligned and how the patient should be repositioned for an optimal image to be obtained.

Figure 2–21

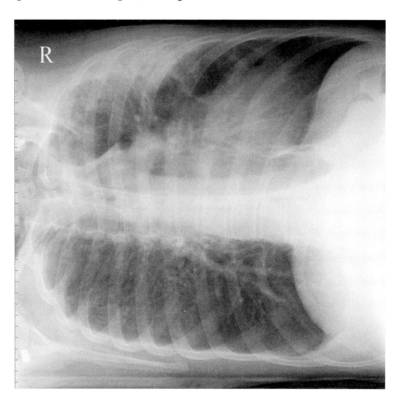

20. (Figure 2-21; AP projection): _____
_____
_____
_____

Figure 2–22

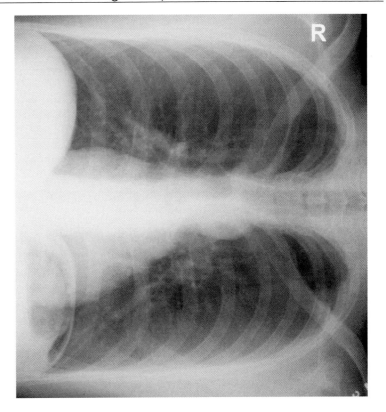

21. (Figure 2-22; AP projection): _____

_____

_____

_____

AP Lordotic Projection

Figure 2–23

1. Identify the labeled anatomy in Figure 2-23.

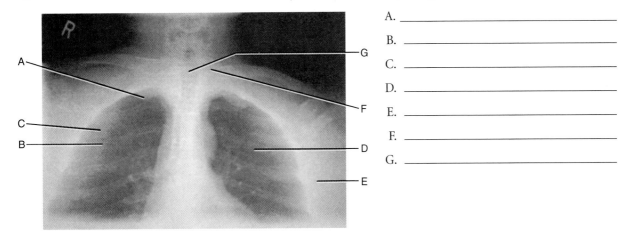

A. _____

B. _____

C. _____

D. _____

E. _____

F. _____

G. _____

2. Define *foreshorten:* _____

3. The lordotic chest image is taken to visualize the _____.

4. On a lordotic chest image with proper positioning, the medial ends of the clavicles are projected onto the (A) _____ thoracic vertebra and the posterior and anterior portions of the first through fourth ribs lie (B) _____ and are nearly (C) _____.

5. Describe three methods that can be used to position the clavicles superior to the lung apices.

   A. _____

   _____

   B. _____

   _____

   C. _____

   _____

6. A lordotic chest image with poor positioning demonstrates the medial clavicles superimposed over the lung apices. What two positional changes can be made to obtain an image with accurate positioning?

   A. _____

   B. _____

7. How must the patient be positioned to draw the lateral borders of the scapulae out of the lung field and the superior angles away from the lung apices?

   _____

8. How can rotation be identified on a lordotic chest image?

   _____

9. On a lordotic chest image with accurate positioning, the (A) _____ is centered within the collimated field. This is accomplished by centering the central ray to the (B) _____ plane halfway between the (C) _____ and (D) _____.

10. What anatomical structures are included on a lordotic chest image with accurate positioning?

   _____

For the following descriptions of lordotic chest images with poor positioning, state how the patient would have been mispositioned or the central ray misaligned for such an image to be obtained.

11. The clavicles are superimposed over the lung apices, and the anterior ribs appear inferior to their corresponding posterior ribs.

_____

_____

12. The lateral borders of the scapulae are demonstrated within the lung field, and the superior scapular angles are demonstrated within the apical region.

_____

13. The right SC joint superimposes the vertebral column, whereas the left joint is demonstrated without superimposing the vertebral column.

_____

For the following lordotic chest image with poor positioning, state what anatomical structures are misaligned and how the patient should be repositioned for an optimal image to be obtained.

Figure 2–24

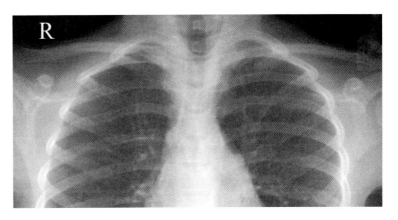

14. (Figure 2-24): _____

_____

_____

PA Oblique Projection (RAO and LAO Positions)

1. Identify the labeled anatomy in Figure 2-25.

Figure 2–25

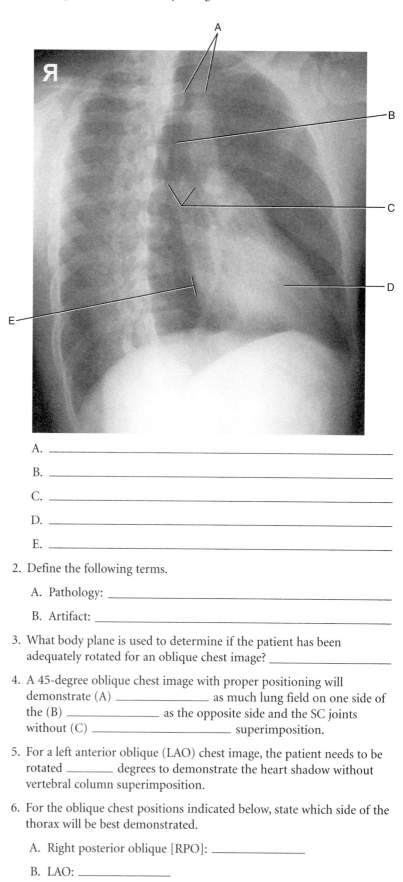

A. _____

B. _____

C. _____

D. _____

E. _____

2. Define the following terms.

A. Pathology: _____

B. Artifact: _____

3. What body plane is used to determine if the patient has been adequately rotated for an oblique chest image? _____

4. A 45-degree oblique chest image with proper positioning will demonstrate (A) _____ as much lung field on one side of the (B) _____ as the opposite side and the SC joints without (C) _____ superimposition.

5. For a left anterior oblique (LAO) chest image, the patient needs to be rotated _____ degrees to demonstrate the heart shadow without vertebral column superimposition.

6. For the oblique chest positions indicated below, state which side of the thorax will be best demonstrated.

A. Right posterior oblique [RPO]: _____

B. LAO: _____

7. The RPO position corresponds with what anterior oblique position? _____

8. Full lung aeration has been obtained on an oblique chest image when _____ posterior ribs are demonstrated above the hemidiaphragms.

9. On an oblique image with accurate positioning, the (A) _____ are centered within the collimated field. This is accomplished by centering the central ray at a level 7½ inches (18 cm) inferior to the (B) _____.

10. What anatomical structures are included on an oblique chest image with accurate positioning?

_____

For the following descriptions of PA oblique chest images with poor positioning, state how the patient would have been mispositioned for such an image to be obtained.

11. A 45-degree oblique image demonstrates less than two times the lung field on one side of the thoracic vertebrae than the other side.

_____

12. A 45-degree oblique image demonstrates more than two times the lung field on one side of the thoracic vertebrae than the other side.

_____

13. A 60-degree LAO image demonstrates superimposition of the vertebral column and heart shadow.

_____

For the following PA oblique chest images with poor positioning, state what anatomical structures are misaligned and how the patient should be repositioned for an optimal image to be obtained.

Figure 2–26

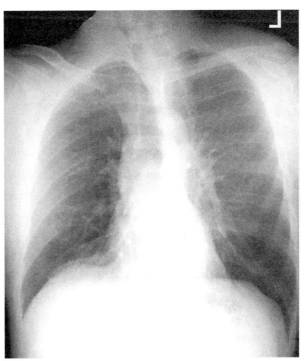

14. (Figure 2-26): _____

_____

_____

_____

_____

Figure 2–27

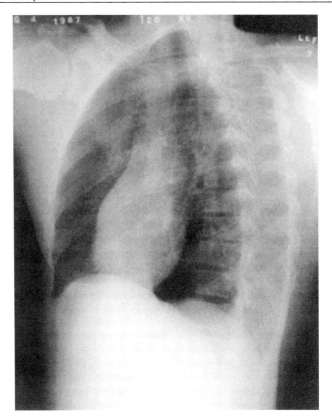

15. (Figure 2-27): _____

_____

_____

_____

Abdomen

1. Describe how the following abdominal images should be hung on a view box or displayed on a CRT monitor.

   A. AP: _____

   B. Left lateral decubitus: _____

2. Define the following terms.

   A. Ascites: _____

   B. Voluntary motion: _____

   C. Involuntary motion: _____

   D. Ambulatory: _____

   E. Peritoneal cavity: _____

3. Describe the location of the psoas major muscles.

   _____

   _____

4. A. Describe the location of the kidneys. _____

   _____

   _____

   B. Which kidney is usually demonstrated inferiorly? _____

   C. What causes the inferior location of this kidney? _____

   _____

5. List four structures that when optimally demonstrated ensure that adequate contrast, density, and penetration have been achieved on an abdominal image.

   A. _____

   B. _____

   C. _____

   D. _____

6. State how the milliampere-seconds (mAs) or kVp level is adjusted for abdominal images of a patient who has a large amount of bowel gas.

   A. mAs: _____

   B. kVp: _____

7. List four possible patient conditions that may require an increase in the routine exposure to obtain adequate image density.

   A. _____

   B. _____

   C. _____

   D. _____

8. State how the mAs or kVp level is adjusted for abdominal images of a patient with one of the conditions listed in question 9.

   A. mAs: _____

   B. kVp: _____

9. State two possible causes of voluntary motion on abdominal images.

A. _____

B. _____

10. List three ways in which voluntary motion can be controlled when abdominal images are taken.

A. _____

B. _____

C. _____

11. State the most common cause of involuntary motion on abdominal images. _____

12. How can involuntary motion be controlled on abdominal images?

_____

13. State whether voluntary or involuntary motion is demonstrated on the following images.

Figure 2–28

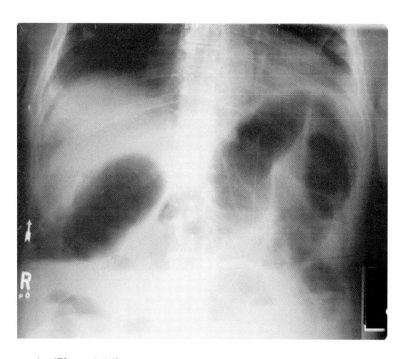

A. (Figure 2-28): _____

Figure 2–29

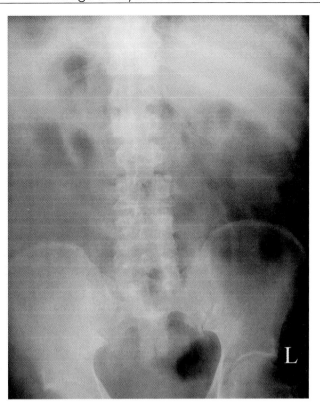

B. (Figure 2-29): _____

14. Complete Table 2-3.

TABLE 2-3 **Abdominal Technical Data**				
Position or Projection	**kVp**	**Grid**	**AEC Chamber(s)**	**SID**
AP projection				
Lateral decubitus position				

AEC, Automatic exposure control; *AP,* anteroposterior; *kVp,* kilovolt peak; *SID,* source–image receptor distance.

15. Complete Table 2-4.

TABLE 2-4 **IR Size, Placement, and Direction**		
Position or Projection	**IR Size**	**Placement and Direction**
PA projection		
Lateral decubitus position		

IR, Image receptor; *PA,* posteroanterior.

AP Projection (Supine and Upright)

16. Identify the labeled anatomy in Figure 2-30.

Figure 2–30

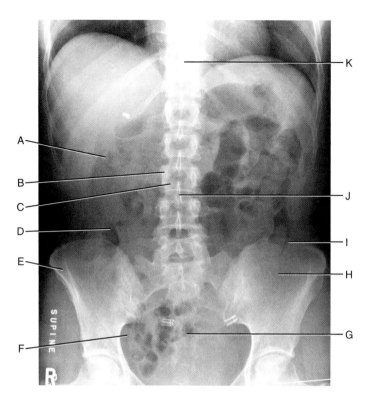

A. _____

B. _____

C. _____

D. _____

E. _____

F. _____

G. _____

H. _____

I. _____

J. _____

K. _____

17. Identify the labeled anatomy in Figure 2-31.

Figure 2–31

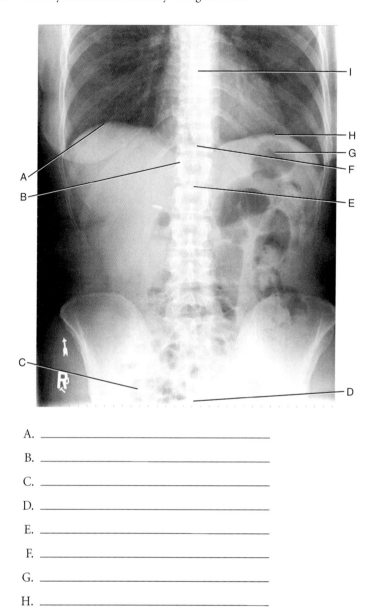

A. _____

B. _____

C. _____

D. _____

E. _____

F. _____

G. _____

H. _____

I. _____

18. Identify the patient condition that is being demonstrated in Figure 2-32.

Figure 2–32

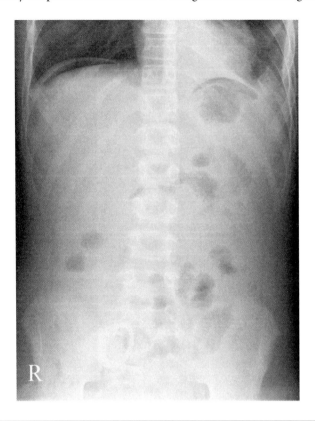

19. How should the patient be positioned to prevent rotation on an AP abdominal image?

_____

_____

20. An AP projection of the abdomen has been obtained when the spinous processes are aligned with the midline of the (A) _____, the distance from the pedicles to the (B) _____ is equal on each side, and the sacrum is aligned with the (C) _____ .

21. A. To best demonstrate intraperitoneal air, how long should the patient be positioned upright before the image is taken?_____

    B. Why is this time delay necessary? _____

    _____

22. Why is it possible for the upper abdominal region to appear rotated, whereas the lower abdominal region demonstrates an AP projection?

    _____

    _____

23. What spinal condition may result in an AP abdominal image that appears rotated? _____

24. How is the patient positioned to ensure that the long axis of the lumbar vertebral column is aligned with the long axis of the IR on an AP abdominal image?

_____

_____

25. From full inspiration to expiration, the diaphragm position moves from (A) _____ (an inferior/a superior) to (B) _____ (an inferior/a superior) position. On full expiration the right side of the diaphragmatic dome will be at the same transverse level as the (C) _____ thoracic vertebra, whereas on inspiration it is found at the (D) _____ thoracic vertebra.

26. A. What respiration is used for an AP abdominal image? _____

   B. Why is this respiration used? _____

27. State why it is important that both of the following structures are demonstrated on a supine abdominal image.

   A. Eleventh thoracic vertebrae: _____

   _____

   B. Symphysis pubis: _____

   _____

28. Why is it necessary to center 1 inch (2.5 cm) more inferiorly on the male patient than the female patient to include the symphysis pubis?

_____

_____

29. For each of the body types listed below, state whether one lengthwise IR or two crosswise IRs should be used for abdominal images.

   A. Hypersthenic: _____

   B. Sthenic: _____

   C. Asthenic: _____

30. When two crosswise IRs are used to image the abdomen, why is it necessary to have at least 2 inches (5 cm) of peritoneal cavity overlap?

_____

31. What anatomical structures are included on the following AP abdominal images?

   A. Supine: _____

   _____

   B. Upright: _____

For the following descriptions of AP abdominal images with poor positioning, state how the patient would have been mispositioned or the central ray misaligned for such an image to be obtained.

32. The distance from the right lumbar vertebral pedicles to the spinous processes is greater than the left pedicles to the spinous processes.

_____

33. The upper abdominal region demonstrates an equal distance from the vertebral pedicles to the spinous processes on each side, and the lower abdominal region demonstrates the sacrum and symphysis pubis without alignment. The sacrum is rotated toward the right pelvic inlet.

_____

_____

34. The supine abdominal image does not include the symphysis pubis or inferior peritoneal cavity.

_____

For the following AP abdominal images with poor positioning, state what anatomical structures are misaligned and how the patient should be repositioned for an optimal image to be obtained.

35. A supine abdominal image was requested.

Figure 2–33

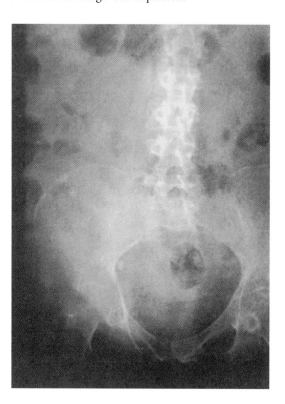

(Figure 2-33): _____

_____

_____

_____

36. A supine abdominal image was requested.

Figure 2–34

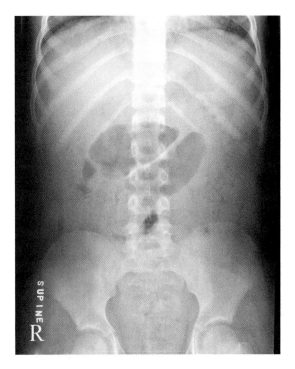

(Figure 2-34): _____

_____

_____

_____

37. An upright abdominal image was requested.

Figure 2–35

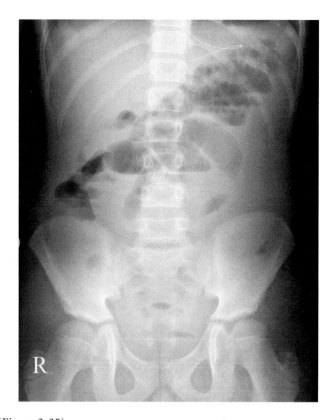

(Figure 2-35): _____

_____

_____

_____

Left Lateral Decubitus Position (AP Projection)

1. Identify the labeled anatomy in Figure 2-36.

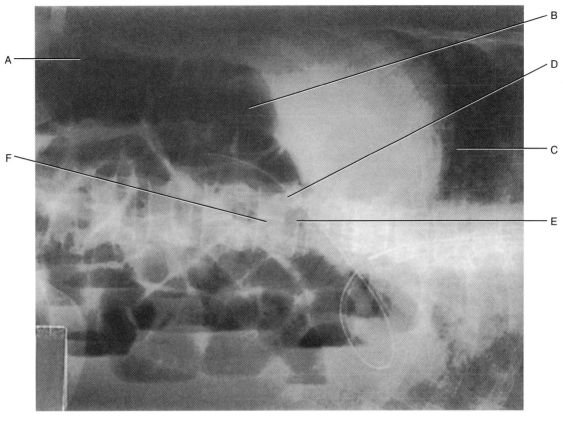

Figure 2–36

A. _____

B. _____

C. _____

D. _____

E. _____

F. _____

2. Define the following terms.

   A. Compensating filter: _____

      _____

   B. Decubitus: _____

3. A patient's requisition requests that a decubitus abdominal image be taken to rule out ascites. Describe how to determine the technique factors to use for this patient.

   _____

   _____

4. How is a compensating filter positioned to obtain uniform image density on a patient with excessive abdominal soft tissue?

   _____

   _____

5. For a decubitus abdominal image, the (A) _____ side of the patient is positioned against the imaging table or cart. Why is this side chosen? (B) _____

   _____

6. How is the patient positioned for a decubitus abdominal image to prevent rotation? _____

   _____

7. Placing a pillow between the patient's knees for a decubitus abdominal image will prevent _____.

   _____

8. To obtain optimal intraperitoneal air demonstration, the patient should remain in the decubitus position for (A) _____ minutes before the image is taken. Why is this time delay necessary?
   (B) _____

   _____

9. Intraperitoneal air is most often found beneath the
   _____ on a decubitus abdominal image with proper positioning.

10. Describe the shape of a patient's body that will result in the intraperitoneal air being demonstrated over the right iliac wing on a properly positioned decubitus abdominal image.

    _____

11. For each of the body types listed below, state whether one lengthwise IR or two crosswise IRs are used for decubitus abdominal images.

    A. Hypersthenic: _____

    B. Sthenic: _____

    C. Asthenic: _____

12. What respiration is used for a decubitus abdominal image? _____

13. What anatomical structures are included on a decubitus abdominal image with accurate positioning?

    _____

    _____

14. State when gonadal shielding is used on female and male patients for imaging the abdomen in a decubitus position.

    A. Female: _____

    B. Male: _____

For the following descriptions of decubitus abdominal images with poor positioning, state how the patient would have been mispositioned or the central ray misaligned for such an image to be obtained.

15. The image demonstrates a greater distance from the left lumbar vertebral pedicles to the spinous processes than the right pedicles to the spinous processes.

    _____

16. The image demonstrates the upper abdominal region with equal distances from the vertebral pedicles to the spinous processes on each side, and the lower abdominal region demonstrates the sacrum and symphysis pubis without alignment. The sacrum is rotated toward the left pelvic inlet.

_____

_____

17. The image demonstrates a clipped right diaphragmatic dome.

_____

For the following decubitus abdominal image with poor positioning (Figure 2-37), state what anatomical structures are misaligned and how the patient should be repositioned for an optimal image to be obtained.

Figure 2–37

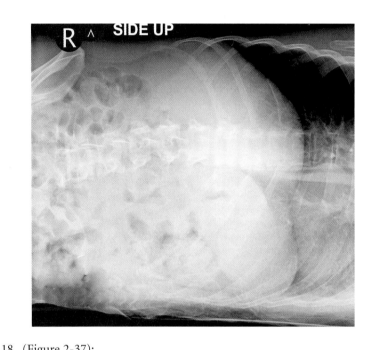

18. (Figure 2-37): _____

_____

_____

_____

Pediatrics

Chest

1. Why is it not necessary to use a long SID when imaging the neonatal or infant chest? _____

_____

2. Adequate contrast and density are present on chest images when what lung structures are clearly visualized? _____

_____

3. Sufficient penetration has been obtained on chest images when _____

_____

are faintly demonstrated.

4. Why do neonatal and infant chest images demonstrate less image contrast than adult chest images?

_____

5. Discuss the importance of the neonate's or infant's face being positioned forward and the cervical vertebrae being in a neutral position when the patient undergoes imaging for endotracheal tube (ET) placement. _____

_____

_____

6. State the purpose of the following tube and catheters.

A. Endotracheal tube: _____

B. Umbilical artery catheter: _____

C. Umbilical vein catheter: _____

7. Complete Table 2-5.

TABLE 2-5 Pediatric Chest Technical Data			
Position or Projection	kVp	Grid	SID
Neonate: Supine or mobile AP projection			
Infant: Supine or mobile AP projection			
Child: PA projection			
Child: AP projection			
Neonate: Cross-table lateral position			
Infant: Cross-table lateral position			
Child: Lateral position			
Neonate: Lateral decubitus position			
Infant: Lateral decubitus position			
Child: Lateral decubitus position			

AP, Anteroposterior; kVp, kilovolt peak; PA, posteroanterior; SID, source–image receptor distance.

8. Complete Table 2-6.

TABLE 2-6 IR Size, Placement, and Direction		
Position or Projection	IR Size	Placement and Direction
Neonate: Supine or mobile AP projection		
Infant: Supine or mobile AP projection		
Child: PA projection		
Child: AP projection		
Neonate: Cross-table lateral position		
Infant: Cross-table lateral position		
Child: Lateral position		
Neonate: Lateral decubitus position		
Infant: Lateral decubitus position		
Child: Lateral decubitus position		

AP, Anteroposterior; IR, image receptor; PA, posteroanterior.

Neonate and Infant
AP Projection (Supine or with Mobile X-Ray Unit)
9. Identify the labeled anatomy in Figure 2-38.

Figure 2–38

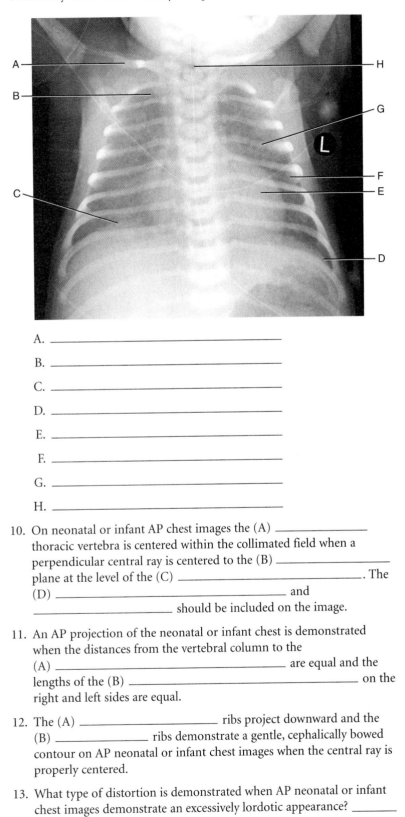

A. _____

B. _____

C. _____

D. _____

E. _____

F. _____

G. _____

H. _____

10. On neonatal or infant AP chest images the (A) _____ thoracic vertebra is centered within the collimated field when a perpendicular central ray is centered to the (B) _____ plane at the level of the (C) _____. The (D) _____ and _____ should be included on the image.

11. An AP projection of the neonatal or infant chest is demonstrated when the distances from the vertebral column to the (A) _____ are equal and the lengths of the (B) _____ on the right and left sides are equal.

12. The (A) _____ ribs project downward and the (B) _____ ribs demonstrate a gentle, cephalically bowed contour on AP neonatal or infant chest images when the central ray is properly centered.

13. What type of distortion is demonstrated when AP neonatal or infant chest images demonstrate an excessively lordotic appearance? _____

14. An AP neonatal chest image taken on full inspiration will demonstrate (A) _____ posterior ribs above the diaphragm, whereas an AP infant chest image will demonstrate at least (B) _____ posterior ribs.

15. What causes the lungs on a neonatal chest image to have a fluffy appearance? _____

_____

16. Explain when the image should be exposed in the following situations to obtain maximum lung expansion.

    A. Neonate breathing without a ventilator:

    _____

    B. Neonate on a conventional ventilator:

    _____

    C. Neonate on a high-frequency ventilator:

    _____

For the following descriptions of neonatal or infant AP chest images with poor positioning, state how the patient would have been mispositioned or the central ray misaligned for such an image to be obtained.

17. The right sternal clavicular end is demonstrated further from the vertebral column than the left sternal clavicular end, and the right lower posterior ribs are longer than the left. The patient's head is turned toward the right side.

_____

_____

18. The chest demonstrates an excessively lordotic appearance. The anterior ribs are projecting upwardly and the posterior ribs are horizontal. The sixth thoracic vertebra is at the center of the image.

_____

_____

19. Seven posterior ribs are demonstrated above the diaphragm for a neonatal AP chest image. The patient was on a conventional ventilator.

_____

_____

20. The patient's chin is superimposed over the airway and apical lung field.

_____

_____

For the following AP neonatal or infant chest images with poor positioning, state what anatomical structures are misaligned and how the patient should be repositioned for an optimal image to be obtained.

Figure 2–39

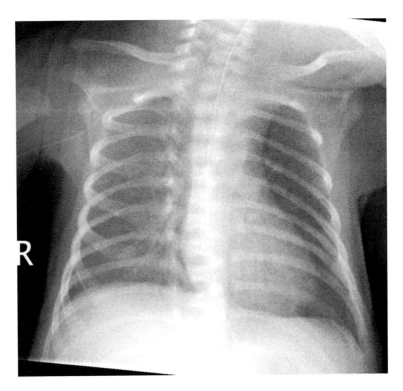

21. (Figure 2-39): _____

_____

_____

_____

Figure 2–40

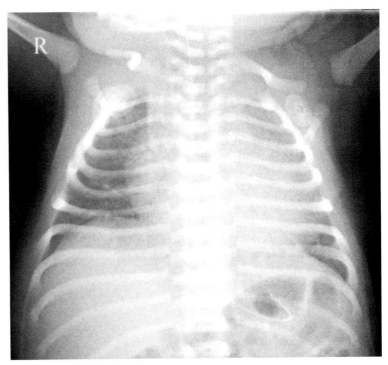

22. (Figure 2-40): _____

_____

_____

_____

_____

_____

Figure 2–41

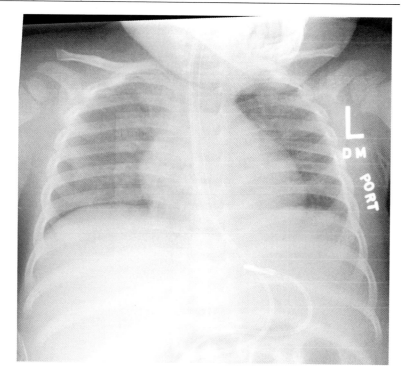

23. (Figure 2-41): _____

_____

_____

_____

Child

PA and AP Projections

1. Identify the labeled anatomy in Figure 2-42.

Figure 2–42

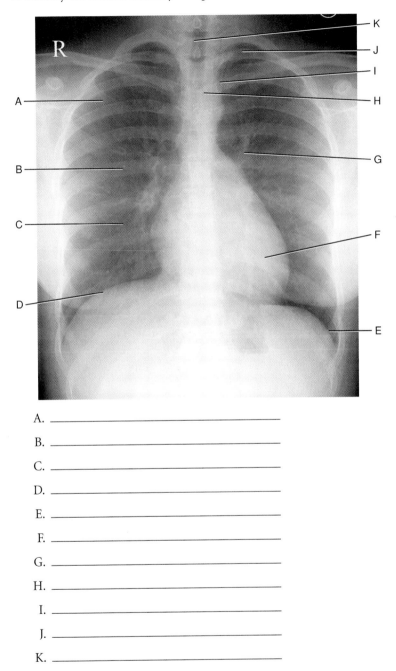

A. _____

B. _____

C. _____

D. _____

E. _____

F. _____

G. _____

H. _____

I. _____

J. _____

K. _____

For the following descriptions of child PA/AP chest images with poor positioning, state how the patient would have been mispositioned or the central ray misaligned for such an image to be obtained.

2. Mobile AP projection: The left sternoclavicular end is visualized without vertebral column superimposition, and the vertebral column is superimposed over the right sternal clavicular end.

_____

_____

3. PA projection: Six posterior ribs are demonstrated above the diaphragm.

_____

_____

4. Mobile AP projection: The manubrium is superimposed over the fifth thoracic vertebra, the posterior ribs demonstrate vertical contour, and more than 1 inch (2.5 cm) of apical lung field is visible above the clavicles.

_____

_____

5. PA projection: The second thoracic vertebra is superimposed over the manubrium.

_____

_____

6. PA projection: The fourth thoracic vertebra is superimposed over the manubrium, and the lateral ends of the clavicles are projecting superiorly.

_____

For the following PA/AP child chest images with poor positioning, state what anatomical structures are misaligned and how the patient should be repositioned for an optimal image to be obtained

Figure 2–43

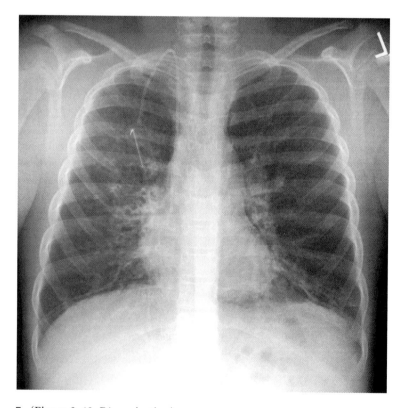

7. (Figure 2-43; PA projection): _____

_____

_____

Figure 2–44

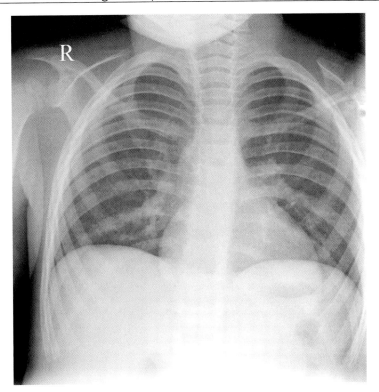

8.   (Figure 2-44; PA projection): _____

_____

Figure 2–45

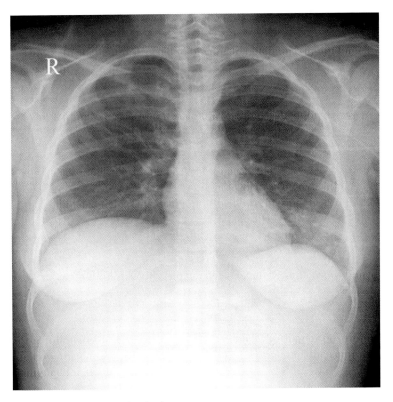

9.   (Figure 2-45; PA projection): _____

_____

_____

Figure 2–46

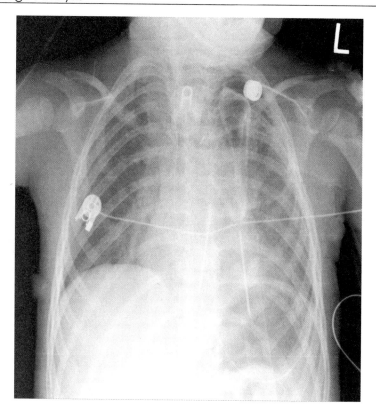

10. (Figure 2-46; AP projection): _____

_____

_____

Figure 2–47

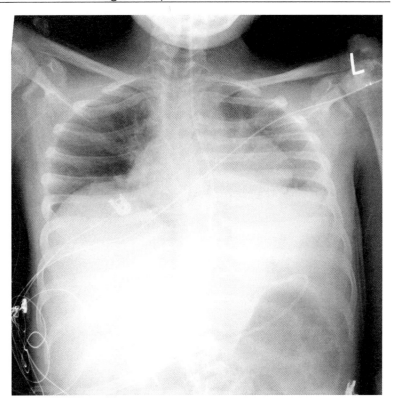

11. (Figure 2-47; AP projection): _____

_____

_____

_____

Neonate and Infant
Cross-table Left Lateral Position (Supine or with Mobile X-Ray Unit)

1. Identify the labeled anatomy in Figure 2-48.

Figure 2–48

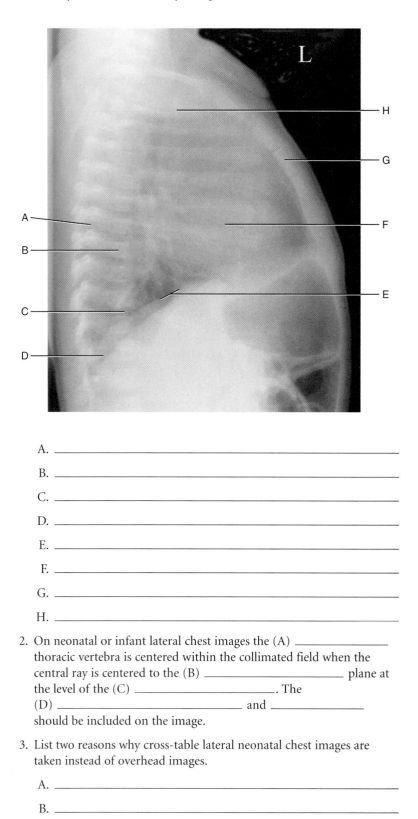

A. _____

B. _____

C. _____

D. _____

E. _____

F. _____

G. _____

H. _____

2. On neonatal or infant lateral chest images the (A) _____ thoracic vertebra is centered within the collimated field when the central ray is centered to the (B) _____ plane at the level of the (C) _____. The (D) _____ and _____ should be included on the image.

3. List two reasons why cross-table lateral neonatal chest images are taken instead of overhead images.

A. _____

B. _____

4. To avoid chest rotation on lateral neonatal and infant chest images, align an imaginary line connecting the shoulders, the posterior ribs, and the posterior pelvic wings _____ to the IR.

5. Explain why the ½-inch (1.25-cm) posterior rib separation demonstrated on optimally positioned adult lateral chest images is not demonstrated on neonatal or infant lateral chest images.

_____

_____

6. On a sufficiently aerated neonatal or infant lateral chest image the hemidiaphragms form a gentle, _____ curve.

For the following descriptions of neonatal or infant lateral chest images with poor positioning, state how the patient would have been mispositioned or the central ray misaligned for such an image to be obtained.

7. The left posterior ribs are demonstrated posterior to the right posterior ribs.

_____

_____

8. The humeral soft tissue is superimposed over the anterior lung apices.

_____

9. The patient's chin is demonstrated within the collimated field.

_____

10. The hemidiaphragms demonstrate an exaggerated cephalic curvature and are positioned high in the thorax.

_____

For the following neonatal or infant lateral chest images with poor positioning state what anatomical structures are misaligned and how the patient should be repositioned for an optimal image to be obtained.

Figure 2–49

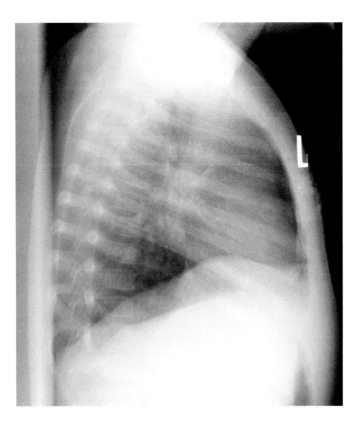

11. (Figure 2-49): _____

_____

_____

_____

Figure 2–50

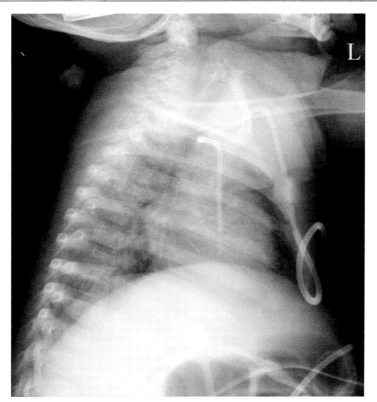

12. (Figure 2-50): _____

_____

_____

_____

Child

Left Lateral Position

1. Identify the labeled anatomy in Figure 2-51.

Figure 2–51

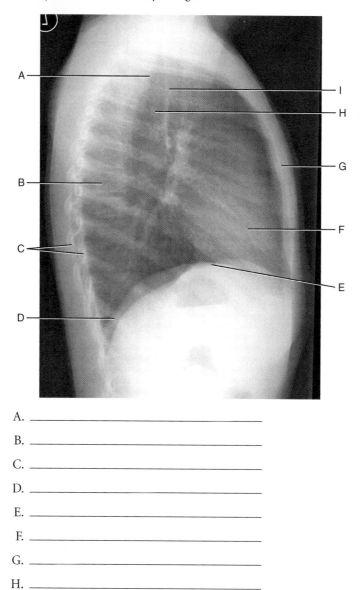

A. _____

B. _____

C. _____

D. _____

E. _____

F. _____

G. _____

H. _____

I. _____

For the following descriptions of child lateral chest images with poor positioning, state how the patient would have been mispositioned or the central ray misaligned for such an image to be obtained.

2. More than ½ inch (1.25 cm) of separation is demonstrated between the posterior ribs. The gastric air bubble is adjacent to the posteriorly located lung.

_____

_____

3. The hemidiaphragms demonstrate an exaggerated cephalic curve, and they do not cover the entire eleventh thoracic vertebra.

_____

4. The humeral soft tissue is superimposed over the anterior lung apices.

_____

For the following lateral child chest images with poor positioning, state what anatomical structures are misaligned and how the patient should be repositioned for an optimal image to be obtained.

Figure 2–52

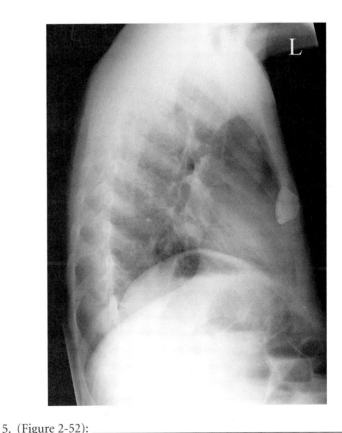

5. (Figure 2-52): _____

_____

_____

_____

Figure 2-53

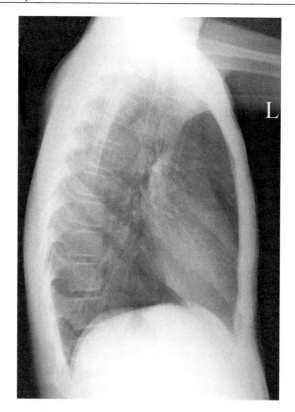

6. (Figure 2-53): _____

_____

_____

Neonate and Infant
Lateral Decubitus Position (AP Projection)
1. Identify the labeled anatomy in Figure 2-54.

Figure 2–54

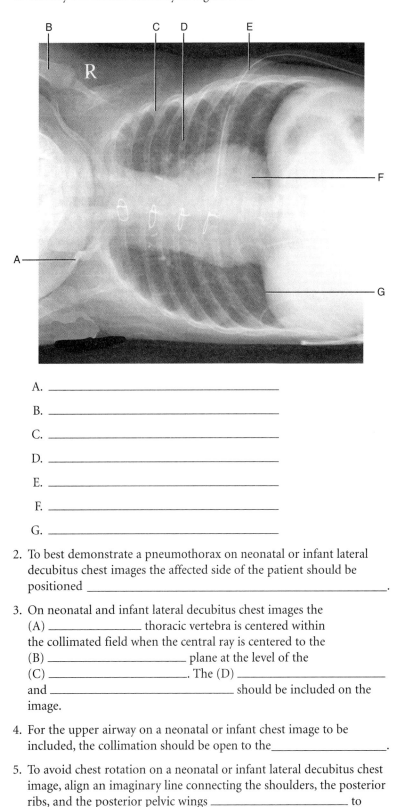

A. _____

B. _____

C. _____

D. _____

E. _____

F. _____

G. _____

2. To best demonstrate a pneumothorax on neonatal or infant lateral decubitus chest images the affected side of the patient should be positioned _____.

3. On neonatal and infant lateral decubitus chest images the (A) _____ thoracic vertebra is centered within the collimated field when the central ray is centered to the (B) _____ plane at the level of the (C) _____. The (D) _____ and _____ should be included on the image.

4. For the upper airway on a neonatal or infant chest image to be included, the collimation should be open to the_____.

5. To avoid chest rotation on a neonatal or infant lateral decubitus chest image, align an imaginary line connecting the shoulders, the posterior ribs, and the posterior pelvic wings _____ to the IR.

6. A lateral decubitus neonatal or infant chest image taken without a lordotic appearance will demonstrate the anterior ribs (A) _____, and the posterior ribs will demonstrate a (B) _____ contour.

7. Full lung is demonstrated on neonatal and infant lateral decubitus images when _____ posterior ribs are demonstrated above the diaphragm.

For the following descriptions of neonatal or infant lateral decubitus chest images with poor positioning, state how the patient would have been mispositioned or the central ray misaligned for such an image to be obtained.

8. The right sternal clavicular end is demonstrated farther from the vertebral column than the left sternal clavicular end, and the right posterior ribs are longer than the left.

   _____

   _____

9. The anterior ribs are projecting cephalically, and the posterior ribs are horizontal.

   _____

   _____

10. The six posterior ribs are demonstrated superior to the diaphragm.

   _____

   _____

11. The image was taken to demonstrate pleural effusion on the right side. Artifact lines are superimposed over the lateral aspect of the right lung.

   _____

   _____

12. The image was taken to demonstrate a left-side pneumothorax. The right arm is superimposed over the upper right lateral lung field.

   _____

   _____

For the following lateral decubitus neonatal or infant chest images with poor positioning, state what anatomical structures are misaligned and how the patient should be repositioned for an optimal image to be obtained.

Figure 2–55

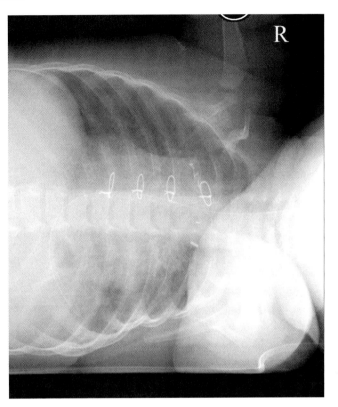

13. (Figure 2-55): _____

_____

_____

_____

_____

Figure 2–56

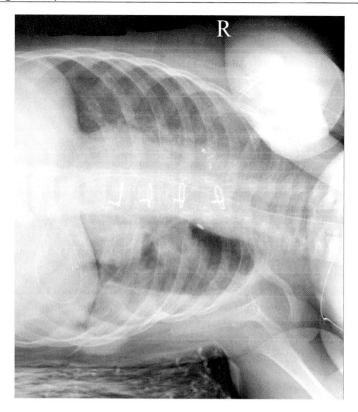

14. (Figure 2-56): _____

_____

_____

Figure 2–57

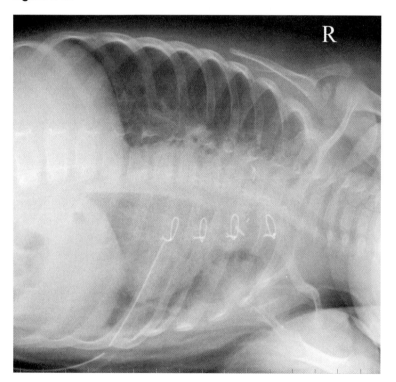

15. (Figure 2-57): _____

_____

_____

_____

_____

Figure 2–60

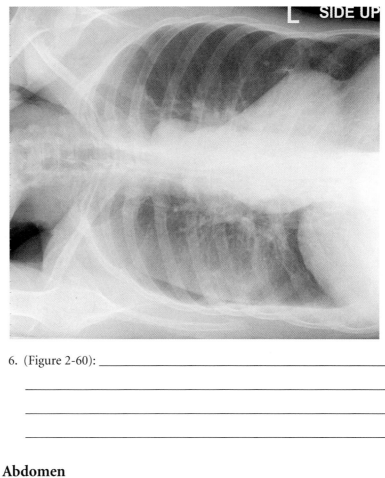

6. (Figure 2-60): _____

_____

_____

_____

Abdomen

1. Contrast, density, and penetration should be sufficient to demonstrate the _____

_____

on neonatal and infant AP abdominal images.

2. Explain why abdominal organs are not well defined on neonatal and infant images.

_____

_____

3. List the positioning procedures (screen-film and digital) that will help demonstrate neonatal and infant abdominal images with sharply defined diaphragms and the gases within the stomach and intestines.

A. _____

B. _____

C. _____

D. _____

E. _____

4. Complete Table 2-7.

TABLE 2-7   Pediatric Abdominal Technical Data

Position or Projection	kVp	Grid	SID
Neonate: AP projection			
Infant: AP projection			
Child: AP projection			
Neonate: Lateral decubitus position			
Infant: Lateral decubitus position			
Child: Lateral decubitus position			

AP, Anteroposterior; *kVp,* kilovolt peak; *SID,* source–image receptor distance.

5. Complete Table 2-8.

TABLE 2-8   IR Size, Placement, and Direction

Position or Projection	IR Size	Placement and Direction
Neonate: AP projection		
Infant: AP projection		
Child: AP projection		
Neonate: Lateral decubitus position		
Infant: Lateral decubitus position		
Child: Lateral decubitus position		

AP, Anteroposterior; *IR,* image receptor.

Neonate and Infant
AP Projection (Supine)

6. Identify the labeled anatomy in Figure 2-61.

Figure 2–61

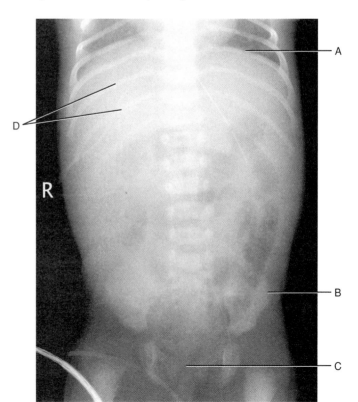

A. _____

B. _____

C. _____

D. _____

7. How is the patient positioned for an AP neonatal or infant abdomen image without rotation?

_____

_____

8. Why are AP abdominal images taken on expiration?

_____

_____

9. A neonatal or infant AP abdominal image taken on expiration will demonstrate the diaphragm domes superior to the _____ posterior rib.

10. On neonatal and infant AP abdominal images the (A) _____ lumbar vertebra is centered within the collimated field when the central ray is centered to the (B) _____ plane at a level (C) _____ inches (D) _____ to the (E) _____ . The (F) _____ should be included on the image.

For the following descriptions of neonatal or infant AP abdominal images with poor positioning, state how the patient would have been mispositioned or the central ray misaligned for such an image to be obtained.

11. The diaphragm is not included on the image.

_____

12. The patient's upper vertebral column is tilted toward the left side.

_____

13. The left inferior posterior ribs are longer than the posterior ribs on the right side.

_____

14. The right iliac wing is wider than the left wing.

_____

15. The diaphragm is at the level of the ninth posterior rib.

_____

For the following AP neonatal or infant abdominal images with poor positioning, state what anatomical structures are misaligned and how the patient should be repositioned for an optimal image to be obtained.

Figure 2–62

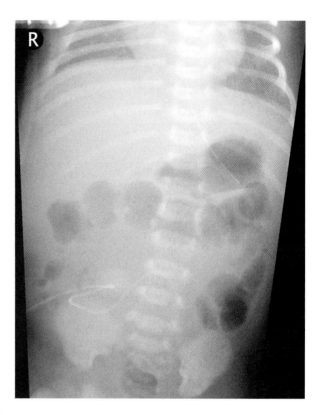

16. (Figure 2-62): _____

_____

_____

_____

Figure 2–63

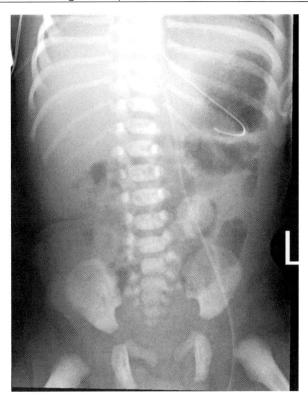

17. (Figure 2-63): _____

_____

_____

_____

Child

AP Projection

1. Identify the labeled anatomy in Figure 2-64.

Figure 2–64

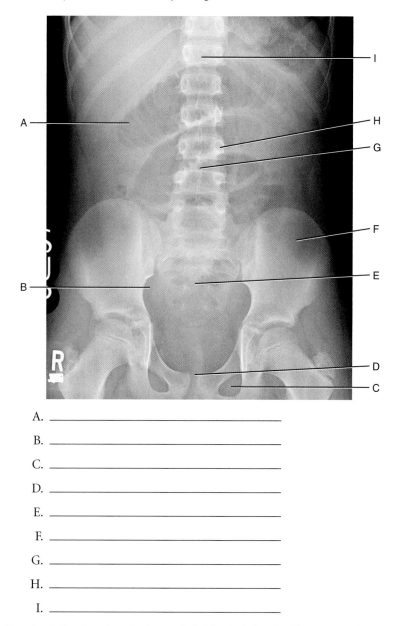

A. _____

B. _____

C. _____

D. _____

E. _____

F. _____

G. _____

H. _____

I. _____

For the following descriptions of child AP abdominal images with poor positioning, state how the patient would have been mispositioned or the central ray misaligned for such an image to be obtained.

2. The distance from the right lumbar vertebral pedicles to the spinous processes is greater than the distance from the left pedicles to the spinous processes.

_____

_____

3. The left inferior posterior ribs are longer than the right, and the left iliac wing is wider than the right.

_____

_____

For the following AP child abdominal images with poor positioning, state what anatomical structures are misaligned and how the patient should be repositioned for an optimal image to be obtained.

Figure 2–65

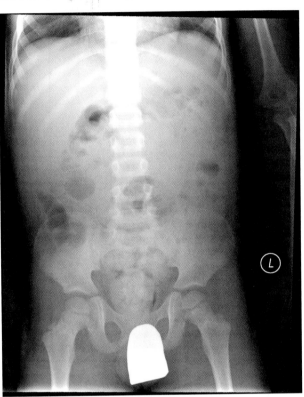

4. (Figure 2-65; Supine abdomen): _____

_____

_____

_____

Figure 2–66

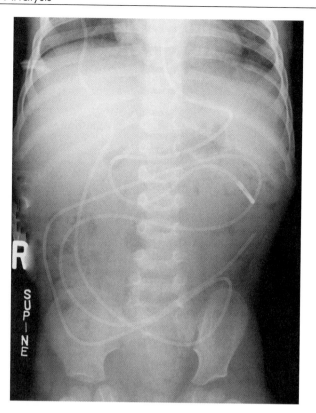

5. (Figure 2-66; Supine abdomen): _____

_____

_____

_____

Figure 2–67

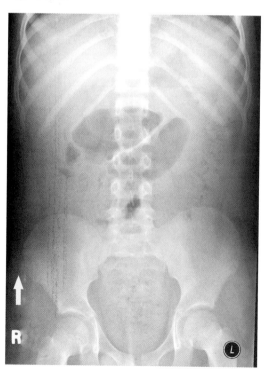

6. (Figure 2-67; Upright abdomen): _____

_____

_____

_____

_____

_____

Neonate and Infant
Left Lateral Decubitus Position (AP Projection)
1. Identify the labeled anatomy in Figure 2-68.

Figure 2–68

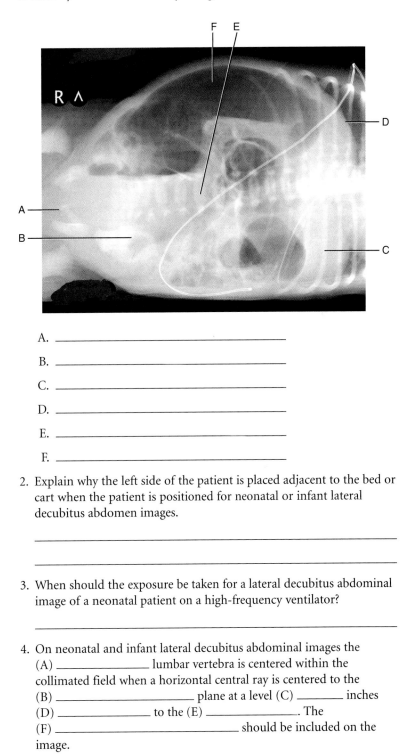

A. _____

B. _____

C. _____

D. _____

E. _____

F. _____

2. Explain why the left side of the patient is placed adjacent to the bed or cart when the patient is positioned for neonatal or infant lateral decubitus abdomen images.

_____

_____

3. When should the exposure be taken for a lateral decubitus abdominal image of a neonatal patient on a high-frequency ventilator?

_____

4. On neonatal and infant lateral decubitus abdominal images the (A) _____ lumbar vertebra is centered within the collimated field when a horizontal central ray is centered to the (B) _____ plane at a level (C) _____ inches (D) _____ to the (E) _____. The (F) _____ should be included on the image.

For the following descriptions of neonatal or infant left lateral decubitus abdominal images with poor positioning, state how the patient would have been mispositioned or the central ray misaligned for such an image to be obtained.

5. The left iliac wing is narrower than the right iliac wing.

_____

_____

6. The diaphragm is not included on the image.

_____

_____

7. The right posterior ribs are longer than the posterior ribs on the left side.

_____

_____

For the following left lateral decubitus neonatal or infant abdominal images with poor positioning, state what anatomical structures are misaligned and how the patient should be repositioned for an optimal image to be obtained.

Figure 2–69

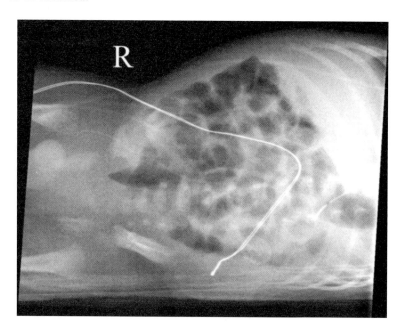

8. (Figure 2-69): _____

_____

_____

Figure 2–70

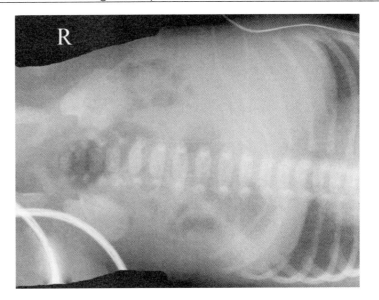

9. (Figure 2-70): _____

_____

_____

Child
Left Lateral Decubitus Position (AP Projection)
1. Identify the labeled anatomy in Figure 2-71.

Figure 2–71

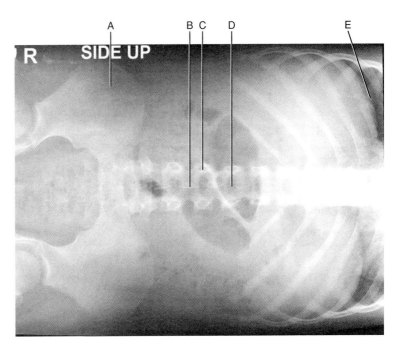

A. _____

B. _____

C. _____

D. _____

E. _____

2. Identify the patient condition demonstrated on the image in Figure 2-72.

Figure 2–72

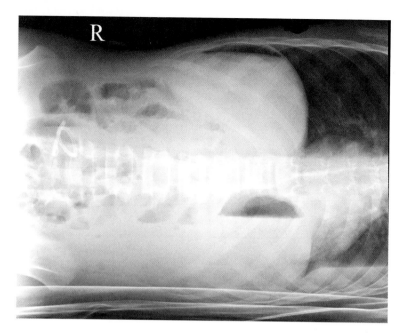

For the following descriptions of child lateral decubitus abdominal images with poor positioning, state how the patient would have been mispositioned or the central ray misaligned for such an image to be obtained.

3. The diaphragm is at the level of the ninth posterior rib. The child was on a conventional ventilator.

_____

_____

4. The distance from the left lumbar vertebral pedicles to the spinous processes is greater than that from the right pedicles to the spinous processes.

_____

_____

For the following child lateral decubitus images with poor positioning, state what anatomical structures are misaligned and how the patient should be repositioned for an optimal image to be obtained.

5. (Figure 2-72): _____

_____

_____

Figure 2–73

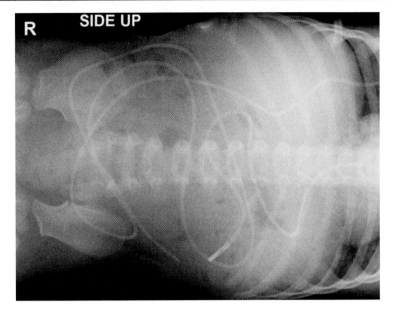

6. (Figure 2-73): _____

_____

_____

CHAPTER 2
STUDY QUESTION ANSWERS
Chest

1. A. As if the patient were in an upright position. Marker is reversed.
   B. As if the patient were in an upright position. Marker is correct.
   C. As if the patient were in an upright position. Marker is correct.
   D. As if the patient were in an upright position. Marker is reversed.
   E. Hang so side of the patient that was positioned upward when the image was exposed is upward on the displayed image. Marker is correct for AP projection and reversed for PA projection.

2. It decreases magnification of the heart and increases the sharpness of the recorded details of the lungs and heart.
3. A. Halt patient respiration.
   B. Halt body movements.
   C. Use a short object–image receptor distance (OID).
   D. Use a 72-inch (183-cm) SID.
4. Vascular lung markings and fluid levels or air within the pleural cavity
5. Thoracic vertebrae and mediastinal structures

6.

Position or Projection	kVp	Grid	AEC Chamber(s)	SID
PA projection	110	Grid	Both outside	72 inch (183 cm)
Lateral position	125	Grid	Center	72 inch (183 cm)
AP projection	70-80	Nongrid		48-50 inch (120-125 cm)
AP projection	80-100	Grid	Both outside	48-50 inch (120-125 cm)
Lateral decubitus position	125	Grid	Center	72 inch (183 cm)
AP axial (lordotic) projection	125	Grid	Both outside	72 inch (183 cm)
Oblique position	125	Grid	Over lung of interest	72 inch (183 cm)

AEC, Automatic exposure control; AP, anteroposterior; kVp, kilovolt peak; SID, source–image receptor distance.

7.

Position or Projection	IR Size	Placement and Direction
PA projection	14 × 17 inch (35 × 43 cm)	Lengthwise: Sthenic or asthenic body
		Crosswise: Hypersthenic body
Lateral position	14 × 17 inch (35 × 43 cm)	Lengthwise
AP projection	14 × 17 inch (35 × 43 cm)	Lengthwise: Asthenic body
		Crosswise: Sthenic or hypersthenic body
Lateral decubitus position	14 × 17 inch (35 × 43 cm)	Crosswise with respect to patient
AP axial (lordotic) projection	14 × 17 inch (35 × 43 cm)	Lengthwise
Oblique position	14 × 17 inch (35 × 43 cm)	Lengthwise

AP, Anteroposterior; IR, image receptor; PA, posteroanterior.

PA Projection

8. A. Right lung apex
   B. Clavicle
   C. Fourth thoracic vertebra
   D. Scapula
   E. Fourth anterior rib
   F. Diaphragm
   G. Costophrenic angle
   H. Heart shadow
   I. Lung
   J. Hilum
   K. Seventh posterior rib
   L. Aortic arch
   M. Superior manubrium
   N. Left SC joint
   O. Air-filled trachea

9. A. Cavity encasing the lungs
   B. Presence of air in pleural cavity
   C. Removal of a lung
   D. Within the abdominal cavity
   E. Spinous process of the seventh cervical vertebra
   F. Narrow end of a cone-shaped object
   G. Image density line that is created when fluid and air within an object separate
   H. Rotation of part toward the front of body
10. A. Should be placed in an upright position
    B. Should be horizontal
11. A. Pleural effusion
    B. Pneumothorax
    C. Pneumectomy
12. A. Transversely
    B. Anteroposteriorly
    C. Vertically
13. Vertical
14. Disease processes, advanced pregnancy, excessive obesity, a slouching patient, or confining clothing
15. A. Hypersthenic
    B. Short and wide
16. A. Asthenic and sthenic
    B. Long and narrow
17. Place a hand along the patient's sides at the level of costophrenic angles. Ask the patient to inhale and observe whether your hands remain within the IR's boundaries.
18. Superolaterally
19. Place the patient's shoulders and arms at equal distances from the IR.
20. A. Sternal ends of clavicles
    B. Right and left corresponding posterior ribs
21. A. Scoliosis
    B. No
    C. On a rotated patient the distances will be uniform down the length of the lung field, but with scoliosis the vertebral column to lateral lung edge distance will vary down the length of the each lung and between each lung.
22. The shoulders are depressed.
23. Place hands on hips and rotate elbows and shoulders anteriorly.
24. A. Midcoronal
    B. Fourth
    C. 1 inch (2.5 cm)
25. A. If the patient's shoulders are not depressed
    B. If the patient's upper midcoronal plane is leaning toward the IR
26. The diaphragm is allowed to move to its lowest position.
27. A. Placing the patient in an upright position
    B. Having the patient perform a deep inspiration
28. It coaxes the patient into a deeper inspiration.
29. 10 or 11

30. A. Pneumothorax
    B. Foreign body
31. A. Higher
    B. Nine
    C. Broader
    D. Shorter
    E. Lighter
32. A. Seventh thoracic vertebra
    B. Horizontal
    C. Midsagittal
    D. Vertebral prominens
33. The apices, lateral lungs, and costophrenic angles
34. Rotated into an RAO position
35. The shoulders were not depressed.
36. The right elbow and shoulder were not rotated anteriorly.
37. The patient's upper midcoronal plane was tilted toward the IR.
38. The patient's upper midcoronal plane was tilted away from the IR.
39. The image was taken on expiration.
40. Eight posterior ribs are demonstrated above the diaphragm, and the clavicles are not on the same horizontal plane. Expose the image after coaxing the patient into a deeper inspiration and depress the shoulders.
41. The vertebral column is superimposed over the right sternal clavicular end, and the left inferior posterior ribs are longer than the right. Rotate the patient toward the left side until the shoulders are at equal distances from the IR.
42. The scapulae are demonstrated in the superolateral lung field, the third thoracic vertebra is superimposed over the manubrium, and the inferior tip of the costophrenic angles are not included in the collimation field. Rotate the shoulders and elbows anteriorly, tilt the patient's upper midcoronal plane toward the IR until it is parallel with the IR, and move the central ray and IR inferiorly by ½ inch (1.25 cm).
43. The fifth thoracic vertebra is superimposed over the manubrium, and only a portion of the tenth posterior rib is seen above the diaphragm. Tilt the upper midcoronal plane away from the IR until it is parallel with the IR, and expose the image after coaxing the patient into a deeper inspiration.

Left Lateral Position

1. A. Lung apex
   B. Scapulae
   C. Thoracic vertebra
   D. Intervertebral foramen
   E. Posterior ribs
   F. Intervertebral disk space
   G. Costophrenic angles

H. Diaphragm

I. Heart shadow

J. Sternum

K. Hili

L. Esophagus

M. Trachea

2. A. Abnormal lateral deviation of the spinal column

B. Half of the diaphragm

C. Variance from the normal or routine

D. Forward curvature of the vertebral column

E. Backward curvature of the vertebral column

3. A. ½ inch (1.25 cm)

B. Posterior

C. Anterior

4. Align the shoulders, posterior ribs, and posterior pelvic wings perpendicular to the IR holder.

5. A. Right

B. It is situated farther from the IR, so diverged x-rays will cause it to magnify.

6. By evaluating the degree of posterior rib and anterior rib superimposition

7. A. Find the gastric air bubble, which is located beneath the left hemidiaphragm.

B. Outline the heart shadow, which is located within the left hemidiaphragm.

8. Beneath the left hemidiaphragm

9. Left

10. Rotate the left side of the patient anteriorly approximately 1 inch (2.5 cm), or rotate the right side of the patient posteriorly approximately 1 inch (2.5 cm).

11. The anterior ribs will be superimposed, whereas the posterior ribs will demonstrate differing degrees of separation.

12. The midsagittal plane is parallel to the IR.

13. Right

14. A. The heart shadow will be more magnified on the right lateral chest image.

B. The left hemidiaphragm will project lower than the right hemidiaphragm on a right lateral chest image.

15. A. Right lateral

B. Left lateral

C. Left lateral

16. Position the humeri vertically.

17. Anteroinferior

18. The eleventh thoracic vertebra will be superimposed by the lung field.

19. A. Take exposure after the second full inspiration.

B. Take exposure with the patient in an upright position.

20. Twelfth

21. A. Midcoronal

B. Eighth

C. Midcoronal

D. Inferior

22. The lung apices, sternum, posterior ribs, diaphragm, and costophrenic angles

23. Patient's humeri were not positioned vertically.

24. The left thorax was rotated anteriorly.

25. If no medical indication explains this relationship, the patient's lower thorax was situated closer to the IR than the upper thorax (midsagittal plane was not parallel with IR).

26. Image A: More than ½ inch (1.25 cm) of separation is present between the posterior ribs. The inferior heart shadow projects into the inferiorly and anteriorly located lung field. Rotate the patient's right side anteriorly approximately ½ inch (1.25 cm).

Image B: The right and left posterior ribs are separated by more than ½ inch (1.25 cm), indicating that the chest was rotated. The superior heart shadow does not extend beyond the sternum and the gastric air bubble is demonstrated adjacent to the posteriorly situated lung, verifying that the right lung is situated anterior to the sternum, and the left lung posteriorly. Rotate the patient's right side posteriorly approximately ½ inch (1.25 cm).

27. The humeral soft-tissue shadows are superimposed over the anterior lung apices. Position the patient's humeri vertically.

28. A. The manubrium is at the level of the third thoracic vertebra. Tilt the upper midcoronal plane toward the IR until the midcoronal plane is parallel with the IR.

B. This image reflects accurate positioning. One might conclude that the left hemidiaphragm is too superior and that the patient's midsagittal plane was tilted, but by evaluating the PA image it can be determined that because the left hemidiaphragm is situated higher than the right on this patient, this positioning is accurate.

AP Projection (Supine or with Mobile X-Ray Unit)

1. A. Right apex

B. Right SC joint

C. Scapula

D. Fifth posterior rib

E. Medial scapular border

F. Diaphragm

G. Costophrenic angle

H. Heart shadow

I. Aortic arch

J. Manubrium

K. Third thoracic vertebra

2. A. Excessive convexity of the thoracic vertebrae

B. Tissues and organs (heart, trachea, and esophagus) that separate the sternum and vertebral column

C. Outline of a shape

3. So the reviewer knows which image was taken first if more than one were taken on the same day

4. So the reviewer will know the accuracy of the air-fluid levels demonstrated

5. The fluid is evenly spread throughout the lung field, so no definite air-fluid line is visible.

6. Kilovoltage

7. A. Used to inflate the lungs; penetration of the upper mediastinal region
   B. Used to remove fluid or air from the pleural space; density and penetration to visualize the radiopaque identification line interruptions at the side hole
   C. Used to allow infusion of substances that are too toxic for peripheral infusion; density and penetration to demonstrate the superior mediastinal region and lungs
   D. Used to measure atrial pressures, pulmonary artery pressure, and cardiac output; density and penetration to visualize the mediastinal structures

8. A. Chest tube
   B. Central venous line
   C. Pulmonary artery line (external electrocardiographic leads are also demonstrated)

9. A. The vertical dimension does not fully expand in the recumbent or seated positions.
   B. Because a low SID is used, resulting in increased magnification.

10. Place the shoulders and anterior superior iliac spines at equal distances from the IR and bed.

11. A. Sternal ends of clavicles
    B. Right and left corresponding posterior ribs

12. Rotation is evident when the distances from the sternal clavicular ends to the vertebral column and the lengths of the right and left corresponding posterior ribs are not equal.

13. Clavicles will be on the same horizontal plane.

14. Poor shoulder positioning will demonstrate decreased lung field superior to the clavicles, whereas poor central ray alignment will demonstrate increased lung field superior to the clavicles.

15. Place back of patient's hands on hips and rotate elbows and shoulders anteriorly.

16. A. Fourth
    B. 1 inch (2.5 cm)
    C. Downward

17. A. More than 1 inch (2.5 cm) of apices will be seen above the clavicles, and the posterior ribs will be vertically shaped.
    B. Less than 1 inch (2.5 cm) of the apices will be seen above the clavicles, and the posterior ribs will be horizontal.

18. Angle the central ray 5 to 10 degrees cephalically.

19. A. 5 degrees caudally
    B. To offset the upward lift of the manubrium, clavicles, and superior ribs

20. 9 to 10

21. Pressure from the abdominal organs prevents the diaphragm from shifting to an inferior position.

22. Instruct the patient to take two full breaths before the image is exposed.

23. The high-frequency ventilator maintains the lung expansion at a steady mean pressure.

24. A. Seventh thoracic
    B. Midsagittal
    C. 4
    D. Jugular notch

25. The lung apices, lateral lungs, and costophrenic angles

26. The patient would have been in a left posterior oblique (LPO) position, or the central ray would have been angled toward the left side of the chest.

27. The central ray was angled too caudally.

28. The central ray was angled too cephalically.

29. The central ray was aligned perpendicular to the IR. It would be best to angle 5 to 10 degrees cephalically.

30. Eight posterior ribs are demonstrated superior to the diaphragm, the clavicles are not horizontal, the left SC joint appears away from the vertebral column, and the left posterior ribs demonstrate greater length than the right. Expose the image after coaxing the patient into a greater inspiration, depress the shoulders, and place an elevating device beneath the left IR border to position the IR parallel with the bed or angle the central ray toward the right side of the patient until it is aligned perpendicular to the IR.

31. More than 1 inch (2.5 cm) of apical lung field is demonstrated above the clavicles, and the posterior ribs have a vertical contour. Angle the central ray cephalically until it is aligned perpendicular to the midcoronal plane.

32. The manubrium is superimposed over the third thoracic vertebra, and less than 1 inch (2.5 cm) is demonstrated above the clavicles. Angle the central ray caudally until it is aligned perpendicular to the midcoronal plane.

Lateral Decubitus Position (AP or PA Projection)

1. A. Diaphragm
   B. Tenth posterior rib
   C. Heart shadow
   D. Lateral scapular border
   E. Clavicle

2. A. To fill with air
   B. Invasion of fluid into the pleural cavity
   C. Penetrable by x-rays

3. A. Mark side positioned away from the table with an R marker and an arrow pointing upward or "word" marker identifying the side of the patient positioned upward.

B. Display so that lateral right side of the chest is upward.

4. When vascular lung markings are seen throughout the lung field
5. A. Air
   B. Fluid
6. Within the side of the chest positioned closer to the table or cart
7. A. Decrease kVp by 8%
   B. Increase mAs by 35%
8. A. Left lateral decubitus
   B. Left lateral decubitus
9. A. Sternal ends of the clavicles
   B. Right and left corresponding posterior ribs
10. A. Posterior ribs
    B. Shoulders
    C. Posterior pelvic wings
11. AP
12. Above the patient's head
13. Fourth
14. A. Midcoronal
    B. Parallel
15. 9 or 10
16. Elevate the patient on a radiolucent sponge or cardiac board.
17. Right side of chest was positioned closer to the IR than left side.
18. Left side of chest was positioned closer to the IR than right side.
19. Patient's upper midcoronal plane was tilted toward the IR.
20. The right sternal clavicular end is superimposed over the vertebral column, and the posterior ribs on the left side demonstrate greater length than those on the right. Rotate the left side away from the IR until the midcoronal plane and IR are parallel.
21. The manubrium is superimposed over the fifth thoracic vertebra. Tilt the upper midcoronal plane toward the IR until it and the IR are parallel.

AP Lordotic Projection
1. A. Lung apex
   B. Posterior fourth rib
   C. Anterior fourth rib
   D. Superior scapular angle
   E. Lateral border scapula
   F. Medial clavicular end
   G. First thoracic vertebra
2. Cause the long axis of an object to appear shorter
3. Lung apices
4. A. First
   B. Horizontally
   C. Superimposed
5. A. Arch the patient's back until the midcoronal plane is at a 45-degree angle to the IR. A perpendicular central ray is used.

B. Have the patient remain completely upright, and use a 45-degree cephalic central ray angle.
   C. Patient's back is arched as much as possible, and the central ray is angled cephalically in the amount necessary to equal 45 degrees.
6. A. Increase the degree of patient arch.
   B. Increase the degree of central ray angulation.
7. Place the back of the patient's hands on hips and rotate the elbows and shoulders anteriorly.
8. When the SC joints are not at equal distances from the vertebral column
9. A. Superior lung field
   B. Midsagittal
   C. Manubrium
   D. Xiphoid
10. The clavicles, lung apices, and two thirds of the lung field
11. The midcoronal plane was at less than a 45-degree angle to IR or central ray was angled cephalically less than needed.
12. The elbows and shoulders were not drawn anteriorly.
13. The patient was rotated in an LPO position.
14. The medial clavicular ends are superimposed over the lung apices, and the anterior ribs are demonstrated inferior to their corresponding posterior rib. Cephalically increase the central ray angulation or have the patient increase the amount of back arch until the angle of the midcoronal plane and IR is 45 degrees.

PA Oblique Projection (RAO and LAO Positions)
1. A. SC joints
   B. Air-filled trachea
   C. Principal bronchi
   D. Heart shadow
   E. Posterior heart shadow
2. A. Change in body tissue that is caused by a disease process
   B. Undesirable structure that is demonstrated on an image
3. Midcoronal
4. A. Twice
   B. Vertebral column
   C. Spinal
5. 60
6. A. Right
   B. Right
7. LAO
8. 10 or 11
9. A. Right and left principal bronchi
   B. Vertebra prominens
10. The apices, costophrenic angles, and lateral chest walls
11. The patient was not rotated enough.
12. The patient was rotated too much.

13. The patient was not rotated enough.

14. Less than two times the lung field is demonstrated on the right side of this thorax than on the right side. Increase the degree of patient obliquity until the midcoronal plane is at a 45-degree angle to the IR.

15. Approximately three times the lung field is demonstrated on the right side of this thorax than on the left side, which indicates that the patient was rotated approximately 60 degrees. An LAO chest image taken to evaluate the lung field should demonstrate only two times the lung field on the right side than the left and would demonstrate the vertebral column superimposed over the heart shadow. Decrease the degree of patient obliquity until the midcoronal plane is at a 45-degree angle to the IR.

Abdomen

1. A. As if the patient were in an upright position. Marker is correct.
   B. So side of the patient that was positioned upward when the image was exposed is upward on the displayed image. Marker is correct.
2. A. Invasion of fluid
   B. Motion that the patient is capable of controlling
   C. Motion that the patient is incapable of controlling
   D. Able to walk
   E. Cavity containing the abdominal structures
3. They are located lateral to the lumbar vertebrae, starting at the first lumbar vertebra and extending to the lesser trochanters.
4. A. They are located lateral to the vertebral column, with the upper poles at approximately the eleventh thoracic vertebra and the lower poles at approximately the third lumbar vertebra.
   B. Right
   C. It is located beneath the liver.
5. A. Psoas major muscle
   B. Kidneys
   C. Inferior ribs
   D. Lumbar transverse processes
6. A. 30% to 50% decrease
   B. 5% to 8% decrease
7. A. Obesity
   B. Bowel obstruction
   C. Soft-tissue masses
   D. Ascites
8. A. Increase 30% to 50%
   B. Increase 5% to 7%
9. A. Patient breathing during exposure
   B. Patient moving during exposure
10. A. Explaining to the patient the importance of holding still
    B. Making the patient as comfortable as possible
    C. Using the shortest exposure time

11. Peristaltic activity
12. Use the shortest possible exposure time.
13. A. Involuntary motion; cortical outlines of ribs and bony structures are sharp
    B. Voluntary motion; cortical outlines of ribs are blurry

14.

Position or Projection	kVp	Grid	AEC Chamber(s)	SID
AP projection	70-80	Grid	All	40-48 inches (100-120 cm)
Lateral decubitus position	70-80	Grid	Center	40-48 inches (100-120 cm)

AEC, Automatic exposure control; *AP*, anteroposterior; *kVp*, kilovolt peak; *SID*, source–image receptor distance.

15.

Position or Projection	IR Size	Placement and Direction
PA projection	14 × 17 inch (35 × 43 cm)	Lengthwise (to patient): Sthenic and asthenic (up to 14 cm width)
		Crosswise: Hypersthenic, sthenic, and asthenic (over 14 cm width)
Lateral decubitus dosition	14 × 17 inch (35 × 43 cm)	Lengthwise (to patient): Sthenic and asthenic (up to 14 cm width)
		Crosswise: Hypersthenic, sthenic, and asthenic (over 14 cm width)

IR, Image receptor; *PA*, posteroanterior.

AP Projection (Supine and Upright)

16. A. Kidney
    B. Pedicle
    C. Third vertebral body
    D. Intestinal gas
    E. Anterior superior iliac spine (ASIS)
    F. Inlet pelvis
    G. Sacrum
    H. Iliac wing
    I. Iliac crest
    J. Spinous process
    K. Eleventh thoracic vertebra
17. A. Diaphragmatic dome
    B. Pedicle
    C. Inlet pelvis
    D. Sacrum
    E. Spinous process
    F. Twelfth vertebral body
    G. Gastric bubble
    H. Diaphragmatic dome
    I. Ninth thoracic vertebra

18. Intraperitoneal air is located directly beneath each diaphragm dome.
19. Position the patient's shoulders and anterior superior iliac spines at equal distances from the IR.
20. A. Vertebral body
    B. Spinous processes
    C. Symphysis pubis
21. A. 10 to 20 minutes
    B. It allows time for the air to rise to the level of the diaphragm.
22. The upper and lower lumbar vertebrae can rotate independently.
23. Scoliosis
24. Align the xiphoid and a point halfway between the patient's anterior superior iliac spines with the collimator's longitudinal light line.
25. A. An inferior
    B. A superior
    C. Eighth or ninth
    D. Eleventh
26. A. Expiration
    B. Because less pressure is placed on the abdominal organs
27. A. Ensures that the kidneys, tip of liver, and spleen are included on the image
    B. Ensures that the inferior border of the peritoneal cavity is included on the image
28. Because the male patient's pelvis is longer
29. A. Two crosswise
    B. One lengthwise
    C. One lengthwise
30. To ensure that no middle peritoneal information is excluded
31. A. The eleventh thoracic spinous process, lateral body soft tissue, iliac wings, and obturator foramen
    B. The diaphragm, lateral body soft tissue, and iliac wings
32. Patient was rotated into an RPO position.
33. The upper abdomen was in an AP projection, whereas the pelvic area was rotated into an LPO position.
34. The central ray and IR were centered too superiorly.
35. The sacrum is not aligned with the symphysis pubis, the distance from the left pedicles to the spinous processes is less than the distance from the right pedicles to the spinous processes, and the lateral soft tissue is not included on the image. Rotate the patient toward the left side until the shoulders and anterior iliac spines are positioned at equal distances from the IR, and expose images of the abdomen using two crosswise IRs instead of one lengthwise.
36. The symphysis pubis is not included on the image. This is a male patient. Center the central ray 1 inch (2.5 cm) superior to the iliac crest and align the IR with the central ray.

37. The domes of the diaphragm are not included on the image. Center the central ray and IR approximately 2 inches (5 cm) superiorly.

Left Lateral Decubitus Position (AP Projection)

1. A. Iliac wing
   B. Intestinal gas
   C. Diaphragmatic dome
   D. Pedicle
   E. Vertebral body
   F. Spinous process
2. A. Filter used to compensate for the differences in part thickness so that uniform image density can be obtained
   B. A lying-down position
3. Measure the patient, and increase the mAs 30% to 50% or the kVp 5% to 8% from the routine technique that would normally be used for this body measurement.
4. Place the thicker end of the filter toward the right side of the patient and the thinner end toward the left side.
5. A. Left
   B. This will position the gastric air bubble away from the abdominal area where the intraperitoneal air would be demonstrated.
6. Align the shoulders, posterior ribs, and posterior pelvic wings perpendicular to the imaging table or cart.
7. Forward rotation of the side positioned farther from the imaging table
8. A. 10 to 20
   B. To allow time for the air to move away from the soft tissue structures and rise to the level of the right diaphragm
9. Right hemidiaphragm
10. Patient with wide hips and narrow waist and thorax
11. A. Two crosswise
    B. One lengthwise
    C. One lengthwise
12. Expiration
13. The right hemidiaphragm, ninth thoracic vertebra, right lateral soft tissue, and right iliac wing
14. A. If two crosswise IRs are used and the upper abdomen is being imaged
    B. All the time
15. The right side of the patient was positioned farther from the IR than the left side.
16. The thorax and upper abdominal region were positioned accurately, whereas the right side of the pelvis and lower abdomen are closer to the IR than the left side.
17. The IR and central ray were positioned too inferiorly.
18. The right iliac wing is narrower than the left iliac wing, and the distance from the right pedicles to

the spinous processes is less than the distance from the left pedicles to the spinous processes. Rotate the patient's right side toward the IR until the shoulders and the anterior superior iliac spines are positioned at equal distances from the IR.

Pediatrics

Chest

1. Heart magnification in pediatric imaging is minimal because the heart OID is short.
2. Internal lines and tubes and lung tissue (air-filled alveolar and linear connecting tissue)
3. The thoracic vertebrae mediastinal structures are faintly demonstrated.
4. Neonates and infants have fewer alveoli, causing the lungs to be denser.
5. Head rotation and cervical flexion and extension cause the ET tip to move superiorly and inferiorly, making it difficult for the reviewer to determine exactly where the tube is positioned.
6. A. Used to inflate the lungs
   B. Used to measure oxygen saturation
   C. Used to deliver fluids and medications
7.

Position or Projection	kVp	Grid	SID
Neonate: Supine or mobile AP projection	65-70		40-48 inches (100-120 cm)
Infant: Supine or mobile AP projection	70-75		40-48 inches (100-120 cm)
Child: PA projection	75-80	Grid (if AP measurement is over 13 cm)	40-48 inches (100-120 cm)
Child: AP projection	70-75		40-48 inches (100-120 cm)
Neonate: Cross-table lateral position	65-70		40-48 inches (100-120 cm)
Infant: Cross-table lateral position	75-80		40-48 inches (100-120 cm)
Child: Lateral position	75-80	Grid (if side-to-side measurement is over 13 cm)	40-48 inches (100-120 cm)
Neonate: Lateral decubitus position	65-70		40-48 inches (100-120 cm)
Infant: Lateral decubitus position	70-75		40-48 inches (100-120 cm)
Child: Lateral decubitus position	75-80	Grid (if AP measurement is over 13 cm)	72 inches (183 cm)

AP, Anteroposterior; *kVp*, kilovolt peak; *PA*, posteroanterior; *SID*, source–image receptor distance.

8.

Position or Projection	IR Size	Placement and Direction
Neonate: Supine or mobile AP projection	8 × 10 inch (18 × 24 cm)	Lengthwise
Infant: Supine or mobile AP projection	8 × 10 inch (18 × 24 cm)	Lengthwise
Child: PA projection	Adjusted to	Lengthwise patient size
Child: AP projection	Adjusted to	Lengthwise patient size
Neonate: Cross-table lateral position	8 × 10 inch (18 × 24 cm)	Lengthwise
Infant: Cross-table lateral position	Adjusted to patient size	Lengthwise
Child: Lateral position	Adjusted to	Lengthwise patient size
Neonate: Lateral decubitus position	8 × 10 inch (18 × 24 cm)	Lengthwise
Infant: Lateral decubitus position	Adjusted to patient size	Lengthwise
Child: Lateral decubitus position	Adjusted to patient size	Lengthwise

AP, Anteroposterior; *IR*, image receptor; *PA*, posteroanterior.

Neonate and Infant

AP Projection (Supine or with Mobile X-Ray Unit)

9. A. Clavicle
   B. Right lung apex
   C. Diaphragm
   D. Costophrenic angle
   E. Heart shadow
   F. Anterior rib
   G. Fourth posterior rib
   H. Air-filled airway
10. A. Fourth
   B. Midsagittal
   C. Mammary line
   D. Upper airway, lungs, mediastinal structures, and costophrenic angles
11. A. Sternal ends of the clavicle
   B. Inferior posterior ribs
12. A. Anterior
   B. Posterior
13. Shape
14. A. Eight
   B. Nine
15. The dense substances of blood, pus, protein, and cells and the less-dense air
16. A. After neonates take a deep breath as observed by watching chest movements
   B. When the manometer's digital bar or analog needle moves to its highest position

C. At any time

17. The patient is rotated toward the right side (RPO position).
18. The central ray was centered too inferiorly.
19. The image was exposed with the ventilator's manometer at a level lower than the highest point.
20. The chin was tucked toward the chest.
21. The left sternal clavicular end is positioned away from the vertebral column, and the left posterior ribs demonstrate greater length than the right posterior ribs. Rotate the patient toward the right side until the midcoronal plane is parallel with the IR.
22. The anterior ribs are projecting upwardly, and the posterior ribs are horizontal. The sixth thoracic vertebra is in the center of the collimated field. Center the central ray approximately 1 inch (2.5 cm) superiorly (at the mammary line).
23. The seventh posterior rib is demonstrated superior to the diaphragm, and the chin is superimposed over the lung apices. If possible, take the exposure after a deeper inhalation and elevate the chin until the cervical vertebrae are in a neutral position.

Child
PA and AP Projections
1. A. Second anterior rib
   B. Sixth posterior rib
   C. Lung
   D. Diaphragm
   E. Costophrenic angle
   F. Heart shadow
   G. Hilum
   H. Superior manubrium
   I. Left sternoclavicular joint
   J. Right lung apex
   K. Air-filled trachea
2. The patient's left side is rotated toward the IR (LPO position).
3. The image was exposed on expiration.
4. The central ray was not perpendicular with the midcoronal plane but was angled caudally.
5. The patient's upper midcoronal plane was tilted away from the IR.
6. The shoulders were elevated.
7. The manubrium is at the level of the third thoracic vertebra, and the clavicles are not horizontal. Tilt the upper midcoronal plane toward the IR until it is parallel with the IR and depress the shoulders.
8. The manubrium is at the level of the fifth thoracic vertebra, and the left side of the thorax has been collimated off the image. Tilt the upper midcoronal plane away from the IR until it is parallel with the IR, and move the central ray medially until it is centered to the midsagittal plane.

9. Eight posterior ribs are demonstrated above the diaphragm, the right sternal clavicular end is visualized away from the vertebral column, and the right posterior ribs demonstrate greater length than the left. Coax the patient into a deeper inhalation and rotate the patient toward the right side until the IR and midcoronal plane are parallel.
10. The manubrium is at the level of the seventh thoracic vertebra, and the posterior ribs are vertical. Angle the central ray cephalically until it is perpendicular to the midcoronal plane.
11. The manubrium is at the level of the second thoracic vertebra, the posterior ribs are horizontal, and five posterior ribs are demonstrated above the diaphragm. Angle the central ray caudally until it is perpendicular to the midcoronal plane and coax the patient into a deeper inhalation.

Neonate and Infant
Cross-table Left Lateral Position (Supine or with Mobile X-Ray Unit)
1. A. Intervertebral foramen
   B. Thoracic vertebra
   C. Intervertebral disk space
   D. Costophrenic angle
   E. Diaphragm
   F. Heart shadow
   G. Sternum
   H. Lung apex
2. A. Fifth
   B. Midcoronal
   C. Mammary line
   D. Apices, costophrenic angles, posterior ribs, and airway
3. A. Less disturbance to the sensitive neonate
   B. Will not result in compression of the lung adjacent to the IR and overinflation of the other lung
4. Perpendicular
5. The OID difference between the right and left lungs is minimal.
6. Cephalic
7. The patient's left side is rotated posteriorly, and the right side is rotated anteriorly.
8. The arms were not elevated to a position near the patient's head.
9. The chin was not tilted upward.
10. The image was taken on expiration.
11. The posterior ribs are demonstrated without superimposition. The right lung is the posterior lung, as indicated by the heart shadow that is demonstrated in the anteriorly and inferiorly located lung. Rotate the right lung anteriorly until an imaginary line connecting the shoulders and the pelvic wings is perpendicular to the IR.
12. The hemidiaphragms demonstrate an exaggerated cephalic curvature, and the humeral soft tissue is

superimposed over the anterior lung apices. Expose the image on full inspiration, and raise the arms until the humeri are next to the patient's head.

Child
Left Lateral Position
1. A. Lung apex
   B. Thoracic vertebra
   C. Posterior ribs
   D. Costophrenic angles
   E. Diaphragm
   F. Heart shadow
   G. Sternum
   H. Esophagus
   I. Trachea
2. The patient's left lung was rotated posteriorly.
3. The image was exposed on expiration.
4. The arms were not elevated.
5. The posterior ribs are not superimposed. The right lung is positioned posterior to the left, as indicated by the left side gastric air bubble that is located beneath the superiorly and anteriorly located left lung. Rotate the right side of the patient anteriorly until an imaginary line connecting the posterior shoulders and posterior iliac wings is aligned perpendicular to the IR.
6. The humeral soft tissue is superimposing the apical lung field. Elevate the humeri until they are positioned superior to the lung field.

Neonate and Infant
Lateral Decubitus Position (AP Projection)
1. A. Clavicle
   B. Humerus
   C. Third anterior rib
   D. Sixth posterior rib
   E. Chest tube
   F. Heart shadow
   G. Diaphragm
2. Up away from the bed or cart
3. A. Fourth
   B. Midsagittal
   C. Mammary line
   D. Airway, lungs, mediastinal structures, and costophrenic angles
4. Patient's bottom lip
5. Perpendicular
6. A. Projecting upwardly
   B. Gentle cephalic bow
7. Eight
8. The patient was rotated toward the right side (RPO position).
9. The central ray was angled too cephalically
10. The image was exposed on expiration.
11. The patient was not elevated on a radiolucent sponge.

12. The right arm was not elevated to a position near the patient's head.
13. The patient's left arm is superimposed over the apical lung region, and the right sternal clavicular end is visible away from the vertebral column. Elevate the left arm until it is next to the patient's head, above the lung field, and rotate the right side of the thorax away from the IR until the shoulders and posterior iliac wings are at equal distances from the IR.
14. The patient's right arm is superimposed over the apical lung region, and the left arm and upper vertebral column is not on the elevating device, resulting in lateral tilting of the upper vertebral column. Elevate the patient's humeri, positioning them next the head, and elevate the entire thorax on the elevating device, placing the upper vertebral column parallel with the device.
15. The upper vertebral column tilts laterally, the left sternal clavicular end is away from the vertebral column, and the left posterior ribs demonstrate greater length than the right posterior ribs. Elevate the patient's head and upper vertebral column until the midsagittal plane is aligned parallel with the bed, and rotate the right side toward the IR until the shoulders and iliac wings are at equal distances from the IR.

Child
Lateral Decubitus Position
(AP or PA Projection)
1. A. Heart shadow
   B. Diaphragm
   C. Eighth posterior rib
   D. Third anterior rib
2. The right side of the patient was positioned closer to the IR than the left side (RAO position).
3. The left side of the patient was positioned closer to the IR than the right side (LPO position).
4. The upper midcoronal plane was tilted posteriorly.
5. The left sternal clavicular end is superimposed over the vertebral column, the posterior ribs on the right side demonstrate the greater length, and the arms are superimposed over the right lateral lung apex. Rotate the patient's right side away from the IR, and elevate the left arm until it is positioned next to the patient's head.
6. The right diaphragm is not included in its entirety. Move the central ray and IR inferiorly approximately 2 inches (5 cm).

Abdomen
1. Diaphragm, bowel gas pattern, and faint outline of bony structures
2. Little intrinsic fat is present to outline the organs.
3. A. Control patient motion.
   B. Halt respiration.

C. Use a short exposure time.

D. Use the shortest possible OID.

E. For digital radiography, use the smallest IR possible to obtain superior resolution.

4.

Position or Projection	kVp	Grid	SID
Neonate: AP projection	65-75		40-48 inches (100-120 cm)
Infant: AP projection	65-75		40-48 inches (100-120 cm)
Child: AP projection	70-80	Grid (if AP measurement is over 5 inches (13 cm)	40-48 inches (100-120 cm)
Neonate: Lateral decubitus position	65-75		40-48 inches (100-120 cm)
Infant: Lateral decubitus position	65-75		40-48 inches (100-120 cm)
Child: Lateral decubitus position	70-80	Grid (if AP measurement is over 5 inches (13 cm)	40-48 inches (100-120 cm)

AP, Anteroposterior; kVp, kilovolt peak; SID, source–image receptor distance.

5.

Position or Projection	IR Size	Placement and Direction
Neonate: AP projection	8 × 10 inch (18 × 24 cm)	Lengthwise
Infant: AP projection	Adjusted to patient size	Lengthwise
Child: AP projection	Adjusted to patient size	Lengthwise
Neonate: Lateral decubitus position	8 × 10 inch (18 × 24 cm)	Lengthwise
Infant: Lateral decubitus position	Adjusted to patient size	Lengthwise
Child: Lateral decubitus position	Adjusted to patient size	Lengthwise

AP, Anteroposterior; IR, image receptor.

Neonate and Infant
AP Projection (Supine)

6. A. Diaphragm
   B. Iliac wing
   C. Symphysis pubis
   D. Posterior ribs

7. Align the shoulders and the posterior pelvic wings at equal distances from the IR.

8. Moves the diaphragm superiorly and puts less pressure on the abdominal organs

9. Eighth

10. A. Fourth
    B. Midsagittal
    C. 2
    D. Superior
    E. Iliac crest
    F. Diaphragm, abdominal structures, and symphysis pubis

11. The central ray was centered too inferiorly.

12. The patient's upper thorax is laterally tilted toward the left side.

13. The patient is rotated toward the left side (LPO position).

14. The patient is rotated toward the right side (RPO position).

15. The image was exposed on inspiration.

16. The central ray is centered to the third lumbar vertebra, the symphysis pubis and the lateral soft tissue are not included in the collimated field, the right posterior ribs demonstrate greater length than the left, and the right iliac wing demonstrates greater width than the left. Center the central ray 1 inch (2.5 cm) inferiorly, collimate to within ½ inch (1.25 cm) of the lateral skinline, and rotate the patient toward the left side until the shoulders and the iliac wings are at equal distances from the IR.

17. The left posterior ribs demonstrate greater length and the left iliac wing greater width than the right side, and the domes of the diaphragm are not included within the collimated field. Rotate the patient toward the right side until the shoulders and iliac wings are at equal distance from the IR, and move the central ray ½ inch (1.25 cm) superiorly, then open the longitudinally collimated field ½ inch (1.25 cm).

Child
AP Projection

1. A. Intestinal gas
   B. Inlet pelvis
   C. Obturator foramen
   D. Symphysis pubis
   E. Sacrum
   F. Iliac wing
   G. Spinous process
   H. 3rd lumbar vertebra pedicle
   I. 12th thoracic vertebra

2. The patient was rotated toward the right side (RPO position).

3. The patient was rotated toward the left side (LPO position).

4. Poor radiation protection practices have been followed. The patient's left arm has been included on the image, longitudinal collimation is inadequate, and the gonadal shield is positioned too superiorly and slightly too laterally. Move the central ray

medially until it is positioned at the midsagittal plane, increase transverse collimation to within ½ inch (1.25 cm) of skinline, longitudinally collimate to symphysis pubis, and move the gonadal shield slightly inferiorly and medially.

5. The symphysis pubis is not included in the collimation field, the central ray is too superior, the right iliac wing is wider than the left, and the right posterior ribs are longer than the left posterior ribs. Center the central ray 2 inches (5 cm) inferiorly, and rotate the patient toward the left side until the shoulders and the iliac wings are at equal distances from the IR.

6. The diaphragm is not included within the collimated field. Move the central ray and IR superiorly approximately 2 inches (5 cm).

Neonate and Infant
Left Lateral Decubitus Position (AP Projection)

1. A. Symphysis pubis
   B. Iliac wing
   C. Posterior rib
   D. Diaphragm
   E. Lumbar vertebra
   F. Intestinal gas
2. To position the gastric bubble away from the elevated diaphragm, where free intraperitoneal air will migrate
3. It does not matter. The level of lung aeration will remain steady.
4. A. Fifth
   B. Midsagittal
   C. 2
   D. Superior
   E. Iliac crest
   F. Diaphragm and abdominal structures
5. The patient was rotated toward the right side (RPO position).
6. The central ray was centered too inferiorly.

7. The patient was rotated toward the right side (RPO position).
8. The diaphragm is not included within the collimated field, the posterior ribs on the right side are longer than those on the left, and the right iliac wing is wider than the iliac wing on the left side. Move the central ray superiorly enough to include a transverse level 1 inch (2.5 cm) inferior to the mammary line, and rotate the patient away from the IR until the shoulders and the iliac wings are at equal distances from the IR.
9. The diaphragm is demonstrated inferior to the ninth posterior rib, and the right pelvic wing is narrower than the left. Expose the patient after exhalation, and rotate the right side toward the IR until the shoulders and the iliac wings are at equal distances from the IR.

Child
Left Lateral Decubitus Position (AP Projection)

1. A. Right ilium
   B. Spinous process
   C. Pedicle
   D. Second vertebral body
   E. Diaphragm
2. Free interperitoneal air under right diaphragm
3. The image was exposed when the ventilator's manometer indicator was at its highest level.
4. The patient was rotated toward the left side (LPO position).
5. The diaphragm is inferior to the ninth posterior rib, indicating that the exposure was taken on inspiration. Expose the image after the patient has exhaled. Free intraperitoneal air is demonstrated adjacent to the right hemidiaphragm.
6. The right iliac wing is wider than the left, and the right posterior ribs are longer than the left posterior ribs. Rotate the patient toward the left side until the shoulders and the iliac wings are at equal distances from the IR.

Image Analysis of the Upper Extremity

LEARNING OBJECTIVES   After completion of this chapter you should be able to:

_____   1. Identify the required anatomy on finger, thumb, hand, wrist, forearm, elbow, and humeral images.

_____   2. Describe how to properly position the patient, image receptor (IR), and central ray on finger, thumb, hand, wrist, forearm, elbow, and humeral images.

_____   3. State how to properly mark and hang finger, thumb, hand, wrist, forearm, elbow, and humeral images.

_____   4. List typical artifacts that are found on finger, thumb, hand, wrist, forearm, elbow, and humeral images.

_____   5. List the image requirements for finger, thumb, hand, wrist, forearm, elbow, and humeral images with accurate positioning.

_____   6. State how to properly reposition the patient when finger, thumb, wrist, forearm, elbow, and humeral images with poor positioning are produced.

_____   7. Discuss how to determine the amount of patient or central ray adjustment required to improve finger, thumb, hand, wrist, forearm, elbow, and humeral images with poor positioning.

_____   8. State the kilovoltage that is routinely used for finger, thumb, hand, wrist, forearm, elbow, and humeral images, and describe what anatomical structures will be visible when the correct technique factors are used.

_____   9. Explain how a joint space is aligned with the central ray and IR to be demonstrated as an open space on an image.

_____   10. Describe which aspects of a phalanx are concave and which are convex.

_____   11. Discuss the differences among fanned, extended, and deviated lateral hand images.

_____   12. State which of the second through fifth metacarpals is the longest and which is the shortest.

_____   13. List the soft-tissue structures that are of interest on wrist images. State where they are located and describe why their visualization is important.

_____   14. Explain how wrist and elbow rotations affect the position of the radial and ulnar styloids.

_____   15. Describe the slant of the distal radial articulating surface.

_____ 16. Discuss how a patient with large, muscular, or thick proximal forearms should be positioned for good posteroanterior (PA) and lateral wrist images to be obtained.

_____ 17. State the carpal bone changes that occur when the wrist is extended, deviated, or ulnar- and radial-deviated in the PA projection and lateral position.

_____ 18. List which carpal bones are situated anteriorly and which are situated posteriorly.

_____ 19. Describe how the positioning procedure should be adjusted if wrist images are ordered with a request that more than one fourth of the distal forearm be included.

_____ 20. State which scaphoid area is most commonly fractured.

_____ 21. Explain how and why the central ray is adjusted if a patient cannot adequately ulnar-flex for the scaphoid position.

_____ 22. Discuss how the degree of central ray angulation needs to be adjusted for the PA, ulnar-deviated scaphoid position if a proximal or distal scaphoid fracture is in question.

_____ 23. Describe what effect the anode-heel effect has on forearm and humeral images.

_____ 24. State how the forearm and humerus are positioned with respect to the x-ray tube to take advantage of the anode-heel effect.

_____ 25. Explain why the IR must extend beyond the wrist and elbow joints when the forearm is imaged and beyond the elbow and shoulder joints when the humerus is imaged.

_____ 26. List palpable structures that are used to identify the location of the elbow and glenohumeral joints.

_____ 27. Explain how the patient is positioned if only one of the joints can be placed in the true position for anteroposterior (AP) and lateral forearm and humeral images.

_____ 28. Describe the effect that elbow deviation has on the demonstration of the capitulum-radial joint on an AP projection of the elbow and soft-tissue structure visualization on a lateral position of the elbow.

_____ 29. State the anatomical structures that are placed in profile on medial and lateral oblique elbow images with accurate positioning.

_____ 30. List the soft-tissue structures on a lateral elbow image that are of interest, and describe why their visualization is important.

_____ 31. Discuss how hand and wrist positioning will affect visualization of the radial tuberosity on lateral elbow images.

_____ 32. State why the patient's humerus is never rotated if a humeral fracture is suspected.

_____ 33. Explain when a grid is needed for humeral images and how the technique factors are adjusted when a grid is added.

STUDY QUESTIONS

Finger

1. Describe how the following upper extremity images would be hung on a view box or displayed on a cathode ray tube (CRT) monitor.

   A. Oblique hand: _____

   B. PA hand: _____

   C. Left wrist: _____

   D. AP forearm: _____

   E. Lateral humerus: _____

2. What is the most frequent cause of recorded detail that lacks sharpness on an image?

   A. _____

   List four methods of controlling this problem.

   B. _____

   C. _____

   D. _____

   E. _____

3. A _____ (high/low) contrast, _____ (high/low) kilovoltage technique will best enhance the bony and soft-tissue structures of the finger.

4. Adequate image contrast, density, and penetration have been obtained on an upper extremity image when the (A) _____ patterns and (B) _____ outlines of the phalanges, metacarpals, and carpal bones are demonstrated.

5. Complete Table 3-1.

TABLE 3-1 **Upper Extremity Technical Data**		
Position or Projection	**kVp**	**SID**
Finger		
Thumb		
PA hand		
PA oblique hand		
Lateral hand		
Wrist		
Forearm		
Elbow		
Humerus		

kVp, Kilovolt peak; *PA*, posteroanterior; *SID*, source–image-receptor distance.

6. Complete Table 3-2. State whether differences exist for screen-film and computed radiography.

TABLE 3-2 IR Size, Placement, and Direction		
Position or Projection	**IR Size**	**Direction, Placement, and Number of Images on IR**
PA, oblique and lateral finger		
AP, oblique and lateral thumb		
PA, oblique and lateral hand	Screen-film	
	Computed radiography	
PA, oblique and lateral wrist	Screen-film	
	Computed radiography	
AP and lateral forearm		
AP and lateral elbow	Screen-film	
	Computed radiography	
AP and lateral humerus		

AP, Anteroposterior; *IR,* image receptor; *PA,* posteroanterior.

PA Projection (Second through Fifth Digits)

7. Identify the labeled anatomy in Figure 3-1.

Figure 3–1

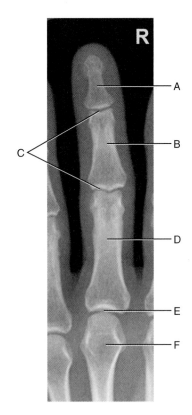

A. _____

B. _____

C. _____

D. _____

E. _____

F. _____

8. Define the following terms.

   A. Long axis: _____

   B. Concave: _____

   C. Medial rotation: _____

   D. Supinate: _____

9. A finger image has been requested for a patient with severe rheumatoid arthritis. The patient has a ring on the affected finger that cannot be removed. What procedure should be followed?

   _____

   _____

10. To prevent finger rotation on a PA finger image, the patient's hand should be positioned _____ against the IR.

11. On a nonrotated PA finger image the midshafts of the phalanges will demonstrate equal (A) _____ and there will be equal (B) _____ width on each side of the phalanges.

12. In which direction is the finger most frequently rotated when rotation occurs on a PA finger image?

    A. _____

    Why?

    B. _____

13. On a rotated PA projection image, the side of the finger that is rolled (A) _____ (farther from/closer to) the IR will demonstrate the greatest phalangeal midshaft concavity and the (B) _____ soft-tissue thickness.

14. On a rotated AP projection image, the side of the finger that is rolled (A) _____ (farther from/closer to) the IR will demonstrate the greatest phalangeal midshaft concavity and the (B) _____ soft-tissue thickness.

15. Which of the finger metacarpals is the longest? _____

16. Which of the finger metacarpals is the shortest? _____

17. The long axis of the affected digit is aligned with the long axis of (A) _____ for a PA finger image to prevent clipping of the distal (B) _____ or proximal (C) _____.

18. How is the patient positioned for a PA finger image to prevent soft-tissue overlap of adjacent fingers onto the affected finger?

    _____.

19. What joint spaces are demonstrated as open spaces on a PA finger image with accurate positioning?

    A. _____

    B. _____

20. To accomplish open joint spaces on a PA finger image, the central ray must be aligned (A) _____ (perpendicular/parallel) to the joint space and the IR must be aligned (B) _____ to the joint space.

21. If the finger is flexed for the PA image, the joint spaces will be (A) _____ and the phalanges will be (B) _____ .

22. On a patient whose finger is flexed, open interphalangeal (IP) joint spaces can be obtained by (A) _____ the hand and elevating the proximal metacarpals until the joint of interest is aligned (B) _____ to the IR.

23. On a PA finger image with accurate positioning, the (A) _____ joint will be centered within the collimated field. This is accomplished by centering a (B) _____ central ray to the (C) _____ joint.

24. Included within the collimated field on a PA finger image with accurate positioning are the (A) _____ and one half of the (B)_____ .

25. Accurate transverse collimation has been obtained when the collimated borders are _____ .

For the following descriptions of PA finger images with poor positioning, state how the patient would have been mispositioned for such an image to be obtained.

26. The image demonstrates unequal soft-tissue width and midshaft concavity on each side of the phalanges. The side of the phalanges with the least amount of concavity is facing the longest finger metacarpal.

    _____

27. The image demonstrates closed IP and metacarpophalangeal (MP) joints, and the distal and middle phalanges are foreshortened.

    _____

For the following PA finger images with poor positioning, state what anatomical structures are misaligned and how the patient should be repositioned for an optimal image to be obtained.

Figure 3–2

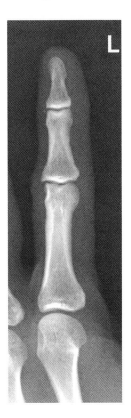

28. (Figure 3-2): _____

    _____

    _____

    _____

    _____

Figure 3–3

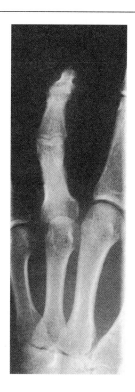

29. (Figure 3-3): _____

_____

_____

_____

_____

Oblique Position

1. Identify the labeled anatomy in Figure 3-4.

Figure 3–4

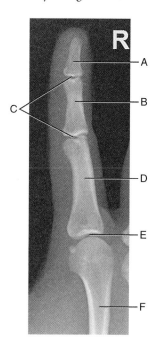

A. _____

B. _____

C. _____

D. _____

E. _____

F. _____

2. What do the following initials stand for?

    A. OID: _____

    B. PIP: _____

    C. IP: _____

    D. MP: _____

3. The affected finger is rotated _____ degrees from the PA projection for an oblique finger image.

4. In which direction are the patient's hand and finger rotated for an oblique position when the third through fifth fingers are imaged?

    A. _____

    For the second finger?

    B. _____

    Why might the second finger be rotated differently?

    C. _____

5. When accurate obliquity has been accomplished, the midshafts of the phalanges will demonstrate (A) _____ as much soft-tissue width and more midshaft phalangeal (B) _____ on one side of the digit than on the opposite side.

6. Why is it important to align the long axis of the affected digit with the long axis of the collimator's light field for an oblique finger image?

    _____

    _____

7. Why should the fingers be slightly spread before an oblique finger image is taken? _____

8. To obtain open IP and MP joint spaces, the finger needs to be fully (A) _____ and positioned (B) _____ to the IR.

9. When imaging the third and fourth fingers, why is it often necessary to position a sponge beneath the distal phalanx?

    _____

10. On an oblique finger image with accurate positioning, the (A) _____ joint will be centered within the collimated field. This is accomplished by centering a (B) _____ central ray to the (C) _____ joint.

11. What anatomical structures are included on an oblique finger image with accurate positioning?

    _____

For the following descriptions of oblique finger images with poor positioning, state how the patient would have been mispositioned for such an image to be obtained.

12. The soft-tissue width and midshaft concavity are nearly equal on each side of the digit.

_____

13. More than twice as much soft-tissue width is present on one side of the phalanges as on the other. One aspect of the midshafts of the phalanges is concave, and the other aspect is slightly convex.

_____

14. The soft tissue from the adjacent digit is superimposed over the affected digit's soft tissue.

_____

15. The image demonstrates closed IP joint spaces, and the distal and middle phalanges are foreshortened.

_____

For the following oblique finger images with poor positioning, state what anatomical structures are misaligned and how the patient should be repositioned for an optimal image to be obtained.

Figure 3–5

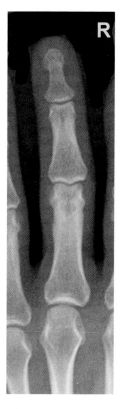

16. (Figure 3-5, Second digit): _____

_____

_____

_____

_____

Figure 3–6

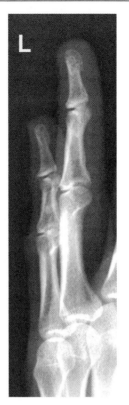

17. (Figure 3-6, Fourth digit): _____

_____

_____

_____

_____

_____

_____

Figure 3–7

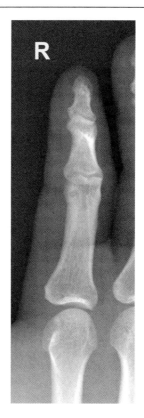

18. (Figure 3-7, Second digit): _____

_____

_____

_____

_____

Lateral Position

1. Identify the labeled anatomy in Figure 3-8.

Figure 3–8

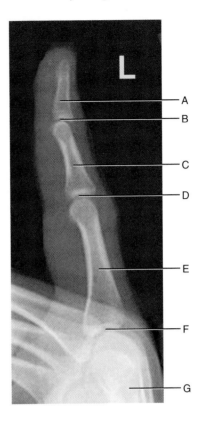

A. _____

B. _____

C. _____

D. _____

E. _____

F. _____

G. _____

2. Define the following terms.

   A. Hyperextend: _____

   B. Internal rotation: _____

   C. External rotation: _____

   D. Convex: _____

3. How many degrees from the PA projection should the finger be rotated for a lateral finger image with accurate positioning? _____

4. On a lateral finger image with accurate positioning, the anterior aspect of the middle and proximal phalangeal midshafts are (A) _____ (concave/convex), and the posterior aspects are (B) _____ (concave/convex).

5. For each of the following fingers, state how the hand is rotated (internally/externally) from the PA projection to place the finger in a lateral position.

   A. Second finger: _____

   B. Third finger: _____

   C. Fourth finger: _____

   D. Fifth finger: _____

6. What determines how the hand is rotated for question 5?

   _____

7. How is the patient's hand positioned for a lateral finger image to prevent soft-tissue overlap of the adjacent fingers onto the affected finger and to best demonstrate the affected finger's proximal phalanx?

   _____

8. On a lateral finger image with accurate positioning, the (A) _____ joint spaces are demonstrated as open spaces and the (B) _____ are demonstrated without foreshortening.

9. On a lateral finger image with accurate positioning, the _____ joint will be centered within the collimated field.

10. What anatomical structures are included on a lateral finger image with accurate positioning?

    _____

11. Describe the positioning error that is demonstrated on the image in Figure 3-9.

Figure 3–9

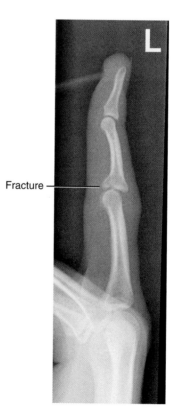

Fracture

_____

_____

For the following descriptions of lateral finger images with poor positioning, state how the patient would have been mispositioned for such an image to be obtained.

12. The proximal phalanges of the unaffected fingers overlap the proximal phalanx of the affected finger.

_____

13. Concavity is demonstrated on both sides of the middle and proximal phalangeal midshafts.

_____

14. The IP joint spaces are closed, and the phalanges are foreshortened.

_____

For the following lateral finger images with poor positioning, state what anatomical structures are misaligned and how the patient should be repositioned for an optimal image to be obtained.

Figure 3–10

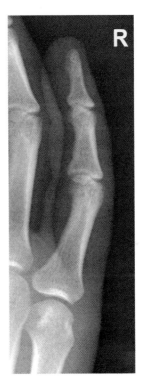

15. (Figure 3-10): _____

_____

_____

_____

Figure 3–11

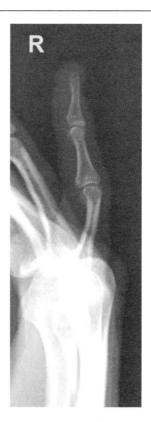

16. (Figure 3-11): _____

_____

_____

_____

_____

_____

Thumb (First Digit)

AP Projection

1. Identify the labeled anatomy in Figure 3-12.

Figure 3–12

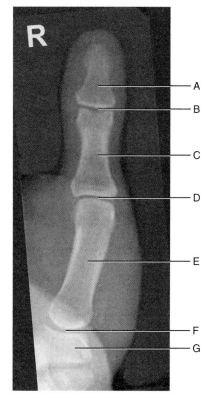

A. _____

B. _____

C. _____

D. _____

E. _____

F. _____

G. _____

2. What does CM stand for? _____

3. The first digit demonstrates no rotation when there is
   (A) _____ soft-tissue (B) _____ and equal
   phalangeal midshaft (C) _____ on each side of the digit.

4. For the thumb to be positioned in an AP projection, the hand is
   (A) _____ (internally/externally) rotated and the
   thumbnail is positioned (B) _____ against the IR.

5. When the thumb is rotated away from an AP projection, the amount
   of phalangeal midshaft concavity increases on the side positioned
   _____ (farther/closer) from/to the IR.

6. Why is it important to align the long axis of the first digit with the
   collimator's longitudinal light line for an AP thumb image? _____

   _____

7. On an AP thumb image with accurate positioning, the (A) _____ (B) _____, and (C) _____ joint spaces should be open and the (D) _____ should be demonstrated without foreshortening.

8. To obtain open joint spaces on an AP thumb image, the patient's thumb is fully _____ and the central ray is accurately aligned and centered to the thumb.

9. How is the hand positioned to prevent the medial palm soft tissue and possibly the fourth and fifth metacarpals from being superimposed over the proximal metacarpal? _____

_____

10. On a PA thumb image with accurate positioning, the _____ joint is closed.

11. On an AP thumb image with accurate positioning, the (A) _____ joint is centered within the collimated field. This is accomplished by centering a (B) _____ central ray to the (C) _____ joint.

12. The MP joint is located at the level where the palm interconnecting skin attaches to the _____.

13. List the anatomical structures that are included within the collimated field on an AP thumb image with accurate positioning. _____

_____

For the following descriptions of AP thumb images with poor positioning, state how the patient would have been mispositioned for such an image to be obtained.

14. The soft-tissue width and the concavity of the phalangeal and metacarpal midshafts on each side are not equal. The side demonstrating the more concavity is facing toward the second through fifth digits, and the thumbnail is facing away from the second through fifth digits.

_____

15. The image demonstrates a foreshortened distal phalanx and a closed distal IP (DIP) joint space.

_____

16. The fifth metacarpal and the medial palm soft tissue are superimposed over the proximal first metacarpal and carpometacarpal (CM) joint.

_____

For the following AP thumb images with poor positioning, state what anatomical structures are misaligned and how the patient should be repositioned for an optimal image to be obtained.

Figure 3–13

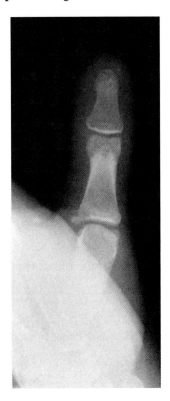

17. (Figure 3-13): _____

_____

_____

_____

Figure 3–14

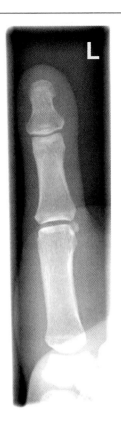

18. (Figure 3-14): _____

_____

_____

_____

_____

Lateral Position

1. Identify the labeled anatomy in Figure 3-15.

Figure 3–15

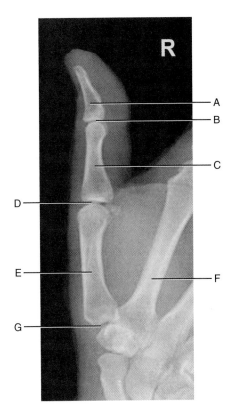

A. _____

B. _____

C. _____

D. _____

E. _____

F. _____

G. _____

2. On a lateral thumb image with accurate positioning, the anterior aspect of the proximal phalanx and the metacarpal midshaft are (A) _____ (concave/convex) and the posterior aspects are (B) _____ (concave/convex).

3. To obtain a lateral image of the thumb, rest the patient's hand flat against the IR and then _____ it until the thumb rolls into a lateral position.

4. How should the thumb be aligned for a lateral thumb image to enable one to collimate tightly without clipping required anatomy? _____

_____

5. How should the thumb be positioned to obtain open joint spaces and demonstrate the phalanges without foreshortening? _____

_____

6. Abducting the thumb will decrease the amount of _____ _____ superimposition of the CM joint.

7. On a lateral thumb image with accurate positioning the (A) _____ joint will be centered within the collimated field. This is accomplished by centering a (B) _____ central ray to the (C) _____ joint, which is located at the level at which the palm interconnecting skin attaches (D) _____.

8. List the anatomical structures that are included within the collimated field on a lateral thumb image with accurate positioning. _____

_____

For the following descriptions of lateral thumb images with poor positioning, state how the patient would have been mispositioned for such an image to be obtained.

9. The image does not demonstrate a lateral position. The second and third proximal metacarpals are superimposed over the first proximal metacarpal.

_____

10. The image does not demonstrate a lateral position. The anterior and posterior aspects of the proximal phalanx and metacarpal midshafts demonstrate concavity. The first proximal metacarpal is demonstrated without superimposition of the second and third proximal metacarpals.

_____

For the following lateral thumb images with poor positioning, state what anatomical structures are misaligned and how the patient should be repositioned for an optimal image to be obtained.

Figure 3–16

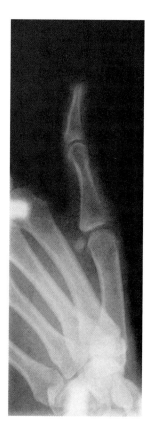

11. (Figure 3-16): _____

_____

_____

_____

Figure 3–17

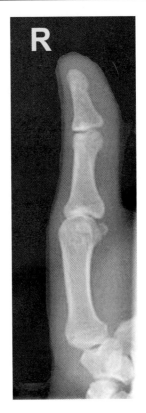

12. (Figure 3-17): _____

_____

_____

_____

Lateral Oblique Position

1. Identify the labeled anatomy in Figure 3-18.

Figure 3–18

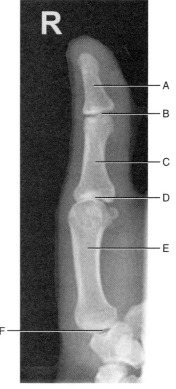

A. _____

B. _____

C. _____

D. _____

E. _____

F. _____

2. The affected thumb is rotated _____ degrees for accurate positioning for an oblique thumb image.

3. The thumb is placed in an oblique position when the patient's hand is (A) _____ and the palm surface is placed (B) _____ against the IR.

4. On an oblique thumb image with accurate positioning, the midshafts of the phalanges will demonstrate (A) _____ as much soft-tissue width and more (B) _____ on the side positioned farther from the IR.

5. On an oblique thumb image with accurate positioning, the (A) _____ joint is centered within the collimated field. This is accomplished by centering a (B) _____ central ray to the (C) _____ joint.

6. What anatomical structures are included on an oblique thumb image with accurate positioning?

_____

7. Accurate transverse collimation has been obtained on a thumb image when the collimated borders are adjacent to the thumb's _____.

For the following description of an oblique thumb image with poor positioning, state how the patient would have been mispositioned for such an image to be obtained.

8. The midshafts of the proximal phalanx and metacarpal demonstrate slight convexity on the posterior surfaces and concavity on the anterior surfaces.

For the following oblique thumb images with poor positioning, state what anatomical structures are misaligned and how the patient should be repositioned for an optimal image to be obtained.

Figure 3–19

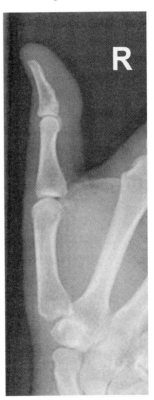

9. (Figure 3-19): _____

Figure 3–20

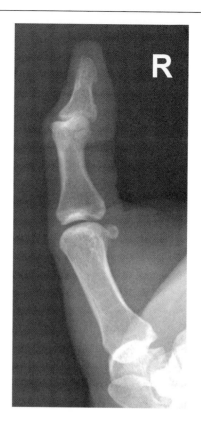

10. (Figure 3-20): _____

_____

_____

_____

Hand

PA Projection

1. Identify the labeled anatomy in Figure 3-21.

Figure 3–21

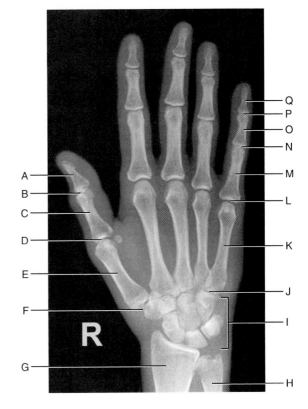

A. _____

B. _____

C. _____

D. _____

E. _____

F. _____

G. _____

H. _____

I. _____

J. _____

K. _____

L. _____

M. _____

N. _____

O. _____

P. _____

Q. _____

2. Define the following terms.

   A. External rotation: _____

   B. Humeral abduction: _____

   C. Pronation: _____

3. A PA hand image has been ordered for a patient who is unable to remove a wedding ring. What procedure should be followed? _____

   _____

4. A PA projection of the hand is demonstrated when there is a uniform (A) _____ outline on each side of the second through fifth digits and equal distance between the (B) _____ heads.

5. To obtain a PA hand projection, (A) _____ the patient's hand and place it (B) _____ against the IR.

6. Why is external rotation seldom the cause of a mispositioned PA hand image?

   _____

7. How is the hand aligned with the collimated field for a PA hand image to obtain maximum collimation? _____

   _____

8. How are the fingers positioned for a PA hand image to prevent soft-tissue overlap of adjacent digits? _____

9. The (A) _____, (B) _____, and (C) _____ joint spaces are demonstrated as open spaces on a PA hand image with accurate positioning.

10. What changes in the joint spaces, phalanges, and metacarpals would be expected on a PA hand image if the hand is in a flexed position when it is imaged? _____

11. On a PA hand image with accurate positioning, the first digit is placed in a(n) _____ position.

12. How will the position of the first digit change if the hand is flexed for a PA hand image? _____

13. On a PA hand image with accurate positioning, the _____ joint space is centered within the collimated field.

14. What anatomical structures are included on an accurately collimated PA hand image?

    _____

    _____

For the following descriptions of PA hand images with poor positioning, state how the patient would have been mispositioned for such an image to be obtained.

15. The image demonstrates superimposed third through fifth metacarpal heads and unequal midshaft concavity of the phalanges and metacarpals.

    _____

16. The image demonstrates soft-tissue overlap of the third, fourth, and fifth digits.

_____

17. The image demonstrates closed IP and CM joints and foreshortened phalanges and metacarpals.

_____

For the following PA hand images with poor positioning, state what anatomical structures are misaligned and how the patient should be repositioned for an optimal image to be obtained.

Figure 3–22

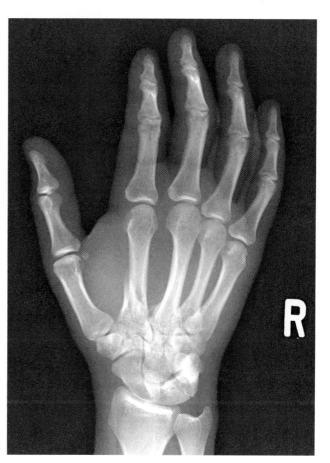

18. (Figure 3-22): _____

_____

_____

_____

Figure 3–23

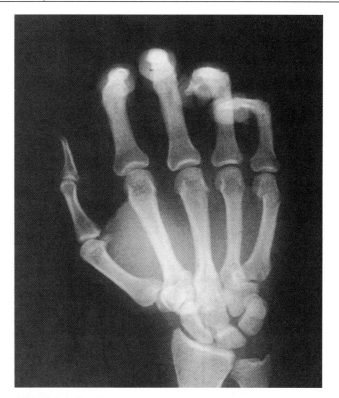

19. (Figure 3-23): _____

_____

_____

_____

20. The PA hand image in Figure 3-22 demonstrates a proximal second metacarpal fracture. If the patient could not move the hand from this position to adequately place it in an AP projection, how should the central ray and IR be adjusted for an optimal PA projection to be obtained?

_____

_____

_____

_____

PA Oblique Projection (External Rotation)

1. Identify the labeled anatomy in Figure 3-24.

Figure 3–24

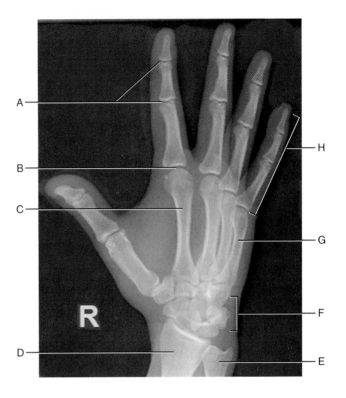

A. _____

B. _____

C. _____

D. _____

E. _____

F. _____

G. _____

H. _____

2. Define the term *superimpose.* _____

3. The hand is rotated (A) _____ degrees (B) _____
   (internally/externally) from the PA projection for an oblique hand
   image.

4. An oblique hand image with accurate positioning demonstrates the
   (A) _____ and (B) _____ metacarpal heads
   without superimposition, whereas the (C) _____,
   (D) _____ , and (E) _____ metacarpal heads
   demonstrate slight superimposition, and the fourth and fifth
   (F) _____ without superimposition.

5. Why is it important to view the hand and not the wrist when
   determining the degree of hand obliquity to use for an oblique hand
   image?

6. How must the fingers be positioned to demonstrate open IP and MP joints on an oblique hand image? _____

_____

7. An oblique hand image is ordered to evaluate the healing of a patient's third metacarpal fracture. Is it acceptable to flex the patient's fingers, using them to prop the hand for the image?

A. _____ (Yes/No)

Why or why not?

B. _____

8. On an oblique hand image with accurate positioning, the _____ joint space is centered to the collimated field.

9. What anatomical structures are included on an accurately collimated oblique hand image?_____

_____

For the following descriptions of oblique hand images with poor positioning, state how the patient would have been mispositioned for such an image to be obtained.

10. The metacarpal heads are demonstrated without superimposition, and the spaces between the metacarpal midshafts are nearly equal.

_____

11. The third through fifth metacarpal midshafts are superimposed.

_____

12. The image demonstrates foreshortened phalanges and closed IP joint spaces.

_____

For the following oblique hand images with poor positioning, state what anatomical structures are misaligned and how the patient should be repositioned for an optimal image to be obtained.

Figure 3–25

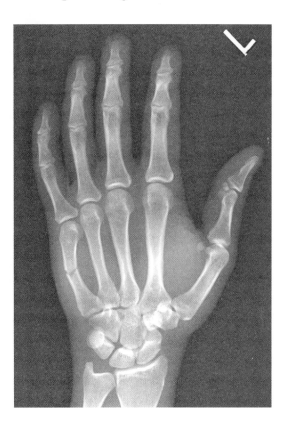

13. (Figure 3-25): _____

_____

_____

_____

Figure 3–26

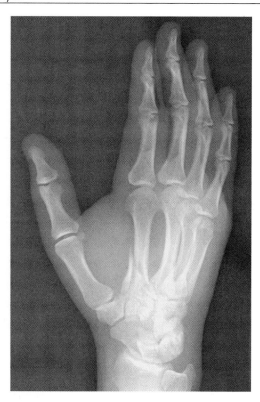

14. (Figure 3-26): _____

    _____

    _____

    _____

15. The PA oblique hand image in Figure 3-25 demonstrates a midshaft fifth metacarpal fracture. If the patient could not move the hand to adequately position it in a PA oblique projection, how should the central ray and IR be adjusted for an optimal PA oblique projection to be obtained?

    _____

    _____

    _____

    _____

16. The PA oblique hand image in Figure 3-26 demonstrates a proximal second metacarpal fracture. If the patient could not move the hand to adequately position it in a PA oblique projection, how should the central ray and IR be adjusted for an optimal PA oblique projection to be obtained?

    _____

    _____

    _____

    _____

Lateromedial Projection ("Fan" Lateral Position)

1. Identify the labeled anatomy in Figure 3-27.

Figure 3–27

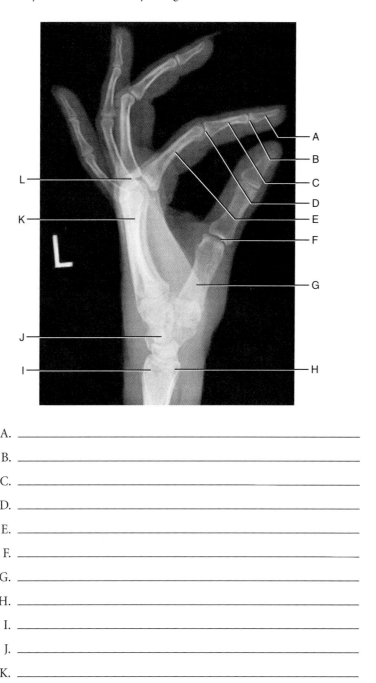

A. _____

B. _____

C. _____

D. _____

E. _____

F. _____

G. _____

H. _____

I. _____

J. _____

K. _____

L. _____

2. Define the following terms.

A. Fan: _____

B. Immobilization prop: _____

C. Palpate: _____

D. Hand flexion: _____

E. Hand extension: _____

3. Why is it difficult to demonstrate the phalanges and metacarpals simultaneously on a fan lateral hand image? _____

_____

4. For a fan lateral hand image, the digits are most effectively fanned by drawing the second and third fingers (A) _____ (anteriorly/posteriorly) and the fourth and fifth fingers (B) _____ (anteriorly/posteriorly).

5. In what projection or position will the first digit be placed for accurate positioning for a lateral hand image?

_____

6. A lateral hand image with accurate positioning will demonstrate superimposed _____.

7. The fifth metacarpal can be distinguished from the second through fourth metacarpals by its length. It is the (A) _____ (longest/shortest) of these metacarpals, and the second metacarpal is the (B) _____ (longest/shortest).

8. How should the thumb be positioned to obtain open joint spaces and demonstrate the phalanges without foreshortening on a lateral hand image?

_____

9. On a lateral hand image with accurate positioning, the _____ joint spaces are centered within the collimated field.

10. What anatomical structures are included on an accurately collimated lateral hand image?

_____

For the following descriptions of lateral hand images with poor positioning, state how the patient would have been mispositioned for such an image to be obtained.

11. The second through fifth metacarpal midshafts are demonstrated without superimposition. The shortest metacarpal is demonstrated anterior to the other metacarpals.

_____

12. The second through fifth metacarpal midshafts are demonstrated without superimposition. The longest metacarpal is demonstrated anterior to the other metacarpals.

_____

13. The image demonstrates superimposed metacarpals and superimposed digits.

_____

For the following lateral hand images with poor positioning, state what anatomical structures are misaligned and how the patient should be repositioned for an optimal image to be obtained.

Figure 3–28

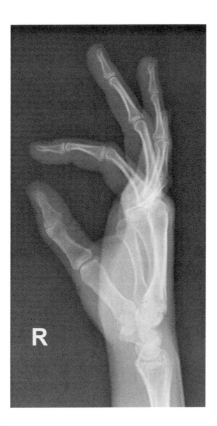

14. (Figure 3-28): _____

_____

_____

_____

Figure 3–29

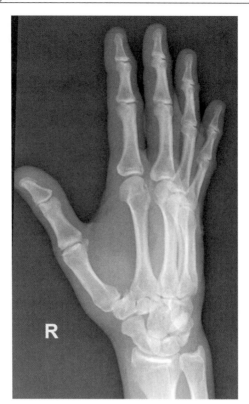

15. (Figure 3-29): _____

_____

_____

_____

Figure 3–30

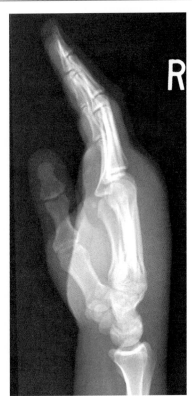

16. (Figure 3-30): _____

_____

_____

_____

Wrist

PA Projection

1. Identify the labeled anatomy in Figure 3-31.

Figure 3–31

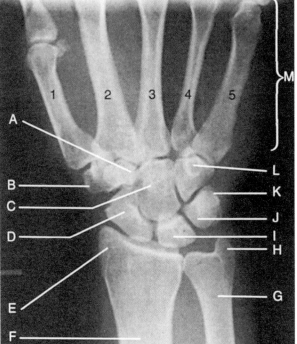

A. _____

B. _____

C. _____

D. _____

E. _____

F. _____

G. _____

H. _____

I. _____

J. _____

K. _____

L. _____

M. _____

2. Define the following terms.

A. Articulation: _____

B. Articular surface: _____

C. Proximal: _____

D. Distal: _____

E. Trapezoid: _____

F. Signet ring configuration: _____

G. Radial wrist deviation: _____

H. Ulnar wrist deviation: _____

3. Describe the shape and location of the scaphoid fat stripe._____

_____

4. Why is the visualization of the scaphoid fat stripe important on a PA wrist image?

_____

5. To demonstrate the ulnar styloid in profile, the elbow is placed in a (A) _____ projection or position and the humerus is positioned (B) _____.

6. How should the radioulnar articulation be demonstrated on a PA wrist image with accurate positioning? _____

7. The (A) _____ (anterior/posterior) margin of the distal radius is demonstrated distal to the (B) _____ (anterior/posterior) margin on a PA wrist image with accurate positioning.

8. How is the forearm positioned for a PA wrist image to obtain open radioscaphoid and radiolunate joint spaces?

_____

9. How is a patient with large muscular or thick proximal forearms positioned for a PA wrist image to prevent demonstrating an excessive amount of the radial articular surface? _____

10. How is the patient positioned for a PA wrist image to obtain open second through fifth CM joint spaces? _____

_____

11. When the hand is placed on a flat surface, the wrist will be (A) _____ (flexed/extended), causing the distal scaphoid to shift (B) _____ (anteriorly/posteriorly).

12. Why is the long axis of the third metacarpal and midforearm aligned with the long axis of the collimated field for a PA wrist image?

A. _____

Where does this alignment position the lunate with respect to the distal radius?

B. _____

13. When the fifth metacarpal and ulna are aligned with the long axis of the collimation field for a PA wrist image, the distal scaphoid shifts (A) _____ (anteriorly/posteriorly) and is (B) _____ (foreshortened/elongated) and the lunate moves (C) _____ (medially/laterally).

14. The distal scaphoid shifts _____ (anteriorly/posteriorly) when the wrist is ulnar-deviated.

15. On a PA wrist image with accurate positioning, the (A) _____ are centered within the collimated field. This is accomplished by centering a (B) _____ central ray to the wrist.

16. What anatomical structures are included on an accurately collimated PA wrist image? _____

_____

17. How should one center the central ray and collimate differently when a PA wrist image is ordered with the request that more than one fourth of the distal forearm be included?_____

_____

For the following descriptions of PA wrist images with poor positioning, state how the patient would have been mispositioned for such an image to be obtained.

18. The ulnar styloid is not demonstrated in profile.

_____

19. The laterally located carpal and metacarpal joints are demonstrated as open spaces, and the medially located carpals and metacarpals are superimposed, closing the medially located carpal joints. The radioulnar joint is closed, and the radial styloid is not in profile.

_____

20. The laterally located carpals and metacarpals are superimposed, the pisiform and hamate hook are well demonstrated, and the radioulnar joint is closed.

_____

21. The posterior margin of the distal radius has been projected too far distal to the anterior margin.

_____

22. The scaphoid is foreshortened and demonstrates a signet ring configuration, the CM joints are obscured, and the lunate is triangular and properly positioned distal to the radius.

_____

23. The scaphoid is elongated, the second through fourth metacarpals are superimposed over the CM joints, and the lunate is triangular and properly positioned distal to the radius.

_____

24. The scaphoid is foreshortened, the lunate is positioned mostly distal to the ulna, the third metacarpal is not aligned with the long axis of the midforearm, and the CM joints are open.

_____

25. The scaphoid is elongated, the lunate is entirely positioned distal to the radius, and the third metacarpal is not aligned with the long axis of the midforearm.

_____

For the following PA wrist images with poor positioning, state what anatomical structures are misaligned and how the patient should be repositioned for an optimal image to be obtained.

Figure 3–32

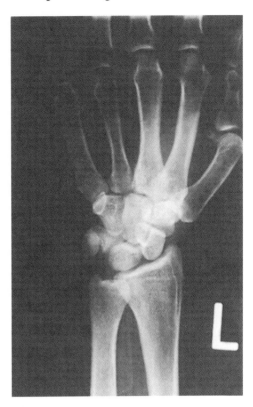

26. (Figure 3-32): _____

_____

_____

_____

Figure 3–33

27. (Figure 3-33): _____

_____

_____

_____

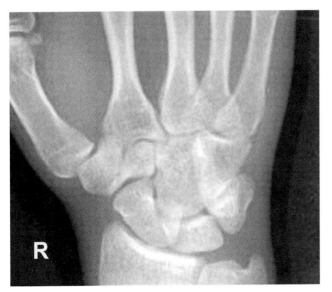

Figure 3–34

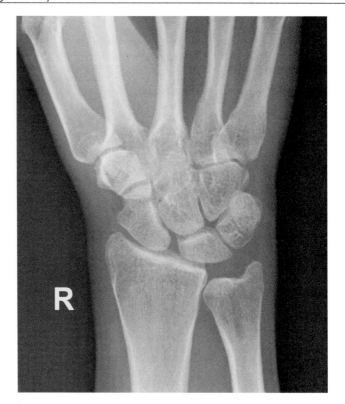

28. (Figure 3-34): _____

_____

_____

_____

Figure 3–35

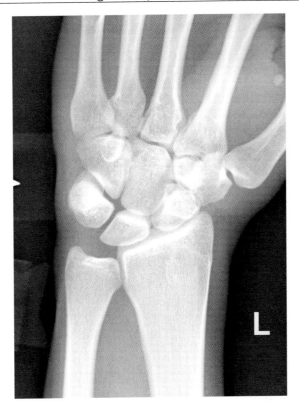

29. (Figure 3-35): _____

_____

_____

_____

PA Oblique Projection (External Rotation)

1. Identify the labeled anatomy in Figure 3-36.

Figure 3–36

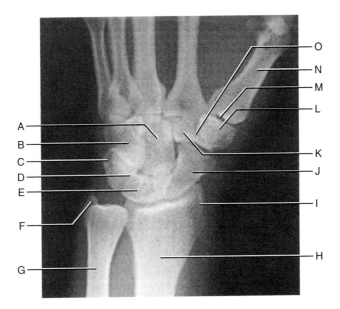

A. _____

B. _____

C. _____

D. _____

E. _____

F. _____

G. _____

H. _____

I. _____

J. _____

K. _____

L. _____

M. _____

N. _____

O. _____

2. Define the term *styloid*. _____

3. What routine degree of patient wrist rotation is required for an oblique wrist image?

A. _____

As a routine, should the wrist be internally or externally rotated from a PA projection?

B. _____

4. What carpal joint space is open on a medial oblique wrist image to indicate that the wrist was adequately rotated? _____

5. For a PA projection image of the wrist, the trapezoid and trapezium are superimposed. Which of these carpal bones is located anteriorly?

_____

6. The long axes of which two anatomical structures should be aligned when positioning the patient for an oblique wrist image to ensure that no radial or ulnar deviation will result?

A. _____

B. _____

7. If the forearm is positioned parallel with the IR for an oblique wrist image, how is the distal radius demonstrated on the resulting image?

_____

8. On a medial oblique wrist image with accurate positioning, the radioulnar joint space is closed. Which surface of the radius is superimposed over the ulna? _____ (anterior/posterior)

9. Where is the ulnar styloid demonstrated on an oblique wrist image with accurate positioning?

A. _____

How must the patient be positioned for this styloid placement to be obtained?

B. _____

10. On an oblique wrist image with accurate positioning, the (A) _____ are centered within the collimated field. This is accomplished by centering a (B) _____ central ray to the wrist.

11. What anatomical structures are included on an accurately collimated oblique wrist image?

_____

For the following descriptions of oblique wrist images with poor positioning, state how the patient would have been mispositioned for such an image to be obtained.

12. The trapezoid and trapezium demonstrate slight superimposition, obscuring the trapeziotrapezoidal joint space, and trapezoid-capitate superimposition is minimal.

_____

13. The scaphoid is foreshortened, and the scaphoid tuberosity is situated next to the radius.

_____

14. The posterior margin of the distal radius is more than ¼ inch (0.6 cm) proximal to the anterior margin.

_____

For the following oblique wrist images with poor positioning, state what anatomical structures are misaligned and how the patient should be repositioned for an optimal image to be obtained.

15. (Figure 3-37): _____

_____

_____

_____

_____

Figure 3–37

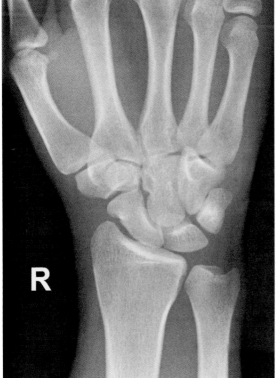

Figure 3–38

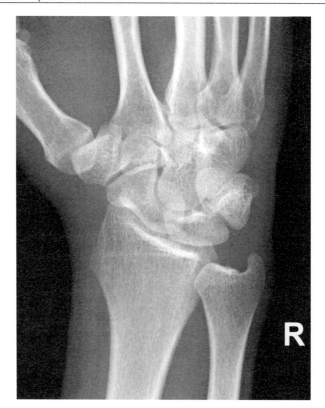

16. (Figure 3-38): _____

_____

_____

_____

Figure 3–39

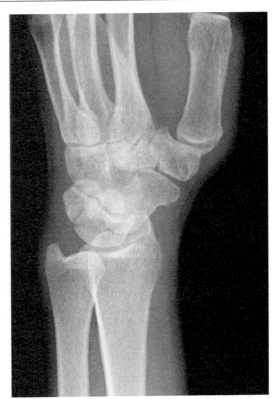

17. (Figure 3-39): _____

_____

_____

_____

Figure 3–40

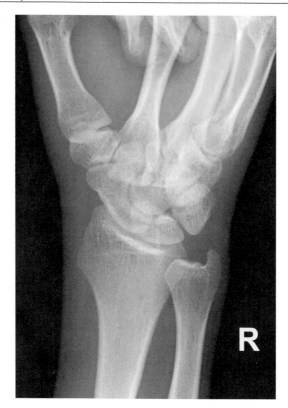

18. (Figure 3-40): _____

_____

_____

_____

_____

_____

Lateral Position (Lateromedial Projection)

1. Identify the labeled anatomy in Figure 3-41.

Figure 3–41

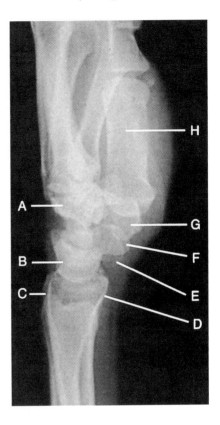

A. _____

B. _____

C. _____

D. _____

E. _____

F. _____

G. _____

H. _____

2. Define the following terms.

A. Dorsal: _____

B. Volar: _____

3. Describe the shape and location of the pronator fat stripe that is demonstrated on a lateral wrist image with accurate positioning.

_____

_____

4. Why is the visualization of the pronator fat stripe on a lateral wrist image of importance? _____

5. What two sets of anatomical structures should be superimposed on a lateral wrist image to indicate that a lateral position has been obtained?

   A. _____ and _____

   B. _____ and _____

6. Which side of the wrist is placed against the IR for a routine lateral wrist image?

   A. _____ (radial/ulnar)

   What projection is this?

   B. _____

   In this projection, is the pisiform or distal scaphoid positioned closer to the IR?

   C. _____

7. The distal scaphoid and pisiform are demonstrated _____ (anterior/posterior) to the capitate and lunate carpal bones on a lateral wrist image with accurate positioning.

8. How are the patient's hand and forearm aligned to prevent radial and ulnar deviation of the wrist for a lateral wrist image? _____
   _____

9. Ulnar deviation of the wrist causes the distal scaphoid to be demonstrated (A) _____ (proximal/distal) to the pisiform, and radial deviation causes the distal scaphoid to be demonstrated (B) _____ (proximal/distal) to the pisiform on a lateral wrist image.

10. If a patient with large muscular or thick proximal forearms is imaged without hanging the proximal forearm off the IR or imaging table, what type of wrist deviation will result? _____

11. For a lateral wrist image, how is the patient positioned so that the wrist is in a neutral position without anterior extension or posterior deviation?
    _____

12. For a lateral wrist image, how are the humerus and elbow positioned to demonstrate the ulnar styloid in profile? _____
    _____

13. For a lateral wrist image, how are the humerus and elbow positioned to demonstrate the ulnar styloid projecting distal to the midline of the ulnar head? _____
    _____

14. Will the elbow and humeral positioning described in question 12 or 13 demonstrate the ulna closer to the lunate on the resulting lateral wrist image? _____
    _____

15. How is the patient positioned to prevent the first proximal metacarpal from being superimposed over the trapezium? _____
    _____

16. On a lateral wrist image with accurate positioning, the
    (A) _____ are centered within the collimated field. This is
    accomplished by centering a (B) _____ central ray to the
    wrist.

17. What anatomical structures are included on an accurately collimated
    lateral wrist image? _____
    _____

18. Accurate transverse collimation has been obtained when the
    collimated borders are _____.

19. State whether the elbow was positioned in an AP projection or lateral
    position for the lateral wrist images in Figure 3-42.

    A. _____

    B. _____

Figure 3–42

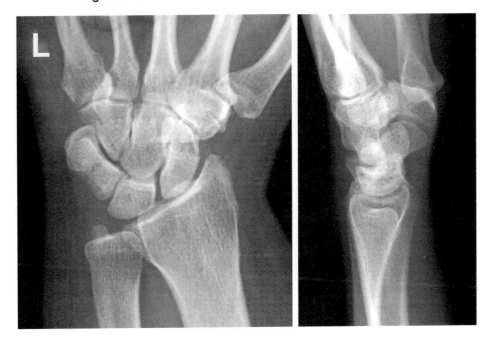

**For the following descriptions of lateral wrist images with poor position-
ing, state how the patient would have been mispositioned for such an
image to be obtained.**

20. The pisiform is demonstrated anterior to the scaphoid, and the ulna is
    demonstrated anterior to the radius.
    _____

21. The pisiform is demonstrated posterior to the distal scaphoid, and the
    radius is anterior to the ulna.
    _____

22. The pisiform is demonstrated distal to the scaphoid, and the
    midcarpal bones are centered within the collimated field.
    _____

23. The distal scaphoid is demonstrated distal to the pisiform.

_____

24. The ulnar styloid is projecting distal to the midline of the ulnar head. (In some facilities, this may not be considered poor positioning.)

_____

25. The first proximal metacarpal is superimposed over the trapezium.

_____

For the following lateral wrist images with poor positioning, identify the anatomical structures that are misaligned, state how the patient should be repositioned for an optimal image to be obtained, and describe the position of the ulnar styloid.

Figure 3–43

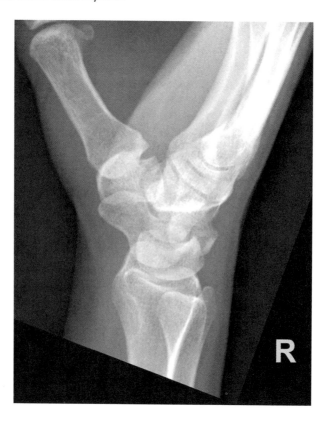

26. (Figure 3-43): _____

_____

Ulnar styloid: _____(Profile/Midline of ulnar head)

Figure 3–44

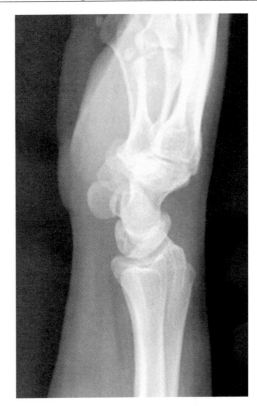

27. (Figure 3-44): _____

_____

Ulnar styloid: _____(Profile/Midline of ulnar head)

Figure 3–45

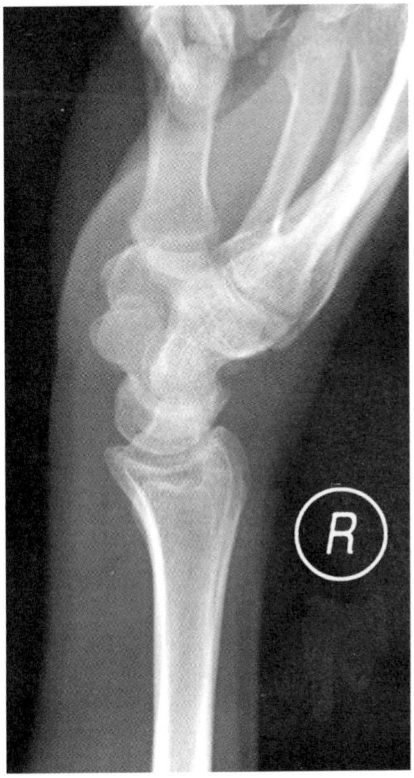

28. (Figure 3-45): _____

_____

_____

_____

Ulnar styloid: _____(Profile/Midline of ulnar head)

Figure 3–46

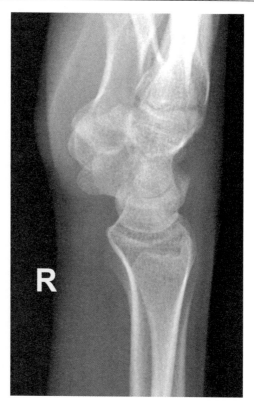

29. (Figure 3-46): _____

_____

Ulnar styloid: _____(Profile/Midline of ulnar head)

Ulnar-Deviation, PA Axial Projection (Scaphoid)

1. Identify the labeled anatomy in Figure 3-47.

Figure 3–47

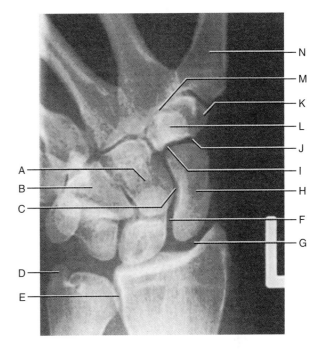

A. _____

B. _____

C. _____

D. _____

E. _____

F. _____

G. _____

H. _____

I. _____

J. _____

K. _____

L. _____

M. _____

N. _____

2. What is the name of the soft-tissue structure demonstrated on an ulnar-deviated PA projection of the wrist that can be used to diagnose joint effusion?

_____

3. Sufficient ulnar deviation of the wrist has been accomplished in the scaphoid position when the long axis of the (A) _____ and (B) _____ are aligned and the lunate is positioned distal to the (C) _____.

4. Why does ulnar deviation of the wrist increase the demonstration of the scaphoid?

_____

5. For an ulnar-deviated PA scaphoid image, how is the patient positioned to obtain open scaphocapitate and scapholunate joint spaces? _____

_____

6. If the wrist is adequately ulnar-deviated for the scaphoid position, how much and in what direction is the central ray angled if a fracture of the scaphoid waist is suspected? _____

7. What central ray angulation is used if the patient is unable to adequately ulnar-deviate?

   A. _____

   Why is this adjustment needed?

   B. _____

8. Where do most fractures occur on the scaphoid? _____

9. How is the central ray angle adjusted for an ulnar-deviated scaphoid image if a fracture of the distal scaphoid is suspected?

   A. _____

   If a proximal scaphoid fracture is suspected?

   B. _____

10. If the central ray is not aligned parallel with the fracture site, will the fracture line be visible on the image? _____ (Yes/No)

11. How is the patient positioned for an ulnar-deviated scaphoid image to obtain an open radioscaphoid joint space? _____

12. On an ulnar-deviated scaphoid wrist image with accurate positioning, the _____ is centered within the collimated field.

13. What anatomical structures are included on an ulnar-deviated scaphoid wrist image with accurate positioning?

_____

_____

14. For the ulnar-deviated scaphoid wrist images in Figure 3-48, state whether a distal, waist, or proximal scaphoid fracture is demonstrated and the degree of central ray angulation that should be used to best demonstrate each.

   A. _____

   B. _____

   C. _____

Figure 3–48

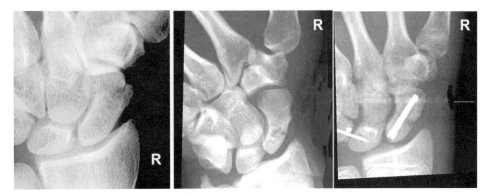

For the following descriptions of ulnar-deviated scaphoid wrist images with poor positioning, state how the patient would have been mispositioned for such an image to be obtained.

15. The scaphocapitate and scapholunate joints are closed, and the lunate is superimposed over a portion of the scaphoid.

_____

16. The scaphotrapezium, scaphotrapezoidal, and CM joint spaces are closed.

_____

For the following ulnar-deviated scaphoid wrist images with poor positioning, state what anatomical structures are misaligned and how the patient should be repositioned for an optimal image to be obtained.

Figure 3–49

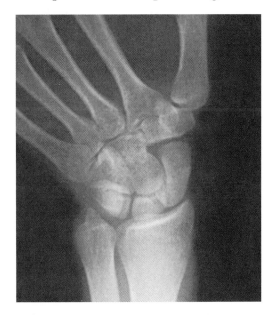

17. (Figure 3-49): _____

_____

_____

_____

Figure 3–50

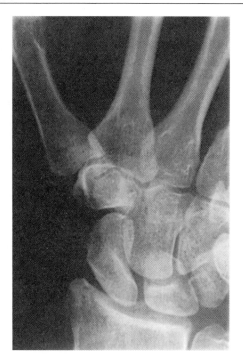

18. (Figure 3-50): _____

_____

_____

_____

Figure 3–51

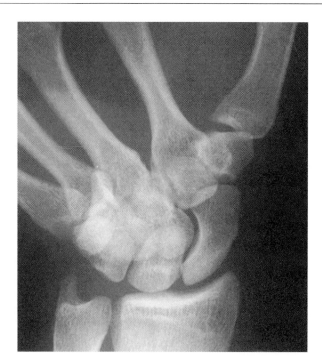

19. (Figure 3-51): _____

_____

_____

_____

Carpal Canal (Tunnel) (Tangential, Inferosuperior Projection)

1. Identify the labeled anatomy in Figure 3-52.

Figure 3–52

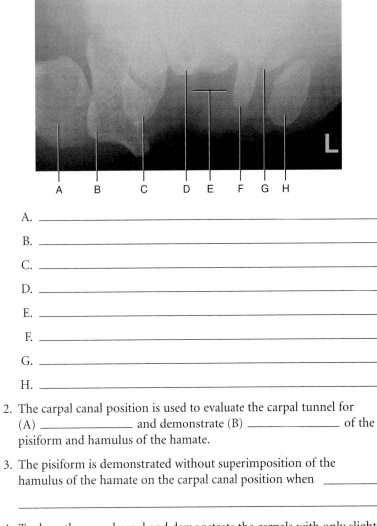

A. _____

B. _____

C. _____

D. _____

E. _____

F. _____

G. _____

H. _____

2. The carpal canal position is used to evaluate the carpal tunnel for (A) _____ and demonstrate (B) _____ of the pisiform and hamulus of the hamate.

3. The pisiform is demonstrated without superimposition of the hamulus of the hamate on the carpal canal position when _____
_____

4. To show the carpal canal and demonstrate the carpals with only slight elongation, the patient's hand is positioned (A) _____ and the central ray angled (B) _____.

5. When imaging a patient who is unable to extend the wrist enough to place the metacarpals to within 15 degrees of vertical, the central ray needs to be (A) _____ (increased/decreased). If a 20-degree angle was required to bring the central ray parallel with the patient's palmar surface in this situation, the angle needed for the carpal canal image would be (B) _____ and the resulting image would show the carpals and carpal canal, although they will be elongated because of the (C) _____
_____.

For the following descriptions of carpal canal wrist images with poor positioning, state how the patient would have been mispositioned for such an image to be obtained.

6. The pisiform is superimposed over the hamulus of the hamate.

   _____

7. The carpal canal is not demonstrated in its entirety, and the carpal bones are foreshortened.

   _____

8. The metacarpal bases obscure the bases of the hamate's hamulus process, pisiform, and scaphoid.

   _____

For the following carpal canal wrist images with poor positioning, state what anatomical structures are misaligned and how the patient should be repositioned for an optimal image to be obtained.

Figure 3–53

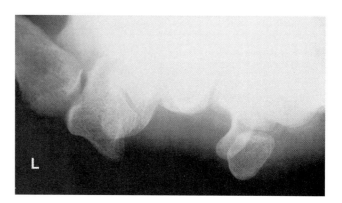

9. (Figure 3-53): _____

   _____

   _____

   _____

Figure 3–54

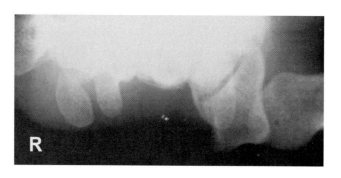

10. (Figure 3-54): _____

   _____

   _____

   _____

Figure 3–55

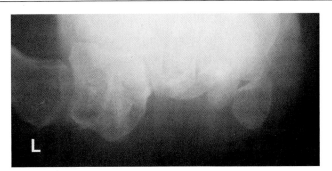

11. (Figure 3-55): _____

_____

_____

_____

Forearm

AP Projection

1. Identify the labeled anatomy in Figure 3-56.

Figure 3–56

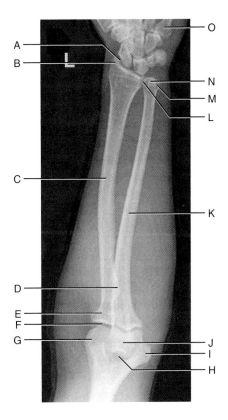

A. _____

B. _____

C. _____

D. _____

E. _____

F. _____

G. _____

H. _____

I. _____

J. _____

K. _____

L. _____

M. _____

N. _____

O. _____

2. Define the following terms.

A. Longitudinal collimation field: _____

B. Transverse collimation field: _____

C. Elbow flexion: _____

3. How is the forearm positioned with respect to the x-ray tube to take advantage of the anode-heel effect? _____

_____

4. Why does the IR need to extend at least 1 inch (2.5 cm) beyond the elbow and wrist joints when the forearm is imaged in an AP projection?

_____

5. How can the location of the elbow joint be determined?

_____

6. On an AP forearm image with accurate positioning, the (A) _____ is centered to the collimated field. This is accomplished by centering a (B) _____ central ray to the (C) _____ .

7. What anatomical structures are included on an AP forearm image with accurate positioning?

_____

8. An AP projection of the distal forearm has been obtained when the radial styloid is demonstrated in profile (A) _____ (medially/laterally) and superimposition of the radius and (B) _____ is minimal.

9. A patient from the emergency room is unable to position the wrist and elbow in an AP projection simultaneously for an AP forearm image. How is this patient positioned for the image? _____

_____

10. What specific anatomical structures must be accurately positioned to place the ulnar styloid distal to the midline of the ulnar head for an AP forearm image?

_____

11. On an AP proximal forearm image with accurate positioning, the radial head and tuberosity are superimposed over the ulna by approximately (A) _____ inch and the (B) _____ are demonstrated in profile.

12. Why is the capitulum-radial joint partially or completely obscured on an AP forearm image?

_____

13. On an AP forearm image with accurate positioning, the radial tuberosity is demonstrated in profile and the radius and ulna are visualized _____ with each other.

14. How is the patient positioned to place the radial tuberosity in profile on an AP forearm image? _____

_____

For the following descriptions of AP forearm images with poor positioning, state how the patient would have been mispositioned for such an image to be obtained.

15. The distal forearm demonstrates superimposition of the first and second metacarpal bases and laterally located carpal bones.

_____

16. The AP proximal forearm demonstrates the ulna without radial head and tuberosity superimposition.

_____

17. The radius is crossing over the ulna, and the radial tuberosity is not demonstrated in profile.

_____

18. The forearm images in Figure 3-57 demonstrate a distal forearm fracture. Evaluate the accuracy of positioning in these two images.

Figure 3–57

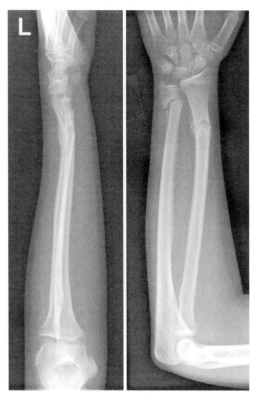

_____

_____

_____

_____

_____

For the following AP forearm image with poor positioning, state what anatomical structures are misaligned and how the patient should be repositioned for an optimal image to be obtained.

Figure 3–58

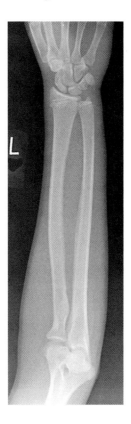

19. (Figure 3-58): _____

_____

_____

_____

20. The AP forearm image in Figure 3-59 demonstrates a midshaft radial fracture. If the patient could not move the forearm to adequately position it in an AP projection, how should the central ray and IR be adjusted for an optimal AP forearm projection to be obtained?

Figure 3–59

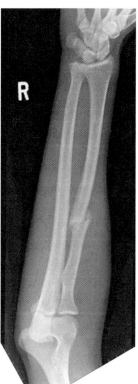

_____

_____

_____

_____

Lateral Position (Lateromedial Projection)

1. Identify the labeled anatomy in Figure 3-60.

Figure 3–60

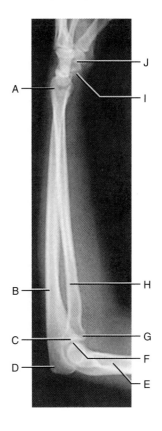

A. _____

B. _____

C. _____

D. _____

E. _____

F. _____

G. _____

H. _____

I. _____

J. _____

2. Define the following terms.

A. Joint effusion: _____

B. Concentric arcs: _____

3. To take advantage of the anode-heel effect, state how the forearm is positioned with respect to the x-ray tube when it is imaged in the lateral position. _____

_____

4. On a lateral forearm image with accurate positioning, the _____ _____ is centered within the collimated field.

5. What anatomical structures are included on an accurately collimated lateral forearm image? _____

6. On a lateral forearm image with accurate positioning, the distal scaphoid is demonstrated (A) _____ to the pisiform and the distal radius and ulna are (B) _____.

7. What side of the arm is placed against the IR for a lateral forearm image? _____

8. On a proximal lateral forearm image with poor positioning, the ulna is demonstrated posterior to the radius. What will the distal scaphoid and pisiform relationship be? _____

9. Describe the placement of the ulnar styloid on a lateral forearm image with accurate positioning.

   A. _____

   How must the patient be positioned to obtain this ulnar styloid positioning?

   B. _____

10. Should the radial tuberosity be demonstrated in profile on a lateral forearm image with accurate positioning?

    A. _____ (Yes/No)

    How is the patient positioned to obtain this positioning?

    B. _____

11. In patients with average-size forearms the elbow joint space is open on a lateral forearm image. What two patient forearm shapes result in a closed elbow joint space?

    A. _____

    B. _____

12. A lateral forearm image with poor positioning demonstrates the capitulum distal to the distal surface of the medial trochlea. What is the radial head and coronoid relationship on this image?

    _____

13. A patient from the emergency room is unable to position the wrist and elbow in a lateral position simultaneously for a lateral forearm image. The requisition states that the examination is being performed to rule out a proximal forearm fracture. How should the patient be positioned for this image?

    _____

    _____

For the following descriptions of lateral forearm images with poor positioning, state how the patient would have been mispositioned for such an image to be obtained.

14. The pisiform is demonstrated anterior to the distal scaphoid, and the ulna is anterior to the radius. The proximal forearm demonstrates accurate positioning.

    _____

15. The pisiform is visible posterior to the distal scaphoid, and the distal surface of the capitulum is demonstrated proximal to the distal surfaces of the medial trochlea.

_____

_____

16. The ulnar styloid is projecting distal to the midline of the ulnar head.

_____

17. The image demonstrates the radial tuberosity in profile anteriorly.

_____

18. The radial head is demonstrated too far posterior on the coronoid process. The distal forearm demonstrates accurate positioning.

_____

For the following lateral forearm image with poor positioning, state what anatomical structures are misaligned and how the patient should be repositioned for an optimal image to be obtained.

Figure 3–61

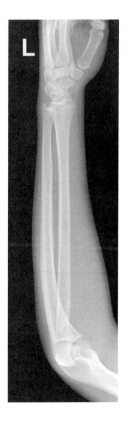

19. (Figure 3-61): _____

_____

_____

_____

20. The lateral forearm image in Figure 3-62 demonstrates a proximal radial fracture. The patient's arm was externally rotated as far as possible. How should the central ray and IR be adjusted for an optimal lateral forearm position to be obtained?

Figure 3–62

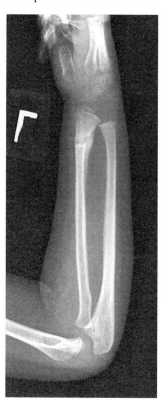

_____

_____

_____

_____

Elbow

AP Projection

1. Identify the labeled anatomy in Figure 3-63.

Figure 3–63

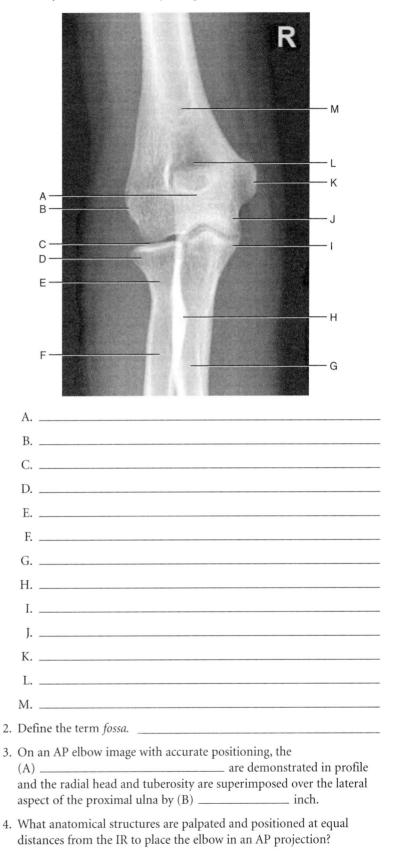

A. _____

B. _____

C. _____

D. _____

E. _____

F. _____

G. _____

H. _____

I. _____

J. _____

K. _____

L. _____

M. _____

2. Define the term *fossa.* _____

3. On an AP elbow image with accurate positioning, the
   (A) _____ are demonstrated in profile
   and the radial head and tuberosity are superimposed over the lateral
   aspect of the proximal ulna by (B) _____ inch.

4. What anatomical structures are palpated and positioned at equal
   distances from the IR to place the elbow in an AP projection?

   _____

5. Which humeral epicondyle rotates out of profile with only a slight degree of elbow rotation? _____

6. On an AP elbow image with accurate positioning, the radial tuberosity is demonstrated in profile (A) _____ (medially/laterally) and the radius and ulna are aligned (B) _____.

7. If the humeral epicondyles are accurately positioned for an AP elbow image, what other structure can be manipulated to change the degree of radial tuberosity visualization?

   _____

8. What two aspects of the positioning procedure need to be accurately set up to demonstrate the capitulum-radial joint space as an open space on an AP elbow image?

   A. _____

   B. _____

9. A poorly positioned AP elbow image demonstrates a closed capitulum-radial joint space. How can one determine if this closure was a result of poor central ray placement or elbow flexion? _____

   _____

   _____

10. How is the patient positioned for an AP elbow image if the elbow is unable to extend at least 30 degrees? _____

    _____

11. On an AP elbow image with accurate positioning, the (A) _____ is centered within the collimated field. This is accomplished by centering a (B) _____ central ray (C) _____ (D) _____ to the medial epicondyle. Why is it easier to palpate the medial epicondyle than the lateral epicondyle? (E) _____

12. What anatomical structures are included on an accurately collimated AP elbow image?

For the following descriptions of AP elbow images with poor positioning, state how the patient would have been mispositioned for such an image to be obtained.

13. The radial head and tuberosity are superimposed over approximately ½ inch (1 cm) of the ulna.

    _____

14. The ulna is demonstrated without radial head superimposition.

    _____

15. The image demonstrates the radius crossing over the ulna, and the radial tuberosity is not shown in profile.

16. The image demonstrates a foreshortened proximal forearm and a closed capitulum-radial joint space.

For the following AP elbow images with poor positioning, state what anatomical structures are misaligned and how the patient should be repositioned for an optimal image to be obtained.

Figure 3–64

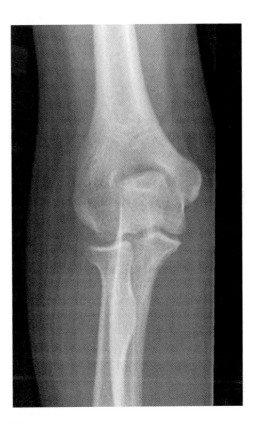

17. (Figure 3-64): _____
_____
_____
_____

Figure 3–65

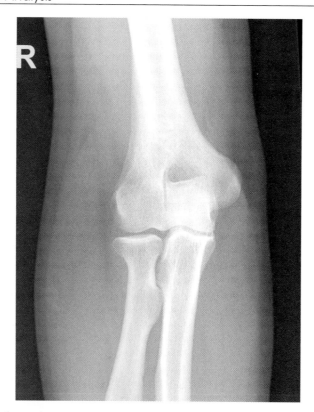

18. (Figure 3-65): _____

_____

_____

Figure 3–66

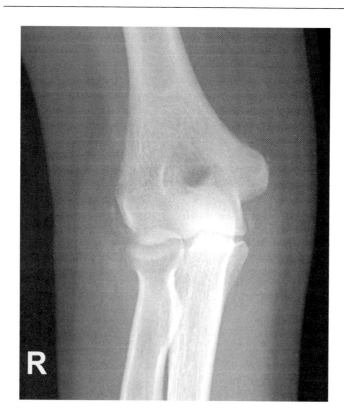

19. (Figure 3-66): _____

_____

_____

_____

Figure 3–67

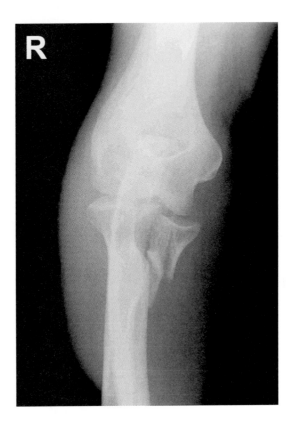

20. The AP image in Figure 3-67 demonstrates a proximal radial fracture. If the patient could not move the arm to adequately position it for an AP projection, how should the central ray and IR be adjusted for an optimal AP elbow projection to be obtained?

_____

_____

_____

AP Oblique Projections (External and Internal Rotation)

1. Identify the labeled anatomy in Figure 3-68.

Figure 3–68

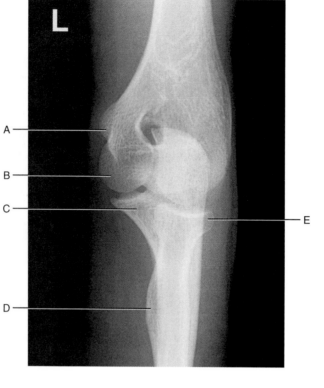

A. _____

B. _____

C. _____

D. _____

E. _____

2. Identify the labeled anatomy in Figure 3-69.

Figure 3–69

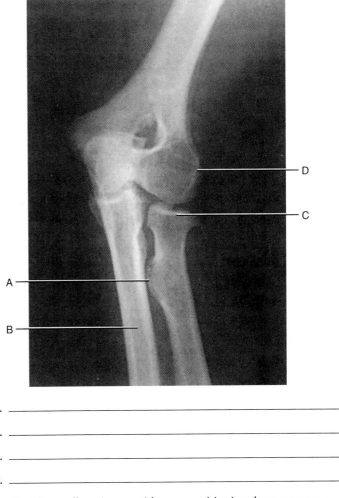

A. _____

B. _____

C. _____

D. _____

3. An AP oblique elbow image with poor positioning demonstrates a closed capitulum-radial joint space. List two possible positioning problems that might have resulted in this image.

A. _____

B. _____

4. Describe the anatomical changes that will occur between the olecranon fossa and the olecranon when the elbow is deviated. _____

_____

5. State whether the forearm or humerus should be placed parallel with the IR to best demonstrate the anatomy listed below in a patient whose arm will not fully extend.

A. Coronoid: _____

B. Radial head: _____

C. Medial trochlea: _____

D. Capitulum: _____

E. Capitulum-radial joint: _____

6. What is the degree of elbow rotation used for AP oblique images?

_____

7. What anatomical structures are demonstrated in profile on an internally rotated AP oblique elbow image with accurate positioning?

_____

_____

8. In which direction is the elbow rotated from the AP projection to obtain an image that demonstrates the radial head and ulna without superimposition? _____

9. What anatomical structures are demonstrated in profile on an externally rotated AP oblique elbow image with accurate positioning?

_____

_____

10. On an AP oblique elbow image with accurate positioning, the (A) _____ is centered within the collimated field. This is accomplished by centering a (B) _____ central ray to the elbow joint located at a level (C) _____ distal to the (D) _____ .

11. What anatomical structures are included on an AP oblique elbow image with accurate positioning? _____

_____

For the following descriptions of AP oblique elbow images with poor positioning, state how the patient would have been mispositioned for such an image to be obtained.

12. The externally rotated AP oblique image demonstrates a closed capitulum-radial joint space. The olecranon is positioned outside the olecranon fossa, and the radial articulating surface is demonstrated.

_____

13. On the internally (medially) rotated AP oblique image, the radial head is demonstrated lateral to the coronoid process, without complete superimposition of the ulna, and the proximal aspect of the olecranon is not demonstrated in profile.

_____

14. On the internally (medially) rotated AP oblique image, a portion of the radial head is demonstrated anterior to the coronoid process, without complete superimposition of the ulna.

_____

15. On the external (lateral) oblique image, a portion of the radial head and tuberosity is superimposed over the ulna.

_____

16. On the externally (laterally) rotated AP oblique image, the coronoid is superimposed over a portion of the radial head, and the radial head and tuberosity are free of superimposition. The radial tuberosity is not demonstrated in profile.

_____

For the following AP oblique elbow images with poor positioning, state what anatomical structures are misaligned and how the patient should be repositioned for an optimal image to be obtained.

Figure 3–70

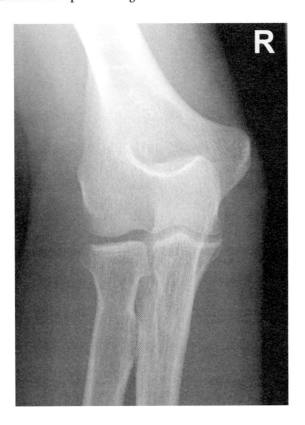

17. (Figure 3-70, External oblique): _____

_____

_____

_____

Figure 3–71

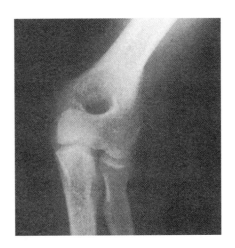

18. (Figure 3-71, External oblique): _____

_____

_____

_____

Figure 3–72

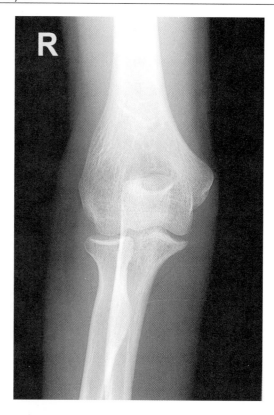

19. (Figure 3-72, Internal oblique): _____

_____

_____

_____

Figure 3–73

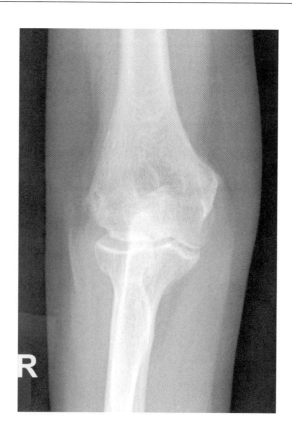

20. (Figure 3-73, Internal oblique): _____

_____

_____

_____

Lateral Position (Lateromedial Projection)
1. Identify the labeled anatomy in Figure 3-74.

Figure 3–74

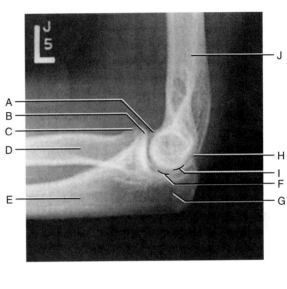

A. _____

B. _____

C. _____

D. _____

E. _____

F. _____

G. _____

H. _____

I. _____

J. _____

2. Define the following instructions.

A. Elevate distal forearm: _____

B. Depress proximal humerus: _____

3. List the three soft-tissue fat pads that may be demonstrated on a lateral elbow image, and describe their locations.

A. _____

B. _____

C. _____

Displacement of these pads may indicate what to the reviewer?

D. _____

4. Why is it important to flex the elbow 90 degrees for a lateral elbow image? _____

_____

5. What three anatomical structures form the three concentric arcs on a lateral elbow image with accurate positioning?

A. _____

B. _____

C. _____

Which of these arcs is the smallest?

D. _____

Which is the largest?

E. _____

How will improper alignment of these arcs affect the elbow joint space?

F. _____

6. Describe the relationship of the radial head and coronoid on a lateral elbow image with accurate positioning.

_____

_____

7. A lateral elbow image with poor positioning demonstrates the radial head positioned posterior on the coronoid process. How would the capitulum and medial trochlea be misaligned on this image?

_____

8. The distal forearm was positioned too low for a lateral elbow image. What will be the relationship between the radial head and coronoid and the capitulum and medial trochlea on the resulting image?

_____

9. A lateral elbow image with poor positioning demonstrates the capitulum too far posterior to the medial trochlea. How will the radial head and coronoid be aligned on this image?

_____

10. The proximal humerus was positioned lower than the distal humerus on a lateral elbow image. What will be the relationship between the radial head and coronoid and the capitulum and medial trochlea on the resulting image?

_____

11. The position of the radial tuberosity on a lateral elbow image is determined by the position of the patient's hand and wrist. For the following hand positions, describe the position of the radial tuberosity.

A. Lateral hand and wrist: _____

B. Supinated hand and wrist: _____

C. Pronated hand and wrist: _____

Which of the radial tuberosity positions above is the desired position for an accurate lateral elbow image?

D. _____

12. On a lateral elbow image with poor positioning, the (A) _____ is centered within the collimated field. This is accomplished by centering a (B) _____ central ray to the elbow joint located (C) _____ inch (D) _____ to the lateral humeral epicondyle.

13. What anatomical structures are included on a lateral elbow image with accurate positioning? _____

_____

For the following descriptions of lateral elbow images with poor positioning, state how the patient would have been mispositioned for such an image to be obtained.

14. The olecranon is positioned within the olecranon fossa, and the posterior fat pad is demonstrated proximal to the olecranon process.

_____

15. The radial tuberosity is positioned in profile anteriorly.

_____

16. The radial head is positioned posterior on the coronoid process, and the distal surface of the capitulum is demonstrated distal to the distal surface of the medial trochlea.

_____

17. The radial head is positioned anterior on the coronoid process, and the distal surface of the capitulum is proximal to the distal surface of the medial trochlea.

_____

18. The radial head is distal to the coronoid process, and the capitulum appears anterior to the medial trochlea.

_____

19. The radial head is proximal to the coronoid process, and the capitulum appears posterior to the medial trochlea.

_____

For the following lateral elbow images with poor positioning, state what anatomical structures are misaligned and how the patient should be repositioned for an optimal image to be obtained.

Figure 3–75

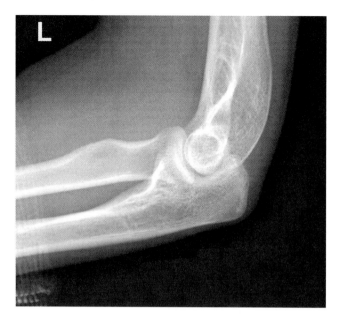

20. (Figure 3-75): _____

_____

_____

_____

Figure 3–76

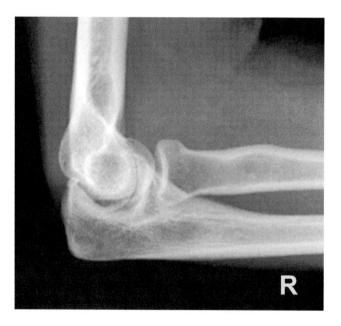

21. (Figure 3-76): _____

_____

_____

_____

Figure 3–77

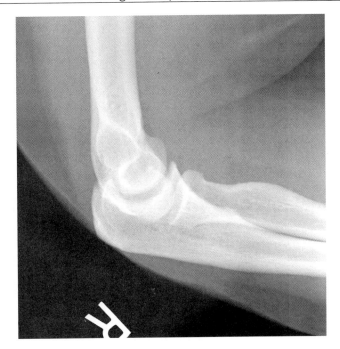

22. (Figure 3-77): _____

_____

_____

_____

Figure 3–78

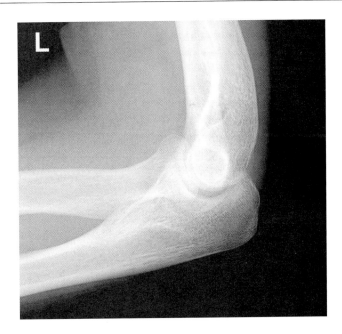

23. (Figure 3-78): _____

_____

_____

_____

Figure 3–79

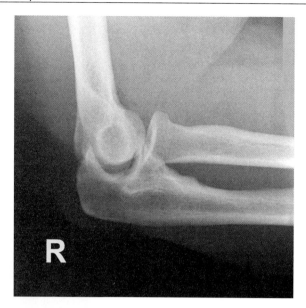

24. (Figure 3-79): _____

_____

_____

_____

25. If the patient is unable to move the arm to adjust for the poor positioning demonstrated in Figure 3-76, how should the central ray and IR be adjusted for an optimal lateral elbow image to be obtained?

_____

_____

_____

_____

Radial Head and Capitulum

1. Identify the labeled anatomy in Figure 3-80.

Figure 3–80

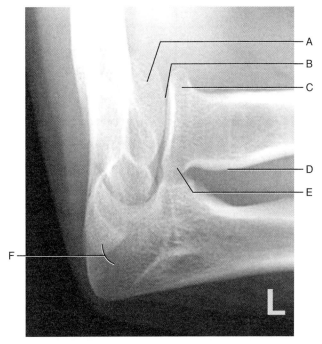

A. _____

B. _____

C. _____

D. _____

E. _____

F. _____

2. A radial head and capitulum image of the elbow with accurate positioning will demonstrate three arcs. The largest and most distally located is the (A) _____; the smaller, center arc is the (B) _____; and the proximal arc is the (C) _____.

3. In what position is the elbow placed to obtain the radial head and capitulum image of the elbow? _____

4. When the distal humerus is in a lateral position, the (A) _____ joint appears as an open space and the radial head is aligned with the (B) _____.

5. The position of the distal forearm for a radial head and capitulum position affects the relationship of what anatomical elbow structures?

_____

_____

6. How can one determine from the image if the forearm was elevated too high for the radial head and capitulum image?

_____

_____

7. A radial head and capitulum image with poor positioning demonstrates the radial head distal to the coronoid process. What is the relationship of the capitulum and medial trochlea on such an image?

_____

8. If accurate humeral positioning and central ray angulation is used for the radial head and capitulum image, the (A) _____ and (B) _____ arcs will be demonstrated without superimposition and the radial head will be superimposed on only the anterior tip of the (C) _____.

9. To accurately separate the arcs of the distal humerus, an imaginary line connecting the humeral epicondyles is positioned (A) _____ to the IR and a (B) _____-degree central ray angulation is directed (C) _____. Will this angle cause the radial head or coronoid to project farther proximally? (D) _____ Will this angle cause the medial trochlea or capitulum to project farther proximally? (E) _____

10. What anatomical structure can be used to determine the portion of the radial head that is positioned in profile on a radial head and capitulum elbow image? _____

11. For each of the following wrist positions, list the location of the radial tuberosity and the aspect of the radial head surface that are demonstrated in profile.

    A. PA wrist: _____

    _____

    B. Lateral wrist: _____

    _____

12. On a radial head and capitulum image of the elbow with accurate positioning, the (A) _____ is centered within the collimated field. Where is the central ray placed to obtain this centering? (B) _____

13. What anatomical structures are included on a radial head and capitulum image of the elbow with accurate positioning? _____

_____

For the following descriptions of radial head-capitulum elbow images with poor positioning, state how the patient would have been mispositioned for such an image to be obtained.

14. The capitulum-radial joint space is closed, the radial head is demonstrated distal to the coronoid process, and the capitulum is demonstrated too far anterior to the medial trochlea.

_____

15. The capitulum-radial joint space is closed, the radial head is demonstrated proximal to the coronoid process, and the capitulum is demonstrated too far posterior to the medial trochlea.

_____

For the following radial head-capitulum elbow images with poor positioning, state what anatomical structures are misaligned and how the patient should be repositioned for an optimal image to be obtained.

Figure 3–81

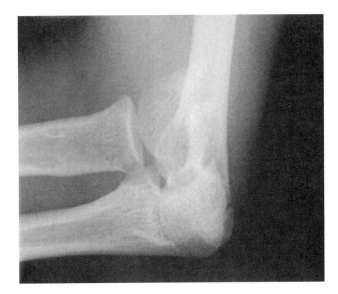

16. (Figure 3-81): _____

_____

_____

_____

Figure 3–82

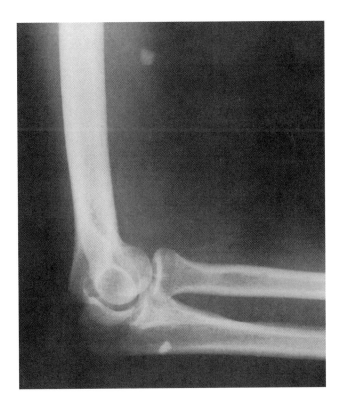

17. (Figure 3-82): _____

_____

_____

_____

18. The capitulum-radial head elbow image in Figure 3-83 demonstrates a radial head and capitulum fracture. Even though the image was obtained with a 45-degree central ray angle the radial head is not anterior enough to the coronoid, nor is the capitulum proximal enough to the medial trochlea, indicating poor patient positioning. If the patient could not move the arm from this position, how should the central ray be adjusted to obtain an optimal capitulum-radial head image?

Figure 3–83

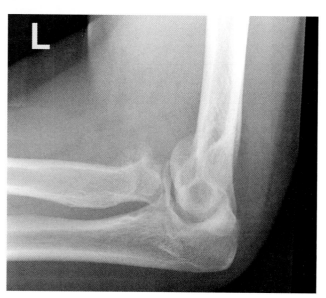

_____

_____

_____

_____

Humerus

AP Projection

1. Identify the labeled anatomy in Figure 3-84.

Figure 3–84

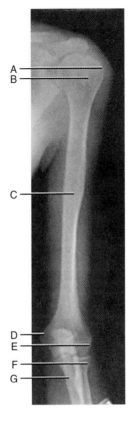

A. _____

B. _____

C. _____

D. _____

E. _____

F. _____

G. _____

2. Define the following terms.

  A. Grid: _____

  B. Grid ratio: _____

  C. Grid cutoff: _____

3. Humeral images can be taken without a grid and still display high image contrast as long as the thickness measurement is below (A) _____ cm. When a grid is used for humeral images, the kilovolt peak (kVp) should be raised above (B) _____.

4. To take advantage of the anode-heel effect, state how the humerus is positioned with respect to the x-ray tube. _____

_____

5. An AP projection of the distal humerus has been obtained when the radial head and tuberosity are superimposed over the ulna by approximately (A) _____ inch and the (B) _____ are demonstrated in profile.

6. On an AP proximal humeral image with accurate positioning, the (A) _____ tubercle is demonstrated laterally in profile, the (B) _____ is demonstrated medially in profile, and the (C) _____ will be visible approximately halfway between the greater tubercle and the humeral head.

7. When the patient is positioned for an AP humeral image, the patient's (A) _____ is externally rotated until an imaginary line connecting the (B) _____ is positioned parallel with the IR.

8. If an AP humeral image is ordered for a patient with a suspected proximal humeral fracture, why is it important not to externally rotate the patient's arm?

   A. _____

   How can the ordered procedure still be performed without adjusting the patient's arm position?

   B. _____

   _____

9. An AP humeral image is ordered for a patient with a humerus that is longer than 17 inches (43 cm). How should the patient's arm be aligned with the IR to include the entire humerus on the same image?

   _____

   _____

10. Why is it necessary to have the IR extend at least 1 inch (2.5 cm) beyond the shoulder and elbow joints when imaging the humerus in the AP projection? _____

    _____

11. Describe how the shoulder and elbow joints can be located to ensure that the IR extends beyond each for an AP humeral image.

    A. Shoulder: _____

    B. Elbow: _____

12. On an AP humeral image with accurate positioning, the _____ is centered within the collimated field.

13. What anatomical structures are included on an AP humeral image with accurate positioning?

    _____

For the following descriptions of AP humeral images with poor positioning, state how the patient would have been mispositioned for such an image to be obtained.

14. The image demonstrates the ulna without radial head and tuberosity superimposition.

    _____

15. The image demonstrates the radial head and tuberosity superimposed over more than ¼ inch (0.6 cm) of the ulna.

For the following AP humeral images with poor positioning, state what anatomical structures are misaligned and how the patient should be repositioned for an optimal image to be obtained.

Figure 3–85

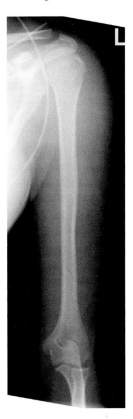

16. (Figure 3-85): _____

_____

_____

_____

Figure 3–86

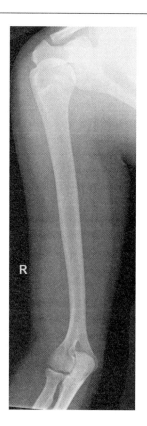

17. (Figure 3-86): _____

_____

_____

_____

Lateral Position

1. Is the image demonstrated in Figure 3-87 a mediolateral or lateromedial projection?

Figure 3–87

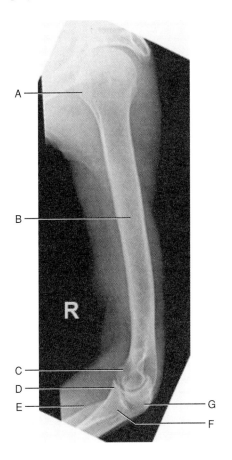

2. Identify the labeled anatomy in Figure 3-87.

A. _____

B. _____

C. _____

D. _____

E. _____

F. _____

G. _____

3. Is the image demonstrated in Figure 3-88 a mediolateral or lateromedial projection?

Figure 3–88

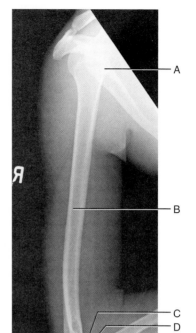

4. Identify the labeled anatomy in Figure 3-88.

A. _____

B. _____

C. _____

D. _____

E. _____

F. _____

5. Will a mediolateral or lateromedial projection of the humerus allow the humerus to be positioned closer to the IR when it is in a lateral position? _____

6. A proximal humeral image with accurate positioning demonstrates the (A) _____ tubercle in profile (B) _____ (medially/laterally).

7. Which projection of the humerus demonstrates the capitulum distal to the medial trochlea and superimposition of the radial head and coronoid process? _____

8. Which projection of the humerus demonstrates the radial head anterior to the coronoid and the capitulum proximal to the medial trochlea?

_____

9. What causes the anatomical structures of the distal humerus to align differently on the two lateral projections of the humerus? _____

_____

10. When positioning the patient for a lateral humeral image, the (A) _____ should be internally rotated until an imaginary line connecting the (B) _____ is positioned perpendicular to the IR.

11. List two alternative positions that can be used to image the humerus in the lateral position in a patient with a suspected fractured proximal humerus.

    A. _____

    B. _____

12. When imaging the proximal humerus, how can one determine if the humeral epicondyles have been accurately positioned for a lateral humeral image?

_____

13. If the patient's humerus is aligned diagonally on the IR and the collimator head or tube column cannot be rotated, a flat contact shield may be used to protect the patient's thorax. Why is it important that these shields be positioned at least 2 inches (5 cm) away from the humeral head? _____

_____

14. On a lateral humeral image with accurate positioning, the _____ is centered within the collimated field.

15. What anatomical structures are included on a lateral humeral image with accurate positioning?

_____

For the following description of a lateral humeral image with poor positioning, state how the patient would have been mispositioned for such an image to be obtained.

16. The mediolateral projection image demonstrates a decrease in image density at the proximal humerus, and the distal humerus displays adequate density.

_____

For the following lateral humeral images with poor positioning, state what anatomical structures are misaligned and how the patient should be repositioned for an optimal image to be obtained.

Figure 3–89

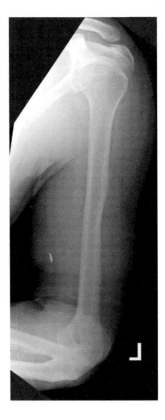

17. (Figure 3-89): _____

_____

_____

_____

18. (Figure 3-90): _____

_____

_____

_____

_____

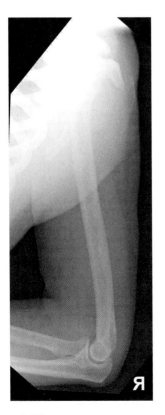

Figure 3–90

CHAPTER 3
STUDY QUESTION ANSWERS

1. A. From the fingertips with the marker correct
   B. From the fingertips with the marker correct
   C. From the fingertips with the marker correct
   D. From the fingertips with the marker correct
   E. From the shoulder with the marker correct for lateromedial and reversed for mediolateral projection
2. A. Patient motion
   B. Explaining the procedure to the patient
   C. Making the patient comfortable
   D. Using a short exposure time
   E. Using immobilization props
3. A. High
   B. Low
4. A. Bony trabecular
   B. Cortical
5. Table 3-1

6. Table 3-2

Position or Projection	kVp	SID
Finger	50-60	40-48 inches (100-120 cm)
Thumb	50-60	40-48 inches (100-120 cm)
PA hand	50-60	40-48 inches (100-120 cm)
PA oblique hand	55-65	40-48 inches (100-120 cm)
Lateral hand	55-65	40-48 inches (100-120 cm)
Wrist	55-65	40-48 inches (100-120 cm)
Forearm	55-65	40-48 inches (100-120 cm)
Elbow	55-65	40-48 inches (100-120 cm)
Humerus	65-75	40-48 inches (100-120 cm)

kVp, Kilovolt peak; *PA*, posteroanterior; *SID*, source–image-receptor distance.

Position or Projection	IR Size	Direction, Placement, and Number of Images on IR
PA, oblique and lateral finger	8 × 10 inches (18 × 24 cm)	Crosswise—three images on IR
AP, oblique and lateral thumb	8 × 10 inches (18 × 24 cm)	Crosswise—three images on IR
PA, oblique and lateral hand	Screen-film	
	10 × 12 inches (24 × 30 cm)	Crosswise—two images on IR
	8 × 10 inches (18 × 24 cm)	Lengthwise—one image on IR
	Computed radiography	
	3-8 × 10 inches (18 × 24 cm)	Lengthwise—one image on IR
PA, oblique and lateral wrist	Screen-film	
	10 × 12 inches (24 × 30 cm)	Crosswise—two images on IR
	8 × 10 inches (18 × 24 cm)	Lengthwise—one image on IR
	Computed radiography	
	3-8 × 10 inches (18 × 24 cm)	Lengthwise—one image on IR
AP and lateral forearm	14 × 17 inches (35 × 43 cm)	Lengthwise—two images on IR
AP and lateral elbow	Screen-film	
	10 × 12 inches (24 × 30 cm)	Crosswise—two images on IR
	Computed radiography	
	2-8 × 10 inches (18 × 24 cm)	Lengthwise—one image on IR
AP and lateral humerus	2-14 × 17 inches (35 × 43 cm)	Lengthwise—one image on IR

AP, Anteroposterior; *IR,* image receptor; *PA,* posteroanterior.

Finger
PA Projection (Second through Fifth Digits)

7. A. Distal phalanx
   B. Middle phalanx
   C. Interphalangeal joints
   D. Proximal phalanx
   E. Metacarpophalangeal joint
   F. Metacarpal head
8. A. Imaginary line that runs lengthwise with structure
   B. Describes a structure that is curved or rounded inward like a cup
   C. Act of rotating the anterior surface of an extremity toward the patient's torso
   D. Act of turning the upper extremity laterally until the palm of the hand is facing anteriorly
9. Shift the ring as far away from the affected area as possible. Note on the requisition that the patient was unable to remove the ring.
10. Flat
11. A. Concavity
    B. Soft-tissue

12. A. Externally into a medial oblique position
    B. The thumb prevents internal rotation.
13. A. Farther
    B. Greater
14. A. Closer
    B. Greater
15. Second
16. Fifth
17. A. The collimator's light line
    B. Phalanx
    C. Metacarpal
18. Spread the fingers apart.
19. A. IP joints
    B. MP joints
20. A. Parallel
    B. Perpendicular
21. A. Closed
    B. Foreshortened
22. A. Supinating
    B. Perpendicular
23. A. Proximal interphalangeal (PIP)
    B. Perpendicular
    C. PIP
24. A. Phalanges
    B. Metacarpal
25. Within ½ inch (1.25 cm) of the finger skinline.
26. The finger was internally rotated into a lateral oblique position.
27. The finger was flexed.
28. Soft-tissue width and concavity is increased on the side of the finger facing the thumb. Rotate the hand and finger internally until they are flat against the IR.
29. The phalanges are foreshortened, the IP and MP joints are closed, and increased concavity is present on the side of the finger facing the third digit. Unflex the finger and internally rotate the hand until the finger and hand are flat against the IR.

Oblique Position

1. A. Distal phalanx
   B. Middle phalanx
   C. Interphalangeal joints
   D. Proximal phalanx
   E. Metacarpophalangeal joint
   F. Metacarpal
2. A. Object-IR distance
   B. Proximal interphalangeal
   C. Interphalangeal
   D. Metacarpophalangeal
3. 45
4. A. Externally
   B. Internally or externally
   C. This rotation will result in the least amount of OID.

5. A. Twice
   B. Concavity
6. So one can tightly collimate without clipping needed anatomical structures
7. To prevent soft-tissue overlap from adjacent fingers
8. A. Extended
   B. Parallel
9. To prevent the finger from tilting toward the IR
10. A. PIP
    B. Perpendicular
    C. PIP
11. The distal, middle, and proximal phalanges and half of the metacarpal
12. The finger was not rotated enough and was too close to a PA projection.
13. The finger was rotated closer to a lateral position than a 45-degree oblique.
14. The fingers were not spread apart.
15. The finger was flexed or tilted toward the IR.
16. Phalangeal concavity and soft-tissue width are equal on each side of the digit. Rotate the hand and finger internally until the finger is at a 45-degree angle to the IR.
17. The anterior aspects of the middle and proximal phalanges demonstrate midshaft concavity, whereas the posterior aspects of these phalanges demonstrate convexity. Internally rotate the hand until the finger is at a 45-degree angle to the IR. The fourth and fifth digits demonstrate superimposition. Have the patient make a fist with the hand and extend the affected fourth digit.
18. The phalanges are foreshortened, and the IP and MP joints are closed. The finger was rotated externally, placing it at a long OID, and the finger was allowed to bend down toward the IR. Rotate the finger and hand internally until the finger is at a 45-degree angle with the IR, and fully extend the finger.

Lateral Position

1. A. Distal phalanx
   B. Distal interphalangeal joint
   C. Middle phalanx
   D. Proximal interphalangeal joint
   E. Proximal phalanx
   F. Metacarpophalangeal joint
   G. Metacarpals
2. A. To extend a structure beyond the normal limit
   B. Act of rotating an extremity toward the torso
   C. Act of rotating an extremity away from the torso
   D. Describes a structure that is outwardly curved
3. 90
4. A. Concave
   B. Convex
5. A. Internally

B. Internally
C. Externally
D. Externally
6. The hand is rotated to obtain the least amount of OID.
7. Flex the hand into a tight fist with the affected finger extended.
8. A. IP
   B. Phalanges
9. PIP
10. The distal, middle, and proximal phalanges and the metacarpal head
11. A device to extend the finger and move the proximal phalanx away from the other phalanges should not be used distal to a fracture, or displacement of the fracture may occur.
12. The hand was not flexed into a tight fist.
13. The finger was not in a lateral position but was in an oblique position.
14. The affected finger was allowed to tilt toward the IR.
15. Twice as much soft tissue and more phalangeal concavity are present on one side of the digit as on the other, there is soft tissue overlap of fourth and fifth fingers, and the DIP and PIP joints are closed. Flex the unaffected fingers into a fist, and increase the degree of external hand obliquity until the finger is in a lateral position. Position the long axis of the finger parallel with the IR.
16. The unaffected fingers are superimposed over the proximal phalanx. Flex the unaffected fingers into a fist while the finger of interest remains extended. Use a positioning device if needed to help extend the finger if no proximal phalanx injury is suspected.

Thumb (First Digit)
AP Projection

1. A. Distal phalanx
   B. Interphalangeal joint
   C. Proximal phalanx
   D. Metacarpophalangeal joint
   E. Metacarpal
   F. Carpometacarpal joint
   G. Carpal bone (trapezium)
2. Carpometacarpal
3. A. Equal
   B. Width
   C. Concavity
4. A. Internally
   B. Directly
5. Closer
6. To allow tight collimation without clipping the required anatomy
7. A. IP
   B. MP
   C. CM
   D. Phalanges

8. Extended
9. Draw the medial palm surface away from the thumb by using the opposite hand or an immobilization device.
10. CM
11. A. MP
    B. Perpendicular
    C. MP
12. Thumb
13. The distal and proximal phalanges, metacarpal, and CM joint
14. The hand was internally rotated more than needed to place the thumb in an AP projection.
15. The thumb was flexed.
16. The medial palm soft tissue was not drawn away from the proximal first metacarpal.
17. The medial palm soft tissue is superimposed over the proximal metacarpal and CM joint. Draw the medial palm away from the proximal metacarpal, using the opposite hand to maintain this positioning.
18. More soft-tissue width and phalanx concavity are present on the side adjacent to the other digits, and the thumbnail is facing away from the second through fifth digits. Decrease the amount of internal rotation until the fingernail is flat against the IR.

Lateral Position

1. A. Distal phalanx
   B. Interphalangeal joint
   C. Proximal phalanx
   D. Metacarpophalangeal joint
   E. First metacarpal
   F. Second metacarpal
   G. Carpometacarpal joint
2. A. Concave
   B. Convex
3. Flex
4. Align the long axis of the thumb with the collimator's longitudinal light line.
5. Align the thumb parallel with the IR.
6. Second proximal metacarpal
7. A. MP
   B. Perpendicular
   C. MP
   D. To the thumb
8. The distal and proximal phalanges, metacarpal, and CM joint
9. The hand was overflexed, and possibly the thumb was not in maximum abduction.
10. The patient's hand was not flexed enough, resulting in underrotation.
11. The proximal second and third metacarpals are superimposed over the proximal first metacarpal. Abduct the thumb and slightly decrease the

amount of hand flexion while maintaining a lateral thumb.

12. Twice as much soft tissue and more phalangeal and metacarpal midshaft concavity are present on the side of the thumb facing the fingers. Increase the amount of hand flexion until the thumb is in a lateral position.

Lateral Oblique Position

1. A. Distal phalanx
   B. Interphalangeal joint
   C. Proximal phalanx
   D. Metacarpophalangeal joint
   E. First metacarpal
   F. Carpometacarpal joint
2. 45
3. A. Extended
   B. Flat
4. A. Twice
   B. Concavity
5. A. MP
   B. Perpendicular
   C. MP
6. The distal and proximal phalanges, metacarpal, and CM joint
7. To within ½ inch (1.25 cm) of skinline
8. The hand was not flat against the IR, causing the thumb to be rotated closer to a lateral position.
9. The anterior aspect of the proximal phalanx and metacarpal demonstrates midshaft concavity, whereas the posterior aspect of the phalanx and metacarpal demonstrates slight convexity. Decrease the degree of hand flexion, positioning the hand flat against the IR.
10. The DIP joint is closed and the distal phalanx is foreshortened. Extend the thumb until it is parallel with the IR.

Hand
PA Projection

1. A. Distal phalanx
   B. Interphalangeal joint
   C. Proximal phalanx
   D. Metacarpophalangeal joint
   E. Metacarpal
   F. Carpometacarpal joint
   G. Radius
   H. Ulna
   I. Carpals
   J. Carpometacarpal joint
   K. Metacarpal
   L. Metacarpophalangeal joint
   M. Proximal phalanx
   N. Proximal interphalangeal joint

   O. Middle phalanx
   P. Distal interphalangeal joint
   Q. Distal phalanx
2. A. Act of rotating an extremity externally, away from the torso
   B. Act of raising the arm so the humerus moves away from the torso
   C. Rotation of the hand internally until the palm's surface is facing posteriorly or down on the surface
3. If it is around the area of interest, shift it as far away as possible. Note on the requisition that the patient was unable to remove the ring.
4. A. Soft-tissue
   B. Metacarpal
5. A. Pronate
   B. Flat
6. The thumb prevents this rotation.
7. The third digit and metacarpal should be aligned with the collimated field's long axis.
8. The fingers should be spread apart.
9. A. IP
   B. MP
   C. CM
10. The joint spaces would be closed, and the phalanges and metacarpals would be foreshortened.
11. Oblique
12. The thumb would move into a lateral position.
13. Third MP
14. The distal, middle, and proximal phalanges, metacarpals, and carpals and 1 inch (2.5 cm) of the forearm
15. The hand was externally rotated into a medial oblique position.
16. The fingers were not separated.
17. The fingers and hand were flexed.
18. The second through fifth metacarpal midshafts are more concave on one side than on the other, and the third through fifth metacarpal heads demonstrate slight superimposition. The IP joint spaces are closed, and the proximal and middle phalanges are foreshortened. Extend and internally rotate the hand, placing it flat against the IR.
19. The second through fifth phalanges are foreshortened, and the IP joint spaces are closed. Extend the hand and place it flat against the IR.
20. Angle the central ray laterally until it is aligned perpendicular to the metacarpals. Prop the IR on an angled sponge until it is perpendicular to the central ray.

PA Oblique Projection (External Rotation)

1. A. Interphalangeal joints
   B. Metacarpophalangeal joint
   C. Second metacarpal

D. Radius
E. Ulna
F. Carpals
G. Fifth metacarpal
H. Phalanges
2. Overlaying of one structure on another
3. A. 45
B. Externally
4. A. Second
B. Third
C. Third
D. Fourth
E. Fifth
F. Metacarpal midshafts
5. Because the wrist will demonstrate more obliquity than the hand when they are rotated
6. They must be extended so they are aligned parallel with the IR.
7. A. Yes, the phalanges are not being evaluated.
B. The reviewer already knows no injury to the fingers is present, as long as no new injury has occurred.
8. MP
9. The distal, middle, and proximal phalanges, metacarpals, and carpals and 1 inch (2.5 cm) of the forearm
10. The hand was not rotated 45 degrees but was closer to a PA projection.
11. The hand was rotated more than 45 degrees.
12. The fingers were flexed toward the IR.
13. The third through fifth metacarpal heads are demonstrated without superimposition, the phalanges are foreshortened, and the IP joints are closed. Externally rotate the hand until it forms a 45-degree angle with the IR, and elevate the distal fingers until they are aligned parallel with the IR.
14. The midshafts of the third through fifth metacarpals are superimposed. The phalanges are foreshortened, and the IP and MP joints are closed. Internally rotate the hand until it forms a 45-degree angle with the IR, and elevate the distal fingers until they are aligned parallel with the IR.
15. Angle the central ray perpendicular to the metacarpals, then adjust it 45-degrees medially. Prop the IR until it is aligned perpendicular to the central ray.
16. Angle the central ray perpendicular to the metacarpals, then adjust it 45-degrees medially. Prop the IR until it is aligned perpendicular to the central ray.

Lateromedial Projection ("Fan" Lateral Position)

1. A. Distal phalanx
B. Distal interphalangeal joint
C. Middle phalanx

D. Proximal interphalangeal joint
E. Proximal phalanx
F. Metacarpophalangeal joint
G. Metacarpal
H. Radius
I. Ulna
J. Carpals
K. Metacarpals
L. Metacarpophalangeal joint
2. A. Spread apart
B. Sponge used to support the patient's position
C. Act of touching a structure through the skin
D. Act of curving the hand into a fist
E. Act of fully opening the hand
3. The thicknesses of the fingers and the metacarpals are so different in this position that uniform image density is difficult to obtain.
4. A. Anteriorly
B. Posteriorly
5. PA projection to a slight oblique
6. Second through fifth metacarpals
7. A. Shortest
B. Longest
8. Depress the thumb until it is parallel with the IR.
9. MP
10. The distal, middle, and proximal phalanges, metacarpals, and carpals and 1 inch (2.5 cm) of the forearm
11. The patient's hand was externally rotated or supinated.
12. The patient's hand was internally rotated or pronated.
13. The patient's fingers were not fanned.
14. The second through fifth metacarpal midshafts are not all superimposed. The fifth metacarpal is demonstrated anteriorly. Internally rotate the hand until the metacarpals are superimposed.
15. The second through fifth metacarpal midshafts are demonstrated without superimposition. The second metacarpal is demonstrated anteriorly. Externally rotate the hand until the metacarpals are superimposed.
16. The second through fifth digits are flexed and superimposed. Fan or spread the fingers as far apart as possible without superimposing the thumb.

Wrist

PA Projection

1. A. Trapezoid
B. Trapezium
C. Capitate
D. Scaphoid
E. Radial styloid
F. Radius
G. Ulna

H. Ulnar styloid
  I. Lunate
  J. Triquetrum
  K. Pisiform
  L. Hamate
  M. Metacarpals
2. A. A joint
  B. Surface on the bone that articulates with another bone surface
  C. Refers to a structure on an extremity that is situated closest to the torso
  D. Refers to a structure on an extremity that is situated farthest from the torso
  E. A four-sided figure where two of the sides are parallel
  F. A figure that demonstrates a small circle inside a larger circle
  G. Act of moving the hand so it moves closer to the radius, causing wrist flexion
  H. Act of moving the hand so it moves closer to the ulna, causing wrist flexion
3. Convex in shape and located lateral to the scaphoid
4. A change in the convexity of this stripe may indicate joint effusion or fracture.
5. A. Lateral
  B. Parallel with the IR
6. As an open space
7. A. Posterior
  B. Anterior
8. Slightly depress the proximal forearm.
9. Allow the proximal forearm to hang off the IR and table enough to slightly depress the proximal forearm.
10. Flex the hand until metacarpals form a 10- to 15-degree angle with the IR.
11. A. Extended
  B. Anteriorly
12. A. To prevent ulnar and radial deviation
  B. One half of the lunate will be distal to it
13. A. Anteriorly
  B. Foreshortened
  C. Medially
14. Posteriorly
15. A. Carpals
  B. Perpendicular
16. The carpal bones, one fourth of the distal ulna and radius, and one half of the proximal metacarpals
17. The central ray centering should be the same, but the longitudinally collimated field should be opened to include the needed amount of forearm.
18. The patient's elbow was not in a lateral position, and the humerus was not parallel with the IR.
19. The patient's wrist was externally rotated (in a medial oblique position).
20. The patient's wrist was internally rotated (in a lateral oblique position).
21. The proximal forearm was elevated.
22. The patient's hand was extended, causing wrist flexion.
23. The patient's hand was overflexed, causing wrist extension.
24. The patient's wrist was in radial flexion.
25. The patient's wrist was in ulnar flexion.
26. The laterally located carpals and metacarpals are superimposed, and the radioulnar articulation is closed. Internally rotate the hand and wrist into a PA projection.
27. The medially located carpals and metacarpals are superimposed, and the radioulnar articulation is closed. Externally rotate the hand and wrist into a PA projection. The carpals are not centered in the collimated field. Move the central ray proximally 1 inch (2.5 cm).
28. The scaphoid is elongated, and the second through fourth CM joints are closed. Decrease hand flexion until the metacarpals are at a 10- to 15-degree angle with the IR.
29. The scaphoid is foreshortened, and the third metacarpal and midforearm are not aligned. Ulnar-flex until the third metacarpal and midforearm are aligned.

PA Oblique Projection (External Rotation)

1. A. Capitate
  B. Hamate
  C. Pisiform
  D. Triquetrum
  E. Lunate
  F. Ulnar styloid
  G. Ulna
  H. Radius
  I. Radial styloid
  J. Scaphoid
  K. Trapezoid
  L. Trapezium
  M. Carpometacarpal joint
  N. First metacarpal
  O. Trapeziotrapezium joint
2. A bony projection
3. A. 45
  B. Externally
4. Trapeziotrapezoidal
5. Trapezium
6. A. Third metacarpal
  B. Midforearm
7. The posterior margin will be projected distal to the anterior margin.
8. Posterior
9. A. In profile

B. The elbow should be placed in a lateral position, and the humerus should be placed parallel with the IR.

10. A. Carpals
    B. Perpendicular

11. The carpal bones, one fourth of the distal forearm, and one half of the proximal metacarpals

12. The patient's wrist was in less than a 45-degree external oblique position.

13. The patient's wrist was in radial flexion.

14. The patient's proximal forearm was depressed.

15. The trapezoid and trapezium are superimposed, the trapeziotrapezoidal joint space is obscured, and the trapezoid demonstrates minimal capitate superimposition. Increase the degree of obliquity until the wrist forms a 45-degree angle with the IR.

16. The scaphoid demonstrates foreshortening, and the long axis of the third metacarpal is not aligned with the midforearm. Ulnar-deviate the wrist until the third metacarpal and midforearm are aligned.

17. The trapezium demonstrates minimal trapezoidal superimposition, the capitate is superimposed by the trapezoid, and the trapeziotrapezoidal joint space is obscured. Decrease the degree of obliquity until the wrist forms a 45-degree angle with the IR.

18. The scaphoid is demonstrated with decreased foreshortening, the second carpometacarpal and scaphotrapezium joints are open, and more than ¼-inch (0.6 cm) of the radial articulating surface is demonstrated. Radial-deviate the wrist until the long axis of the third metacarpal and midforearm are aligned, decrease the amount of hand flexion until the metacarpals are at a 10- to 15-degree angle with the IR, and depress the proximal forearm until the forearm is parallel.

Lateral Position (Lateromedial Projection)

1. A. Capitate
   B. Lunate
   C. Ulnar styloid
   D. Radius
   E. Pisiform
   F. Distal scaphoid
   G. Trapezium
   H. First metacarpal

2. A. Posterior surface
   B. Anterior surface

3. It is convex in shape and is located next to the anterior surface of the distal radius.

4. Changes in the shape and visualization of this stripe may indicate a fracture.

5. A. Distal scaphoid and pisiform
   B. Radius and ulna

6. A. Ulnar
   B. Lateromedial
   C. Pisiform

7. Anterior

8. Align the long axes of the third metacarpal and the midforearm parallel with the IR.

9. A. Distal
   B. Proximal

10. Radial

11. Position the first metacarpal next to the second metacarpal and align it with the forearm.

12. Position the humerus parallel with the IR and the elbow in a lateral position.

13. Position the humerus against the patient's body without abduction, and position the elbow in an AP projection.

14. The position described in question 13, when the elbow is in an AP projection and the humerus is not abducted

15. Depress the distal first metacarpal until it is at the same level as the second metacarpal.

16. A. Carpals
    B. Perpendicular

17. The carpal bones, one fourth of the distal ulna and radius, and one half of the proximal metacarpals

18. Within ½ inch (1.25 cm) of skinline

19. A. AP projection
    B. Lateral position

20. The patient's wrist was externally rotated (or supinated).

21. The patient's wrist was internally rotated (or pronated).

22. The wrist was in radial deviation.

23. The wrist was in ulnar deviation

24. The humerus was not abducted but was placed against the patient, and the elbow was in an AP projection.

25. The distal first metacarpal was elevated.

26. The distal scaphoid is demonstrated anterior to the pisiform. Externally rotate the wrist until it is lateral. The ulnar styloid is in profile.

27. The distal scaphoid is demonstrated posterior to the pisiform. Internally rotate the wrist until it is lateral. The ulnar styloid is seen distal to the midline of the ulnar head.

28. The first metacarpal is not situated adjacent to the second metacarpal, and the wrist is in extension. Place the wrist in a neutral position by positioning the first metacarpal adjacent to the second metacarpal and aligning the first metacarpal and midforearm. The ulnar styloid is in profile.

29. The trapezium is superimposed by the proximal first metacarpal. Lower the first metacarpal until it is at the same level as the second metacarpal. The ulnar styloid is in profile.

Ulnar-Deviation, PA Axial Projection (Scaphoid)

1. A. Capitate
   B. Hamate
   C. Scaphocapitate joint
   D. Ulnar styloid
   E. Radioulnar articulation
   F. Scapholunate joint
   G. Radioscaphoid joint
   H. Scaphoid
   I. Scaphotrapezoidal joint
   J. Scaphotrapezium joint
   K. Trapezium
   L. Trapezoid
   M. CM joint
   N. First metacarpal
2. Scaphoid fat stripe
3. A. First metacarpal
   B. Radius
   C. Radius
4. In ulnar flexion the scaphoid has the space it needs to move posteriorly and will demonstrate a decrease in foreshortening.
5. Position the patient's wrist in a 25-degree external (medial) oblique position.
6. 15 degrees proximally
7. A. 20 degrees proximally
   B. Without ulnar deviation, the distal scaphoid is positioned anteriorly and the scaphoid demonstrates increased foreshortening.
8. Waist
9. A. Increase 5 to 10 degrees
   B. Decrease 5 to 10 degrees
10. No
11. Elevate (5 to 6 degrees) the distal forearm
12. Scaphoid
13. The carpal bones, radioulnar joint, and proximal first through fourth metacarpals
14. A. Distal fracture. The first metacarpal is not aligned with the ulna, so the starting central ray angulation should be 20 degrees. This amount should then be increased by 5 to 10 degrees to a maximum angle of 25 degrees. A 25-degree angle should be used.
    B. Proximal fracture. The first metacarpal and ulna are aligned, so the starting central ray angulation should be 15 degrees. This amount should then be decreased by 5-degrees because the fracture is close to the waist. A 10-degree angle should be used.
    C. Waist fracture. The first metacarpal is aligned with the ulna. A 15-degree central ray angulation should be used.
15. The wrist was medially oblique more than needed.
16. The patient's hand and fingers were flexed.
17. The scapholunate joint is closed, the capitate and hamate demonstrate a small degree of superimposition, and the ulnar styloid is not demonstrated in profile. Decrease the degree of medial wrist obliquity and position the elbow in a lateral position.
18. The scaphocapitate joint space is closed, and the capitate and hamate are demonstrated without superimposition. Increase the degree of medial obliquity until the wrist forms a 25-degree angle with the IR.
19. The scaphotrapezium, scaphotrapezoid, and carpometacarpal joints are closed. Extend the fingers and place the hand flat against the IR.

Carpal Canal (Tunnel) (Tangential, Inferosuperior Projection)

1. A. First metacarpal
   B. Trapezium
   C. Scaphoid
   D. Capitate
   E. Carpal canal
   F. Hamulus of hamate
   G. Triquetrium
   H. Pisiform
2. A. Narrowing
   B. Fractures
3. The patient's hand is rotated 10 degrees internally until the fifth metacarpal is aligned perpendicular to the IR.
4. A. Vertically
   B. 25 degrees proximally
5. A. Increased
   B. 35 degrees
   C. Acute angle between the central ray and IR.
6. The patient's wrist and distal forearm were either in a PA projection or in slight external rotation.
7. The angle between the central ray and metacarpals was too great.
8. The angle between the central ray and metacarpals was too small.
9. The pisiform is superimposed over the hamulus of the hamate. Internally (toward the radius) rotate the hand until the fifth metacarpal is vertical.
10. The metacarpal bases obscure the bases of the hamate's hamulus process, pisiform, and scaphoid. Increase the central ray angle until it is within 15 degrees of the metacarpals, or increase the amount of wrist hyperextension by pulling the fingers posteriorly until the metacarpals are vertical.
11. The carpal canal is not demonstrated in its entirety, and the carpal bones are foreshortened. Decrease the central ray angle until it is within 15 degrees of the metacarpals.

Forearm

AP Projection

1. A. Radioscaphoid joint
   B. Radial styloid
   C. Radius
   D. Radial tuberosity
   E. Radial head
   F. Capitulum-radial joint
   G. Lateral epicondyle
   H. Olecranon fossa
   I. Medial epicondyle
   J. Olecranon
   K. Ulnar midshaft
   L. Radioulnar articulation
   M. Ulnar head
   N. Ulnar styloid
   O. Fifth metacarpal base
2. A. Long axis of the collimated field
   B. Axis that runs perpendicular to the longitudinal axis
   C. Bending of the elbow
3. Position the wrist at the anode end and the elbow at the cathode end of the tube.
4. So they will still be included on the image when they are projected by the diverged beams used to record them
5. It is located ¾ inch (2 cm) distal to the medial epicondyle.
6. A. Forearm midshaft
   B. Perpendicular
   C. Midforearm
7. The radius, ulna, wrist and elbow joints, and forearm soft tissue
8. A. Medially
   B. Ulna
9. The joint that is closer to the area of interest or near the fracture site should be positioned into an AP projection, whereas the other joint is positioned as close to an AP projection as possible.
10. Humerus and elbow
11. A. ¼ inch (0.6 cm)
    B. Humeral epicondyles
12. Because the diverged x-ray beams, used to record this joint, do not align parallel with the joint
13. Parallel
14. Supinate the hand and wrist, placing them in an AP projection.
15. The elbow was accurately positioned, but the hand and wrist were internally rotated.
16. The wrist and hand were accurately positioned, but the elbow was externally rotated.
17. The elbow is accurately positioned, but the hand was pronated.
18. The lateral position and PA projection of the forearm reflect accurate positioning. When forearm images are obtained in a patient with a fracture where the patient is unable to position the distal and proximal forearm in a true position simultaneously, the joint closer to the fracture site should be placed in the true position. For these images the wrist joint demonstrates accurate positioning.
19. The radial head is demonstrated without being superimposed over the ulna. Internally rotate the elbow until an imaginary line connecting the humeral epicondyles is aligned parallel with the IR while maintaining the same wrist positioning.
20. The radial head is demonstrated without superimposition over the ulna. Align the central ray perpendicular to an imaginary line connecting the humeral epicondyles (this will require the central ray to be adjusted toward the medial surface). Prop the IR as needed to align it perpendicular to the central ray.

Lateral Position (Lateromedial Projection)

1. A. Ulnar styloid
   B. Ulna
   C. Coronoid
   D. Olecranon
   E. Humerus
   F. Elbow joint
   G. Radial head
   H. Radius
   I. Pisiform
   J. Distal scaphoid
2. A. Invasion of fluid into the joint
   B. Arcs that have the same center
3. Position the wrist at the anode end and the elbow at the cathode end of the tube.
4. Forearm midpoint
5. The radius, ulna, wrist and elbow joints, and forearm soft tissue
6. A. Distal
   B. Superimposed
7. Ulnar (medial)
8. Distal scaphoid will be anterior to the pisiform.
9. A. It will be demonstrated in profile posteriorly.
   B. Place the elbow in a lateral position and abduct the humerus, positioning it parallel with the IR.
10. A. No
    B. Supinate the hand to place the tuberosity in profile anteriorly, and pronate the hand to place the tuberosity in profile posteriorly.
11. A. Thick or muscular proximal forearm
    B. Thick or muscular distal forearm
12. Radial head will be too posterior to the coronoid.
13. Place the elbow and proximal forearm in a lateral position and allow the distal forearm to rotate as close to a lateral position as the patient will allow.

14. The patient's hand and wrist were externally rotated.
15. The patient's hand and wrist were internally rotated, and the proximal humerus was depressed more than the distal humerus.
16. The patient's elbow was not in a lateral position, but was closer to an AP projection.
17. The patient's wrist and hand were in external rotation.
18. The proximal humerus was elevated.
19. The radial head is posterior to the coronoid, and the distal scaphoid is anterior to the pisiform. Depress the proximal humerus until the humerus is parallel with the IR, and externally rotate the wrist until it is in a lateral position.
20. Adjust the central ray posteriorly until it is aligned with an imaginary line connecting the distal radius and ulna. Prop the IR as needed to align it perpendicular to the central ray.

Elbow

AP Projection

1. A. Olecranon
   B. Lateral epicondyle
   C. Capitulum-radial joint
   D. Radial head
   E. Radial neck
   F. Radius
   G. Ulna
   H. Radial tuberosity
   I. Coronoid
   J. Medial trochlea
   K. Medial epicondyle
   L. Olecranon fossa
   M. Humerus
2. A hollowed or depressed area on a bone.
3. A. Medial and lateral humeral epicondyles
   B. ¼ inch (0.6 cm)
4. Medial and lateral humeral epicondyles
5. Lateral
6. A. Medially
   B. Parallel with each other
7. The wrist and hand position
8. A. Central ray accurately centered to joint
   B. Forearm aligned parallel with the IR
9. Find where the central ray was positioned by diagonally connecting the corners on the collimated elbow image. The two lines connect where the central ray was located. Determine if the olecranon is within the olecranon fossa.
10. Do two AP views—one with the humerus parallel with the IR and one with the forearm parallel with the IR.
11. A. Elbow joint
    B. Perpendicular
    C. ¾ inch (2 cm)
    D. Distal
    E. Because it protrudes more than the lateral epicondyle
12. The elbow joint, one fourth of the proximal forearm and distal humerus, and the lateral soft tissue
13. The patient's arm was internally (medially) rotated.
14. The patient's arm was externally (laterally) rotated.
15. The hand was pronated.
16. The distal forearm was elevated.
17. The humeral epicondyles are not in profile, and the radial head, neck, and tuberosity are superimposed over the ulna by more than ¼ inch (0.6 cm). Externally rotate the elbow until the humeral epicondyles are at equal distances to the IR.
18. The humeral epicondyles are not in profile, and the radial head demonstrates less than ¼ inch (0.6 cm) of superimposition. Internally rotate the elbow until the humeral epicondyles are at equal distances from the IR.
19. The capitulum-radial joint is closed, and the radial articulating surface is demonstrated. If the patient's condition allows, fully extend the elbow. If the patient is unable to extend the elbow, take two partial AP exposures; one with the humerus parallel and one with the forearm parallel with the IR.
20. Angle the central ray laterally until it is aligned perpendicular to an imaginary line connecting the humeral epicondyles. Prop the IR as needed to align it perpendicular to the central ray and parallel with the humeral epicondyle line.

AP Oblique Projections (Internal and External Rotation)

1. A. Medial epicondyle
   B. Medial trochlea
   C. Coronoid
   D. Radial tuberosity
   E. Radial head
2. A. Radial tuberosity
   B. Ulna
   C. Radial head
   D. Capitulum
3. A. The forearm was not positioned parallel with the IR.
   B. The central ray was not centered to the elbow joint.
4. The olecranon will move away from the olecranon fossa with elbow flexion.
5. A. Forearm
   B. Forearm
   C. Humerus
   D. Humerus
   E. Forearm

6. 45 degrees
7. The coronoid process, trochlear notch, and medial aspect of the trochlea
8. Laterally
9. The capitulum and radial head, neck, and tuberosity
10. A. Elbow joint (capitulum-radial joint)
    B. Perpendicular
    C. ¾ inch (2 cm)
    D. Medial epicondyle
11. The elbow joint, one fourth of the proximal humerus and distal forearm, and the lateral soft tissue
12. The distal forearm was elevated.
13. The patient's arm was rotated less than 45 degrees.
14. The patient's arm was rotated more than 45 degrees.
15. The patient's arm was rotated less than 45 degrees.
16. The patient's arm was rotated more than 45 degrees.
17. A small portion of the radial head and tuberosity is superimposed over the ulna. Increase the degree of external obliquity until the humeral epicondyles are at a 45-degree angle to the IR.
18. The capitulum-radial head joint is closed, and a small portion of the radial head is superimposed over the ulna. If the patient's condition allows, fully extend the arm, and if the patient is unable to fully extend the arm, position the forearm parallel with the IR. Increase the degree of external obliquity until the humeral epicondyles are at a 45-degree angle to the IR.
19. The radial head is demonstrated lateral to the coronoid process without complete superimposition of the ulna. Increase the degree of internal obliquity until the humeral epicondyles are at a 45-degree angle to the IR.
20. The radial head is demonstrated lateral to the coronoid process without complete superimposition of the ulna, the capitulum-radial joint is closed, and the articulating surface of the radial head is demonstrated. Increase the degree of internal obliquity until the humeral epicondyles are at a 45-degree angle with the IR. If the patient's condition allows, fully extend the arm, and if the patient is unable to fully extend the arm, position the forearm parallel with the IR.

Lateral Position (Lateromedial Projection)

1. A. Medial trochlea
   B. Coronoid
   C. Radial head
   D. Radius
   E. Ulna
   F. Trochlear notch
   G. Olecranon process
   H. Capitulum
   I. Trochlear sulcus
   J. Humerus
2. A. Situate the distal forearm at a level that is higher than the proximal forearm.
   B. Situate the proximal humerus at a level that is lower than the distal humerus.
3. A. Anterior fat pad, anterior to the distal humerus
   B. Posterior fat pad, within the olecranon fossa
   C. Supinator fat stripe, seen parallel to the anterior aspect of the distal radius
   D. Joint effusion and elbow injury
4. The posterior fat pad can be used as a diagnosing tool only when the elbow is flexed 90 degrees and the olecranon is out of the fossa.
5. A. Capitulum
   B. Trochlear sulcus
   C. Medial aspect of the trochlea
   D. Trochlear sulcus
   E. Medial trochlea
   F. It will close it.
6. The radial head should align with the most anterior and proximal aspects of the coronoid.
7. The capitulum would be distal to the medial trochlea.
8. The radial head would be distal to the coronoid, and the capitulum would be anterior to the medial trochlea.
9. The radial head will be proximal to the coronoid.
10. The radial head will be anterior to the coronoid, and the capitulum will be proximal to the medial trochlea.
11. A. Superimposed by the radius
    B. In profile, anteriorly
    C. In profile, posteriorly
    D. Superimposed by the radius
12. A. Elbow joint
    B. Perpendicular
    C. ¾ inch (2 cm)
    D. Distal
13. The elbow joint, one fourth of the proximal forearm and distal humerus, and the surrounding soft tissue
14. The patient's arm was in extension.
15. The patient's hand and wrist were supinated.
16. The patient's proximal humerus was elevated.
17. The patient's proximal humerus was depressed.
18. The patient's distal forearm was not adequately elevated.
19. The patient's distal forearm was elevated more than needed.
20. The radial head is proximal to the coronoid (capitulum is posterior to the medial trochlea), and the radial tuberosity is seen anteriorly. Depress the distal forearm until the humeral epicondyles

are aligned perpendicular to the IR, and internally rotate the distal forearm until the wrist is in a lateral position.

21. The radial head is distal to the coronoid (capitulum is anterior to the medial trochlea). Elevate the distal forearm until the humeral epicondyles are aligned perpendicular to the IR.

22. The radial head is distal and posterior to the coronoid (capitulum is distal and anterior to the medial trochlea). Elevate the distal forearm and depress the proximal humerus until the humeral epicondyles are aligned perpendicular to the IR.

23. The radial head is proximal and anterior to the coronoid (capitulum is posterior and proximal to the medial trochlea), and the radial tuberosity is visible posteriorly. Depress the distal forearm and elevate the proximal humerus until the humeral epicondyles are aligned perpendicular to the IR, and externally rotate the distal forearm until the wrist is in a lateral position.

24. The radial head is distal and anterior to the coronoid (capitulum is anterior and proximal to the medial trochlea). Elevate the distal forearm and proximal humerus until the humeral epicondyles are aligned perpendicular to the IR.

25. Adjust the central ray angle posteriorly until it is aligned parallel with a line connecting the humeral epicondyles. Prop the IR as needed to align it perpendicular to the central ray and to a line connecting the humeral epicondyles.

Radial Head and Capitulum

1. A. Capitulum
   B. Capitulum-radial joint
   C. Radial head
   D. Radial tuberosity
   E. Coronoid
   F. Medial trochlea
2. A. Medial aspect of the trochlea
   B. Trochlear sulcus
   C. Capitulum
3. Lateral position
4. A. Capitulum-radial
   B. Coronoid process
5. Radial head and coronoid and the capitulum and medial trochlea
6. The radial head will be proximal to the coronoid, and the capitulum will be posterior to the medial trochlea.
7. The capitulum will be anterior to the medial trochlea.
8. A. Capitulum
   B. Medial trochlea
   C. Coronoid process

9. A. Perpendicular
   B. 45
   C. Proximally
   D. Radial head
   E. Capitulum
10. Radial tuberosity
11. A. The radial tuberosity will be in profile posteriorly, the lateral surface of the radial head will be in profile anteriorly, and the medial surface will be in profile posteriorly.
    B. The radial tuberosity will not be in profile but will be superimposed by the radius. The anterior surface of the radial head will appear in profile anteriorly, and the posterior surface will appear in profile posteriorly.
12. A. Radial head
    B. ¾ inch (2 cm) distal to the lateral epicondyle
13. The proximal forearm, distal humerus, and surrounding soft tissue
14. The patient's distal forearm was positioned too close to the IR.
15. The patient's distal forearm was positioned too far away from the IR.
16. The capitulum-radial joint space is closed, the radial head is demonstrated distal to the coronoid process, and the capitulum is demonstrated too far anterior to the medial trochlea. Elevate the distal forearm until the humeral epicondyles are aligned perpendicular to the IR.
17. The capitulum-radial joint space is closed, and the radial head is too distal to the coronoid process (capitulum is too anterior to the medial trochlea). The radial head is not anterior enough to the coronoid (capitulum is not proximal enough to the medial trochlea). Elevate the distal forearm, and depress the proximal humerus.
18. First align the central ray parallel with a line connecting the humeral epicondyles, than adjust the central ray 45-degrees proximally (toward the humerus). Prop the IR as needed to align it perpendicular to the humeral epicondyles.

Humerus
AP Projection

1. A. Greater tubercle
   B. Lesser tubercle
   C. Humeral midshaft
   D. Medial epicondyle
   E. Lateral epicondyle
   F. Radial head
   G. Ulna
2. A. Device placed between the patient and the IR to absorb scatter radiation
   B. Number used to express a grid's scatter-eliminating ability

C. Unwanted absorption, by the grid, of primary radiation

3. A. 13
   B. 70

4. Position the elbow at the anode end of the x-ray tube and the shoulder at the cathode end.

5. A. ¼ inch (0.6 cm)
   B. Humeral epicondyles

6. A. Greater
   B. Humeral head
   C. Lesser tubercle

7. A. Arm
   B. Humeral epicondyles

8. A. Forced external rotation may result in an increased risk of radial nerve damage.
   B. Rotate the patient 35 to 45 degrees toward the affected side for the proximal humerus, and rotate the patient toward the affected side until the humeral epicondyles are parallel with the IR when the distal humerus is of interest.

9. Abduct the humerus and place it diagonally on the IR.

10. To ensure that the joints will be included after the beam's divergence projects the elbow joint distally and the shoulder joint proximally

11. A. Locate at the same level as the coracoid
    B. Locate ¾ inch (2 cm) distal to the epicondyles

12. Humeral midshaft

13. The humerus, shoulder and elbow joints, and lateral humeral soft tissue

14. The patient's arm was externally rotated.

15. The patient's arm was internally rotated.

16. The greater tubercle and the humeral epicondyles are not in profile, and the radial head is superimposed over more than ¼ inch (0.6 cm) of the ulna. Externally rotate the arm until the humeral epicondyles are at equal distances to the IR.

17. The greater and lesser tubercles are nearly superimposed, and the ulna is demonstrated without radial superimposition. Internally rotate the arm until the humeral epicondyles are at equal distances from the IR.

Humerus
Lateral Position

1. Lateromedial
2. A. Lesser tubercle
   B. Humeral shaft
   C. Capitulum
   D. Coronoid
   E. Radial tuberosity
   F. Radial head
   G. Medial trochlea

3. Mediolateral

4. A. Lesser tubercle
   B. Humeral shaft
   C. Capitulum
   D. Radial head
   E. Radial tuberosity
   F. Capitulum-radial joint
   G. Medial trochlea

5. Mediolateral

6. A. Lesser
   B. Medially

7. Lateromedial

8. Mediolateral

9. The effect of the x-ray's divergence on the anatomical structure positioned farthest from the IR

10. A. Arm
    B. Humeral epicondyles

11. A. Transcapular Y position
    B. Transthoracic lateral position

12. The lesser tubercle will be in profile medially.

13. They will be magnified and may be superimposed over the area of interest.

14. Humeral midshaft

15. The humerus, elbow and shoulder joints, and lateral soft tissue

16. The patient's torso was not in a PA projection but was rotated toward the affected humerus.

17. The lesser tuberosity is not in profile, and the capitulum is demonstrated posterior to the medial trochlea. Move the distal humerus away from the IR until the humeral epicondyles are perpendicular to the IR.

18. The image demonstrates a lateral position, as indicated by the optimal distal humerus positioning. The density is lighter at the proximal humerus than at the distal humerus, preventing proximal humerus visualization. Rotate the torso away from the proximal humerus into a PA projection.

Image Analysis of the Shoulder

LEARNING OBJECTIVES

After completion of this chapter you should be able to:

_____ 1. Identify the required anatomy on shoulder, clavicular, acromioclavicular (AC) joint, and scapular images.

_____ 2. Describe how to properly position the patient, image receptor (IR), and central ray on shoulder, clavicular, AC joint, and scapular images.

_____ 3. State how to properly mark and hang shoulder, clavicular, AC joint, and scapular images.

_____ 4. List the typical artifacts that are found on shoulder, clavicular, AC joint, and scapular images.

_____ 5. List the image requirements for shoulder, clavicular, AC joint, and scapular images with accurate positioning.

_____ 6. State how to properly reposition the patient when shoulder, clavicular, AC joint, and scapular images show poor positioning.

_____ 7. Discuss how to determine the amount of patient or central ray adjustment that is required to improve shoulder, clavicular, AC joint, and scapular images with poor positioning.

_____ 8. State the kilovoltage routinely used for shoulder, clavicular, AC joint, and scapular images, and describe what anatomical structures are visible when the correct technique factors are used.

_____ 9. Explain when it is necessary to use a grid for shoulder images.

_____ 10. Discuss why a compensating filter is needed on anteroposterior (AP) shoulder and clavicular images.

_____ 11. State where the humerus might be positioned if a shoulder dislocation is demonstrated on AP and scapular Y shoulder images.

_____ 12. Describe the position of the scapula when the patient's torso is in an AP projection.

_____ 13. Discuss how the visualization of the proximal humerus changes as the humeral epicondyles are placed at different angles to the IR.

_____ 14. Explain how the scapula is affected when the humerus is abducted.

_____ 15. State how the central ray angulation can be adjusted to offset longitudinal scapular foreshortening on a kyphotic patient.

_____ 16. List the anatomical structures that form the Y on a scapular Y shoulder image.

_____ 17. State how the lateral and medial borders of the scapula can be identified.

_____ 18. Describe why the clavicle is often imaged in the AP projection instead of the posteroanterior (PA) projection.

_____ 19. Discuss why non–weight- and weight-bearing images are often required when AC joints are imaged.

_____ 20. Explain why the image density on an AP scapular image varies so greatly.

_____ 21. Describe how the shoulder is retracted to obtain an AP projection of the scapula.

_____ 22. Discuss what anatomical structures must move to allow the humerus to abduct.

_____ 23. Explain why a patient with a fractured scapula may be able to abduct the humerus without moving the scapula.

_____ 24. Describe the effect of humeral abduction on the degree of patient obliquity needed to position the scapula in a lateral position.

_____ 25. State which long axis of the scapular body is placed parallel with the IR as the humerus is abducted.

_____ 26. State where scapular fractures most often occur.

STUDY QUESTIONS

1. Describe how the following shoulder images should be hung on a view box or displayed on a cathode ray tube (CRT) monitor.

   A. Inferosuperior (axial) shoulder: _____

   B. Left axial clavicle: _____

   C. Right scapular Y shoulder: _____

2. List anatomical structures that are demonstrated on shoulder images if proper image density and penetration were demonstrated. _____

   _____

3. Complete Table 4-1.

TABLE 4-1 **Shoulder Technical Data**				
Position or Projection	**kVp**	**Grid**	**AEC Chamber(s)**	**SID**
AP projection, shoulder				
Inferosuperior (axial) projection, shoulder				
Posterior oblique position (Grashey), shoulder				
Anterior oblique position, (scapular Y), shoulder				
AP axial projection (Stryker), shoulder				
Tangential projection (outlet), shoulder				
AP and axial projections, clavicle				
AP projections, AC joint				
AP projection, scapula				
Lateral position, scapula				

AC, Acromioclavicular; *AEC,* automatic exposure control; *AP,* anteroposterior; *kVp,* kilovolt peak; *SID,* source–image receptor distance.

4. When an exposure is set for shoulder images that adequately demonstrates the glenohumeral joint, the acromion process and lateral clavicular end are often overexposed. How can the technologist provide an image that adequately demonstrates all of these structures?

5. When should a grid be used for the axial lateral position?

6. Complete Table 4-2.

TABLE 4-2 IR Size, Placement, and Direction		
Position or Projection	**IR Size**	**Placement and Direction**
AP projection, shoulder		
Inferosuperior (axial) projection, shoulder		
Posterior oblique position (Grashey), shoulder		
Anterior oblique position (scapular Y), shoulder		
AP axial projection (Stryker), shoulder		
Tangential projection (outlet), shoulder		
AP and axial projections, clavicle		
AP projections, AC joint		
AP projection, scapula		
Lateral position, scapula		

AC, Acromioclavicular; *AP,* anteroposterior; *IR,* image receptor.

Shoulder: AP Projection

1. Identify the labeled anatomy on Figure 4-1.

Figure 4–1

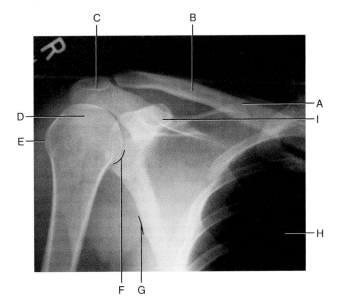

A. _____

B. _____

C. _____

D. _____

E. _____

F. _____

G. _____

H. _____

I. _____

2. Define the following terms.

   A. Overexposed: _____

   B. Shoulder retraction: _____

   C. Shoulder dislocation: _____

3. If an arrow marker is used to indicate internal and external humeral rotation on an AP shoulder image, how is it positioned on the IR for each of the following images?

   A. Internal rotation: _____

   B. External rotation: _____

4. Where is the medial end of the clavicle located on an AP shoulder image with accurate positioning? _____

5. How can the technologist position the patient to prevent rotation on an AP shoulder image?

   _____

6. What is the degree of scapular obliquity on an AP shoulder image?

   A. _____

   What portion of the scapula is situated anteriorly?

   B. _____

7. A nondislocated shoulder demonstrates slight superimposition of the humeral head and _____.

8. Which shoulder dislocation is the most common? _____ (Anterior/Posterior)

9. How is the patient positioned to demonstrate the scapular body without longitudinal foreshortening on an AP shoulder image?

   _____

10. If the scapula is longitudinally foreshortened, the superior scapular angle is projected inferiorly or superiorly to the _____.

11. How can longitudinal scapular foreshortening be avoided when obtaining an AP shoulder image in a kyphotic patient? _____

   _____

12. When the shoulder is demonstrated without humeral abduction, the glenoid cavity faces (A) _____, whereas on humeral abduction the glenoid cavity shifts (B) _____.

13. The lateral humeral epicondyle is aligned with the (A) _____ and the medial epicondyle is aligned with the (B) _____ of the proximal humerus.

14. State how the humeral epicondyles are positioned in reference to the IR to place the anatomical structures as described on the following AP shoulder images.

   A. Greater tubercle is partially in profile laterally: _____

   B. Lesser tubercle is in profile medially: _____

   C. Greater tubercle is in profile laterally: _____

   D. Humeral head is in profile medially: _____

15. How is the patient's arm positioned for an AP shoulder image if a shoulder dislocation or humeral fracture is suspected? _____

   _____

16. The (A) _____ is centered within the collimated field on an AP shoulder image with accurate positioning. This is accomplished by centering a (B) _____ central ray 1 inch (2.5 cm) (C) _____.

17. What anatomical structures are demonstrated within the collimated field on an AP shoulder image with accurate positioning? _____

   _____

18. Describe the location of the palpable coracoid process.

   _____

   _____

For the following descriptions of AP shoulder images with poor positioning, state how the patient would have been mispositioned for such an image to be obtained.

19. The glenoid cavity is nearly in profile with only a small amount of the articulating surface demonstrated, the superolateral border of the scapula is superimposed by the thorax, and the medial clavicular end has been rolled away from the vertebral column.

   _____

20. The scapular body is drawn from beneath the thorax and is transversely foreshortened, the glenoid cavity is demonstrated on end, and the medial clavicular end is superimposed over the vertebral column.

   _____

21. The superior scapular angle is demonstrated superior to the clavicle, and the acromion process and humeral head demonstrate no superimposition.

   _____

22. A neutral shoulder image demonstrates the greater tubercle in profile laterally and the humeral head in profile medially.

   _____

   _____

23. A neutral shoulder image demonstrates the lesser tubercle in profile medially.

   _____

   _____

For the following AP shoulder images with poor positioning, state what anatomical structures are misaligned and how the patient should be repositioned for an optimal image to be obtained.

Figure 4–2

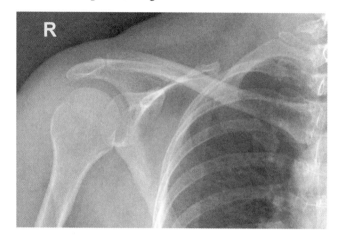

24. (Figure 4-2): _____

_____

_____

_____

Figure 4–3

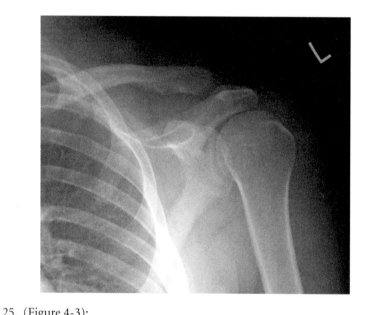

25. (Figure 4-3): _____

_____

_____

_____

Figure 4–4

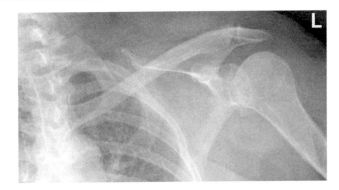

26. (Figure 4-4): _____

_____

_____

_____

Shoulder: Inferosuperior (Axial) Projection

1. Identify the labeled anatomy in Figure 4-5.

Figure 4–5

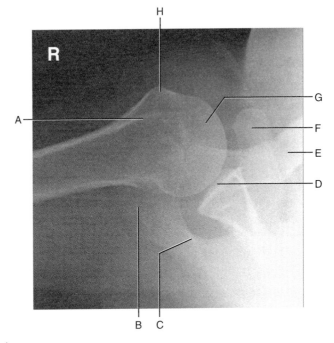

A. _____

B. _____

C. _____

D. _____

E. _____

F. _____

G. _____

H. _____

2. On an axial shoulder image with accurate positioning, the (A) _____ and (B) _____ margins of the glenoid cavity are nearly superimposed and the lateral edge of the coracoid process base is (C) _____ with the glenoid cavity, indicating accurate central ray and (D) _____ alignment.

3. Humeral abduction of the arm is obtained by combined movements of the (A) _____ and (B) _____.

4. On a patient who has no trouble abducting the humerus to a 90-degree angle with the body, the glenoid cavity is placed at a _____ angle with the lateral body surface.

5. Describe how and at what angle to the body's lateral surface the central ray should be aligned on a patient who is able to abduct the humerus to a 90-degree angle with the body for an axial shoulder image. _____

_____

6. How should the angle between the lateral body surface and the central ray be adjusted if the patient can abduct the humerus to only a 45-degree angle with the body?

A. _____

Why is this change required?

B. _____

_____

7. How is the IR positioned for an axial shoulder image?

_____

_____

8. When is the humeral shaft foreshortened on an axial shoulder image?

_____

9. Describe the anatomical structures of the proximal humerus that are demonstrated anteriorly and posteriorly in profile on an axial shoulder image when the humerus is positioned as stated below.

A. Arm externally rotated until the humeral epicondyles are at a 45-degree angle with the floor: _____

_____

B. Arm externally rotated until the humeral epicondyles are perpendicular to the floor: _____

_____

C. Arm externally rotated until the humeral epicondyles are parallel with the floor: _____

_____

10. What is the name of the proximal humerus compression fracture that is better demonstrated on an axial shoulder image when the patient's arm is placed in exaggerated external rotation?

A. _____

How must the humeral epicondyles be positioned to demonstrate this fracture on an axial shoulder image?

B. _____

11. The _____ is centered within the collimated field on an axial shoulder image with accurate positioning.

12. To align the central ray with the glenohumeral joint, center a (A) _____ central ray to the midaxillary region at the same transverse level as the (B) _____.

13. What anatomical structures are included on an axial shoulder image with accurate positioning?

_____

14. For an axillary shoulder image, elevation of the shoulder on a sponge or washcloth prevents clipping of the _____ aspect of the humerus and shoulder.

15. Turning and tilting the patient's head away from the affected shoulder prevents clipping of the (A) _____, (B) _____, and (C) _____.

16. How were the humeral epicondyles positioned for the axial shoulder image in Figure 4-6?

Figure 4–6

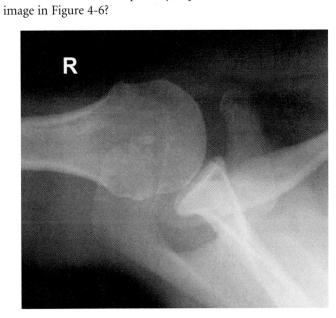

A. _____

How were the humeral epicondyles positioned for the axial shoulder image in Figure 4-7?

Figure 4–7

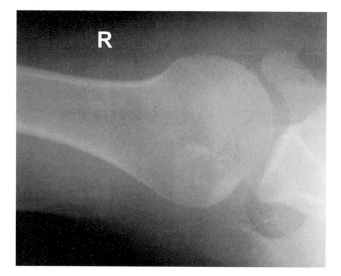

B. _____

For the following descriptions of axial shoulder images with poor positioning, state how the patient would have been mispositioned or the central ray aligned for such an image to be obtained.

17. The glenohumeral joint space is obscured, and the inferior glenoid cavity is demonstrated lateral to the coracoid process base.

_____

18. The glenohumeral joint space is obscured, and the inferior glenoid cavity is demonstrated medial to the lateral edge of the coracoid process base.

_____

19. The greater tubercle is demonstrated in profile posteriorly.

_____

20. The acromion process, scapular spine, and posterior aspect of the proximal humerus were not included on the image.

_____

For the following axial shoulder images with poor positioning, state what anatomical structures are misaligned and how the patient should be repositioned for an optimal image to be obtained.

Figure 4–8

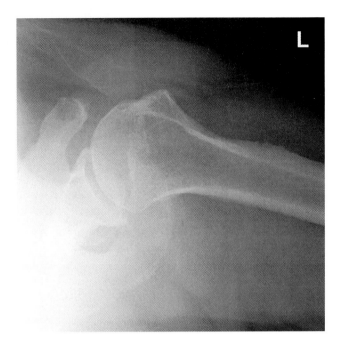

21. (Figure 4-8): _____

_____

_____

_____

Figure 4–9

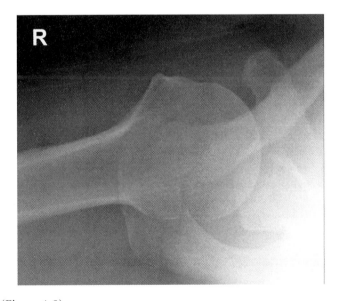

22. (Figure 4-9): _____

_____

_____

_____

Figure 4–10

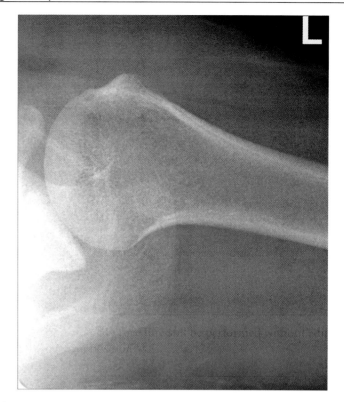

23. (Figure 4-10): _____

_____

_____

_____

Shoulder: Posterior Oblique Position (Grashey Method)

1. Identify the labeled anatomy in Figure 4-11.

Figure 4–11

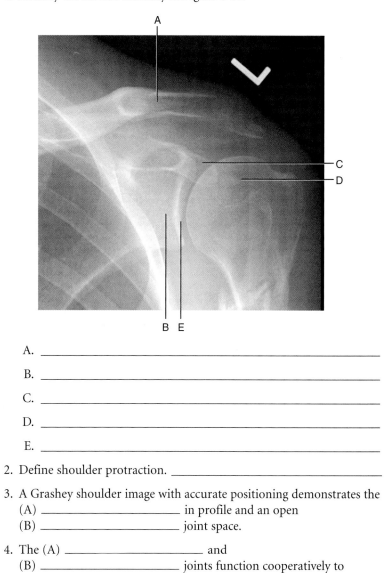

A. _____

B. _____

C. _____

D. _____

E. _____

2. Define shoulder protraction. _____

3. A Grashey shoulder image with accurate positioning demonstrates the
   (A) _____ in profile and an open
   (B) _____ joint space.

4. The (A) _____ and
   (B) _____ joints function cooperatively to
   allow the shoulder to be protracted.

5. The scapular body is positioned parallel with the IR for the Grashey
   method by aligning an imaginary line connecting the
   (A) _____ and (B) _____
   perpendicular to the IR.

6. A 45-degree oblique is routinely used for the Grashey method. List three situations in which the patient requires more than 45 degrees of obliquity to obtain a Grashey image with accurate positioning.

   A. _____

   B. _____

   C. _____

7. Where is the coracoid process positioned with reference to the humeral head on a Grashey shoulder image with accurate rotation?

   A. _____

   _____

   How will this relationship change if the patient is overrotated for the Grashey shoulder image?

   B. _____

   Underrotated?

   C. _____

8. How is the clavicle positioned on a Grashey shoulder image with accurate rotation that was exposed with the patient recumbent?

   _____

9. On a Grashey shoulder image with accurate positioning, the (A) _____ is centered within the collimated field. This is accomplished by centering a (B) _____ central ray 1 inch (2.5 cm) (C) _____ and (D) _____ to the (E) _____.

10. What anatomical structures are demonstrated within the collimated field on a Grashey shoulder image with accurate positioning? _____

   _____

For the following descriptions of Grashey shoulder images with poor positioning, state how the patient would have been mispositioned for such an image to be obtained.

11. The glenohumeral joint space is closed, approximately ½ inch (1.25 cm) of the coracoid process is superimposed over the humeral head, and the clavicle demonstrates excessive transverse foreshortening.

   _____

12. The glenohumeral joint space is closed, the lateral tip of the coracoid process is not superimposed over the humeral head, and the clavicle demonstrates little foreshortening.

   _____

13. Recumbent patient: The glenohumeral joint is closed, and the clavicle is superimposed over the scapular neck.

   _____

For the following Grashey shoulder images with poor positioning, state what anatomical structures are misaligned and how the patient should be repositioned for an optimal image to be obtained.

Figure 4–12

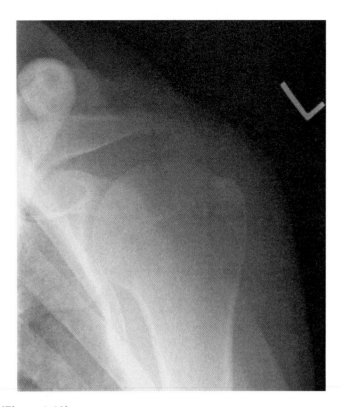

14. (Figure 4-12): _____

_____

_____

Figure 4–13

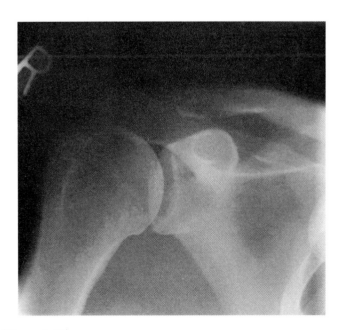

15. (Figure 4-13): _____

_____

_____

Shoulder: Anterior Oblique Position (Scapular Y)

1. Identify the labeled anatomy in Figure 4-14.

Figure 4–14

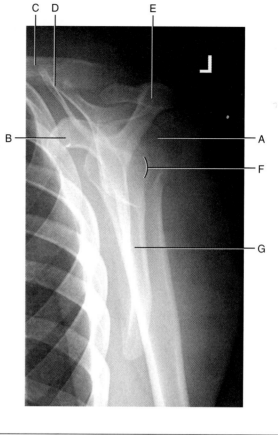

A. _____

B. _____

C. _____

D. _____

E. _____

F. _____

G. _____

2. Why is an anterior oblique position chosen over a posterior oblique position when obtaining a scapular Y image?

A. _____

B. _____

3. What anatomical structures make up the arms of the Y formation demonstrated on a scapular Y shoulder image?

A. _____

What anatomical structure makes up the leg of the Y formation?

B. _____

What anatomical structure is located at the converging point of the arms and leg of the Y?

C. _____

4. A scapular Y image with accurate positioning is obtained when the (A) _____ and (B) _____ borders of the scapula are superimposed and the (C) _____ is demonstrated without scapular body superimposition.

5. Allowing the arm to dangle freely for the scapular Y position places what border of the scapula parallel with the IR when the patient is accurately positioned? _____

6. The scapular body is placed in a lateral position for the scapular Y shoulder image by rotating the patient until the (A) _____ scapular border and a point midway between the (B) _____ and (C) _____ are superimposed.

7. List two indications for the scapular Y position:

   A. _____

   B. _____

8. For an anterior oblique scapular Y shoulder image the patient is rotated toward the (A) _____ (affected/unaffected) shoulder. For a posterior oblique scapular Y shoulder image the patient is rotated toward the (B) _____ (affected/unaffected) shoulder.

9. How can one distinguish the medial and lateral scapular borders from each other on a scapular Y shoulder image with poor positioning?

   _____

10. If the patient is overrotated or underrotated for a scapular Y shoulder position, how can one determine from the image how the patient should be repositioned?

    _____

11. Where are the humeral head and shaft positioned on a nondislocated scapular Y shoulder image?_____

    _____

12. If the patient's shoulder is dislocated, should the Y formation desired on the scapular Y shoulder image be visualized? _____ (Yes/No)

13. Where is the humeral head positioned on the scapular Y shoulder image if the shoulder is dislocated anteriorly?

    A. _____

    _____

    If the shoulder is dislocated posteriorly?

    B. _____

    _____

    Which of these possible dislocations is most commonly seen?

    C. _____

14. How can the patient be positioned to prevent longitudinal foreshortening of the scapula on a scapular Y shoulder position?

    _____

    _____

15. What spinal condition results in longitudinal scapular foreshortening on a scapular Y shoulder image?

   A. _____

   How can the central ray be adjusted to offset this foreshortening when obtaining an anterior oblique image?

   B. _____

   When obtaining a posterior oblique image?

   C. _____

16. On a scapular Y shoulder image with accurate positioning, the (A) _____ is centered within the collimated field. This is accomplished by centering a (B) _____ central ray to the (C) _____ border of the scapula halfway between the (D) _____ and (E) _____ .

17. What anatomical structures are demonstrated on a scapular Y shoulder image with accurate positioning? _____

   _____

For the following descriptions of anterior oblique scapular Y shoulder images with poor positioning, state how the patient would have been mispositioned for such an image to be obtained.

18. The vertebral and lateral borders of the scapular body are demonstrated without superimposition, the lateral scapular border is demonstrated next to the ribs, and the medial border appears laterally.

   _____

19. The lateral and medial borders of the scapula are demonstrated without superimposition, the thicker scapular border is demonstrated laterally, and the thinner scapular border is demonstrated next to the ribs.

   _____

20. The scapular body, acromion process, and coracoid process demonstrate a Y formation, but the superior scapular angle is demonstrated superior to the coracoid process and the scapular spine is demonstrated superior to the acromion process.

   _____

For the following scapular **Y** shoulder images with poor positioning, state what anatomical structures are misaligned and how the patient should be repositioned for an optimal image to be obtained.

Figure 4–15

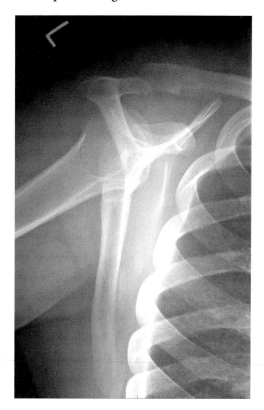

21. (Figure 4-15): _____

_____

_____

Figure 4–16

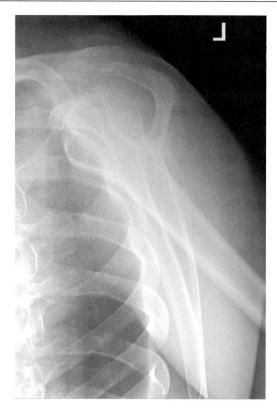

22. (Figure 4-16): _____

_____

_____

Figure 4–17

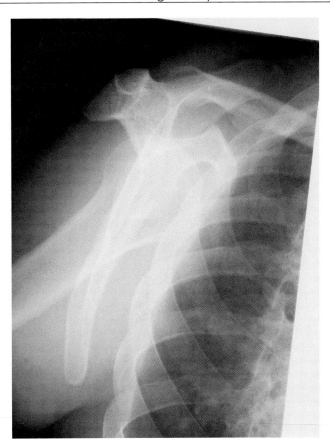

23. (Figure 4-17): _____

_____

_____

Figure 4–18

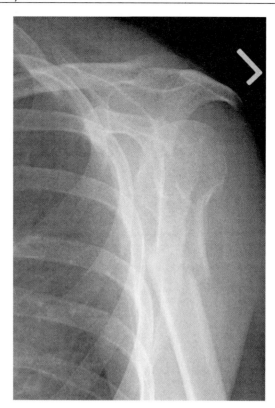

24. (Figure 4-18, Trauma): _____

_____

_____

Shoulder: AP Axial Projection (Stryker "Notch" Method)

1. Identify the labeled anatomy in Figure 4-19.

Figure 4–19

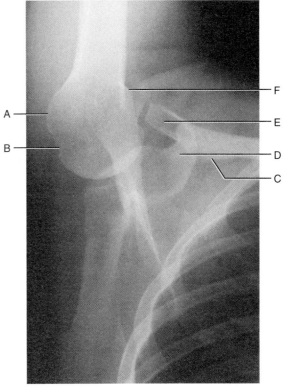

A. _____

B. _____

C. _____

D. _____

E. _____

F. _____

2. A Stryker notch image of the shoulder demonstrates an AP body position when the coracoid is visualized directly _____ to the conoid tubercle of the clavicle.

3. The Stryker notch image is performed to diagnose the presence of the (A) _____ defect of the shoulder. When present, the defect is demonstrated on the (B) _____ aspect of the humeral head.

4. For the Stryker notch image the affected arm is elevated until the humerus is (A) _____, and then the elbow is flexed and the palm of the hand is placed (B) _____.

5. Accurate humeral positioning and a 10-degree (A) _____ central ray angle places the posterolateral aspect of the (B) _____ and the (C) _____ tubercle in profile laterally and the (D) _____ tubercle in profile medially.

6. The (A) _____ is centered to the collimated field for a Stryker notch image. What anatomical structures are demonstrated on a Stryker notch image with accurate positioning?
(B)_____

For the following descriptions of Stryker notch shoulder images with poor positioning, state how the patient would have been mispositioned for such an image to be obtained.

7. The coracoid process is seen inferior to the clavicle, and the humeral shaft demonstrates increased foreshortening.

8. The lesser tubercle is seen in profile medially, but the greater tubercle and posterolateral humeral head are obscured.

9. The posterolateral humeral head is obscured, and the humeral shaft demonstrates increased foreshortening.

For the following Stryker notch shoulder images with poor positioning, state what anatomical structures are misaligned and how the patient should be repositioned for an optimal image to be obtained.

Figure 4–20

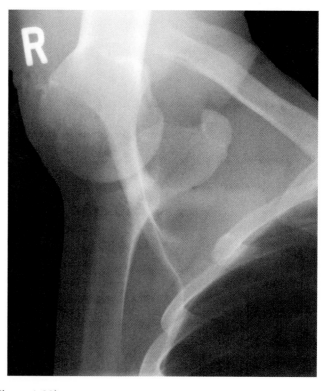

10. (Figure 4-20): _____
_____
_____

Figure 4–21

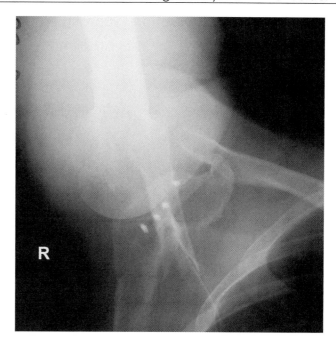

11. (Figure 4-21): _____

_____

_____

Figure 4–22

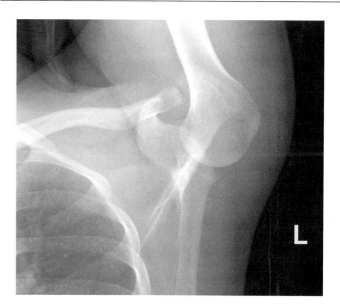

12. (Figure 4-22): _____

_____

_____

Shoulder: Tangential Projection (Supraspinatus "Outlet")

1. Identify the labeled anatomy in Figure 4-23.

Figure 4–23

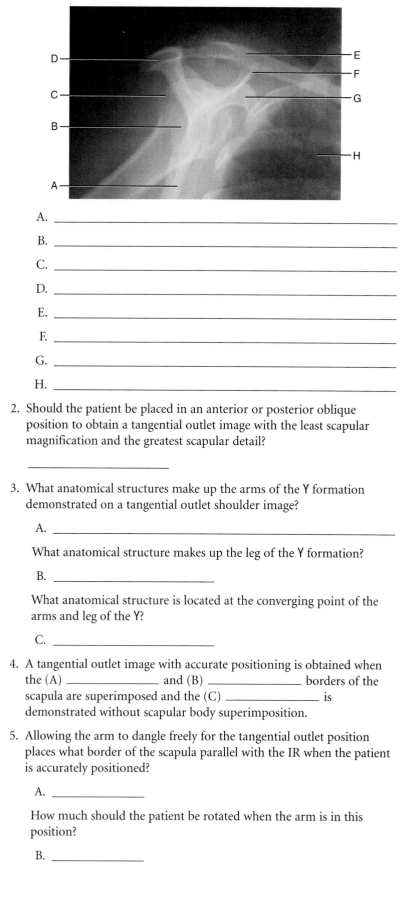

A. _____

B. _____

C. _____

D. _____

E. _____

F. _____

G. _____

H. _____

2. Should the patient be placed in an anterior or posterior oblique position to obtain a tangential outlet image with the least scapular magnification and the greatest scapular detail?

_____

3. What anatomical structures make up the arms of the Y formation demonstrated on a tangential outlet shoulder image?

A. _____

What anatomical structure makes up the leg of the Y formation?

B. _____

What anatomical structure is located at the converging point of the arms and leg of the Y?

C. _____

4. A tangential outlet image with accurate positioning is obtained when the (A) _____ and (B) _____ borders of the scapula are superimposed and the (C) _____ is demonstrated without scapular body superimposition.

5. Allowing the arm to dangle freely for the tangential outlet position places what border of the scapula parallel with the IR when the patient is accurately positioned?

A. _____

How much should the patient be rotated when the arm is in this position?

B. _____

6. How can one distinguish the medial and lateral scapular borders from each other on a tangential outlet shoulder image with poor positioning? _____

_____

7. The tangential outlet image is taken to identify osteophyte formation on the _____ surfaces of the lateral clavicle and acromion angle.

8. On a tangential outlet shoulder image with accurate positioning, the lateral clavicle and acromion are demonstrated approximately (A) _____ inch(es) (B) _____ to the humeral head and supraspinous fossa, and the superior scapular angle is at the level of the (C) _____ aspect of the clavicle. This positioning is obtained when the (D) _____ plane is vertical and the central ray is angled (E) _____.

9. The (A) _____ is placed in the center of the collimated field for a tangential outlet image when the central ray is centered to the (B) _____.
The (C) _____
should be included within the collimated field.

For the following descriptions of tangential outlet shoulder images with poor positioning, state how the patient would have been mispositioned for such an image to be obtained.

10. The vertebral and lateral borders of the scapular body are demonstrated without superimposition, the lateral scapular border is demonstrated next to the ribs, and the medial border appears laterally.

_____

11. The lateral clavicle and acromion process are demonstrated less than ½ inch (1.25 cm) superior to the humeral head and supraspinous fossa, and the superior scapular spine appears superior to the clavicle.

_____

For the following tangential outlet shoulder images with poor positioning, state what anatomical structures are misaligned and how the patient should be repositioned for an optimal image to be obtained.

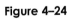
Figure 4–24

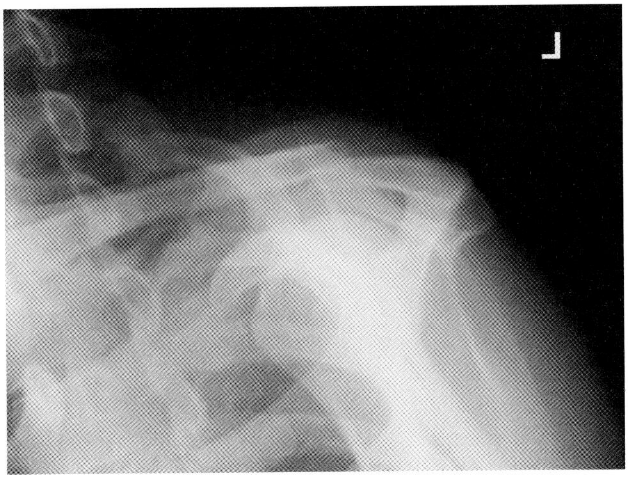

12. (Figure 4-24): _____

_____

_____

_____

_____

Figure 4–25

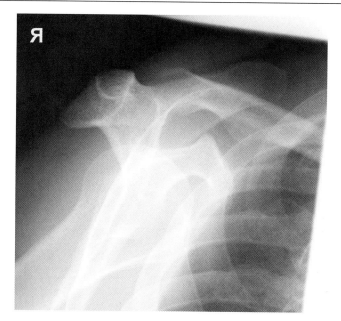

13. (Figure 4-25): _____

_____

_____

Clavicle: AP Projection

1. Identify the labeled anatomy in Figure 4-26.

Figure 4–26

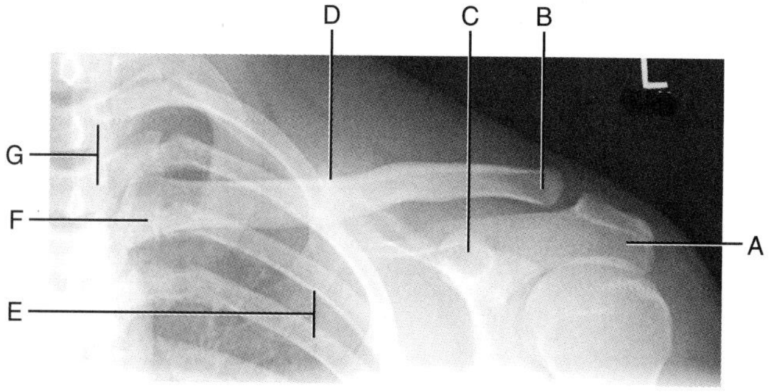

A. _____

B. _____

C. _____

D. _____

E. _____

F. _____

G. _____

2. Where is the compensating filter positioned for an AP clavicular image to demonstrate uniform density of the clavicle?

_____

3. What projection demonstrates the clavicle with the least magnification?

A. _____

Why is it uncommon for this projection to be used?

B. _____

4. Where is the medial end of the clavicle located with respect to the vertebral column on an AP clavicular image with accurate positioning? _____

_____

5. How can the technologist position the patient to prevent rotation on an AP clavicular image?

_____

6. What patient mispositioning causes inferosuperior clavicular foreshortening on an AP clavicular image? _____

7. On an AP clavicular image with accurate positioning, the (A) _____ is centered within the collimated field. This is accomplished by centering a (B) _____ central ray halfway between the (C) _____ and (D) _____ ends of the clavicle.

8. What anatomical structures are demonstrated on an AP clavicular image with accurate positioning? _____

_____

For the following descriptions of AP clavicular images with poor positioning, state how the patient would have been mispositioned for such an image to be obtained.

9. The medial clavicular end is superimposed over the vertebral column, and the vertebral border of the scapula is positioned away from the thoracic cavity.

_____

10. The medial clavicular end is placed 1 inch (2.5 cm) away from the vertebral column, and the lateral border of the scapula is mostly superimposed by the thoracic cavity.

_____

11. The lateral clavicular end is superimposed over the scapular spine, and the superior scapular angle is projected above the midclavicle.

_____

For the following AP clavicular images with poor positioning, state what anatomical structures are misaligned and how the patient should be repositioned for an optimal image to be obtained.

Figure 4–27

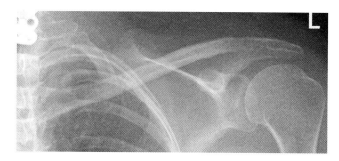

12. (Figure 4-27): _____

_____

_____

Figure 4–28

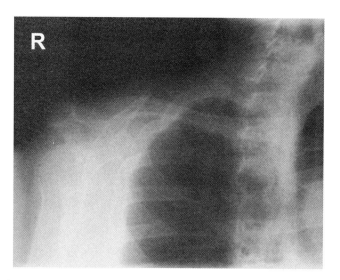

13. (Figure 4-28): _____

_____

_____

Clavicle: AP Axial Projection

1. Identify the labeled anatomy in Figure 4-29.

Figure 4–29

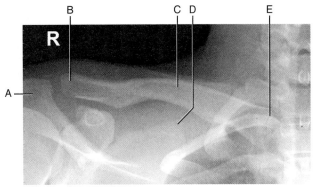

A. _____

B. _____

C. _____

D. _____

E. _____

2. Why is it necessary to use a compensating filter to obtain uniform density for an AP axial clavicular position? _____

_____

3. When evaluating an AP axial clavicular image, how can one determine if an AP has been obtained? _____

_____

4. What are the degree and direction of central ray angulation used for the AP axial clavicular image? _____

5. Where do most fractures of the clavicle occur? _____

6. When the central ray is angled correctly, the (A) _____ and (B) _____ thirds of the clavicle are demonstrated superior to the (C) _____ on an AP axial clavicular image.

7. On an AP axial clavicular image with accurate positioning, the (A) _____ is demonstrated within the collimated field. This is accomplished by centering the central ray halfway between the (B) _____ and (C) _____ ends of the clavicle.

8. What anatomical structures are demonstrated on an AP axial clavicular image with accurate positioning? _____

_____

For the following descriptions of AP axial clavicular images with poor positioning, state how the patient would have been mispositioned or the central ray aligned for such an image to be obtained.

9. The medial clavicular end is drawn away from the vertebral column, the vertebral and lateral borders of the scapula are superimposed by the thoracic cavity, and the clavicle is transversely foreshortened.

_____

10. The lateral and middle thirds of the clavicle are superimposed over the scapula.

For the following AP axial clavicular image with poor positioning, state what anatomical structures are misaligned and how the patient should be repositioned for an optimal image to be obtained.

Figure 4–30

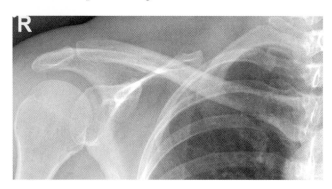

11. (Figure 4-30): _____

_____

_____

AC Joint: AP Projection

1. Identify the labeled anatomy in Figure 4-31.

   A. _____

Figure 4–31

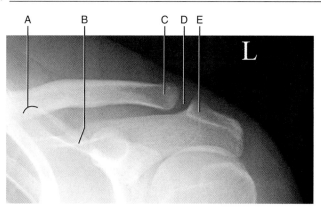

   B. _____

   C. _____

   D. _____

   E. _____

2. Define the following terms.

   A. Weight-bearing: _____

   B. Unilateral: _____

   C. Bilateral: _____

3. Why is it necessary to use an "arrow" or "word" marker on the weight-bearing AC joint image?

   A. _____

   How is the arrow marker placed on the IR?

   B. _____

4. A nonrotated AC joint image demonstrates approximately
   (A) _____ inch of space between the
   (B) _____ and lateral clavicle.

5. How is the patient positioned to ensure that an AP AC joint image is obtained?

   _____

   _____

6. Why are weight- and non–weight-bearing AP AC joint images often requested?

   _____

   _____

7. How is an AC ligament injury identified on an AP AC joint image?

   _____

   _____

8. How much weight does the patient hold in each arm for the weight-bearing AC joint image?

   _____

9. What mispositioning causes inferosuperior clavicular foreshortening on an AP AC joint image?

   A. _____

   How can this foreshortening be identified on an AP AC joint image?

   B. _____

10. On an AP AC joint image with accurate positioning, the
    (A) _____ is centered within the collimated field. This is accomplished by centering the central ray ½ inch (1 cm)
    (B) _____ to the (C) _____.

11. What anatomical structures are demonstrated on an AP AC joint image with accurate positioning?

    _____

12. Why is it necessary to place the central ray at the same area when weight- and non–weight-bearing images are requested? _____

    _____

For the following description of an AP AC joint image with poor positioning, state how the patient would have been mispositioned for such an image to be obtained.

13. The left AC joint is closed, and the scapular body demonstrates an increased amount of thoracic superimposition.

    _____

For the following AC joint image with poor positioning, state what anatomical structures are misaligned and how the patient should be repositioned for an optimal image to be obtained.

Figure 4–32

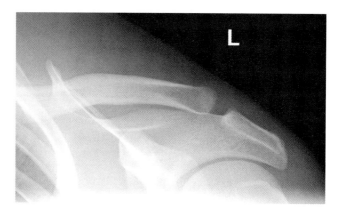

14. (Figure 4-32): _____

_____

_____

Scapula: AP Projection

1. Identify the labeled anatomy in Figure 4-33.

Figure 4–33

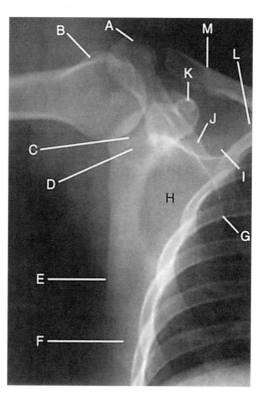

A. _____

B. _____

C. _____

D. _____

E. _____

F. _____

G. _____

H. _____

I. _____

J. _____

K. _____

L. _____

M. _____

2. Define the following terms.

   A. Image density: _____

   B. Density of structure: _____

3. Even though the AP thickness is approximately the same across the scapula, why is the image density not uniform over all parts of the scapula?

   _____

   _____

4. If a breathing technique cannot be used for the AP scapular image, what respiration should be used? _____

5. List the two dimensions that are foreshortened on a scapular image with poor positioning.

   A. _____

   B. _____

6. What degree of scapular rotation is demonstrated when the patient is positioned in an AP projection with the humerus resting against the side?

   A. _____

   Which scapular dimension is foreshortened in this position?

   B. _____

7. How is the patient positioned for an AP projection of the scapula to be obtained?

   A. _____

   _____

   What effect does the position you described in A have on the shoulder when the image is obtained with the patient in a supine position?

   B. _____

   What effect does the position have on the visualization of the glenoid cavity on an AP scapular image?

   C. _____

8. What scapular dimension is foreshortened when the patient's midcoronal plane is poorly positioned? _____

9. On an AP scapular image with accurate positioning, the (A) _____ is centered within the collimated field. This is accomplished by centering a (B) _____ central ray (C) _____ inches (D) _____ to the palpable coracoid process.

10. What anatomical structures are included on an AP scapular image with accurate positioning? _____
_____

For the following descriptions of AP scapular images with poor positioning, state how the patient would have been mispositioned for such an image to be obtained.

11. The glenoid cavity is not in profile, and approximately ½ inch (1 cm) of it is demonstrated. _____
_____

12. An image of a patient who was very mobile demonstrates the inferior scapular angle and inferolateral scapular border with thoracic cavity superimposition. _____
_____

For the following AP scapular images with poor positioning, state what anatomical structures are misaligned and how the patient should be repositioned for an optimal image to be obtained.

Figure 4–34

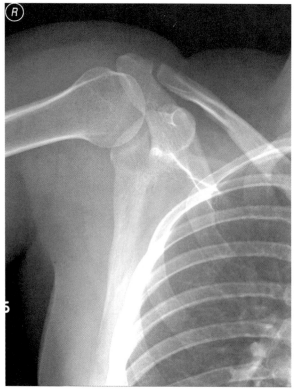

13. (Figure 4-34): _____
_____
_____
_____
_____

Figure 4–35

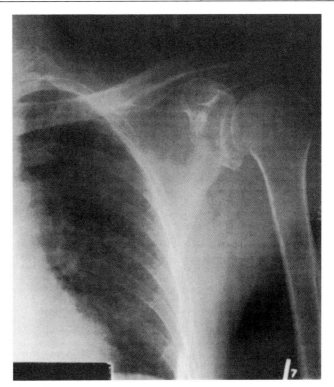

14. (Figure 4-35): _____

_____

_____

Scapula: Lateral Position (Lateromedial or Mediolateral Projection)

1. Identify the labeled anatomy in Figure 4-36.

Figure 4–36

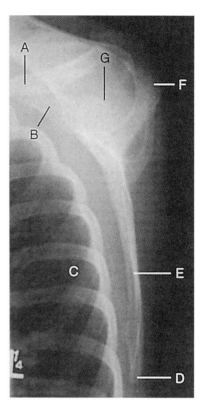

A. _____

B. _____

C. _____

D. _____

E. _____

F. _____

G. _____

2. A lateral scapular image demonstrates superimposed
   (A) _____ and (B) _____ scapular borders
   and the (C) _____ without scapular body
   superimposition.

3. The lateral scapula is imaged with the patient placed in a posterior or
   anterior oblique position. For the posterior oblique position, the
   patient is rotated (A) _____ (toward/away from) the
   affected scapula. In the anterior oblique position, the patient is rotated
   (B) _____ the affected scapula.

4. What patient positioning procedure determines the degree of
   obliquity needed to place the scapula in a lateral position?

   _____

5. Which border of the scapula has a thick, rough-appearing cortical
   outline? _____

6. How is rotation identified on a lateral scapular image with poor positioning?

_____

7. Most scapular fractures occur at the (A) _____ and (B) _____ of the scapula.

8. What humeral position with respect to the body places the long axis of the scapula parallel with the IR for a lateral scapular image?

_____

9. What humeral position with respect to the body places the lateral border of the scapula parallel with the IR for a lateral scapular image?

_____

10. What humeral position with respect to the body demonstrates a Y formation that is similar to that obtained on the scapular Y position of the shoulder for a lateral scapular image?

   A. _____

   What border of the scapula is positioned parallel with the IR for this humeral position?

   B. _____

11. The higher the humerus is elevated for a lateral scapular image the (A) _____ (more/less) the patient needs to be rotated to obtain accurate positioning. Why? (B) _____

_____

_____

12. On a lateral scapular image with accurate positioning, the (A) _____ is centered within the collimated field. This is accomplished by centering a (B) _____ central ray 1 inch (2.5 cm) (C) _____ to the vertebral border halfway between the (D) _____ and (E) _____ angles.

13. What anatomical structures are included on a lateral scapular image with accurate positioning? _____

_____

For the following descriptions of lateral scapular images with poor positioning, state how the patient would have been mispositioned for such an image to be obtained.

14. The lateral and vertebral borders of the scapula are demonstrated without superimposition, the thick border is next to the ribs, and the thin border is demonstrated laterally.

_____

15. The lateral and vertebral borders of the scapula are demonstrated without superimposition, the lateral border is demonstrated laterally, and the vertebral border appears next to the ribs.

_____

For the following lateral scapular images with poor positioning, state what anatomical structures are misaligned and how the patient should be repositioned for an optimal image to be obtained.

Figure 4–37

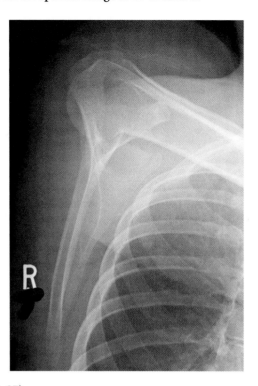

16. (Figure 4-37): _____

_____

_____

Figure 4–38

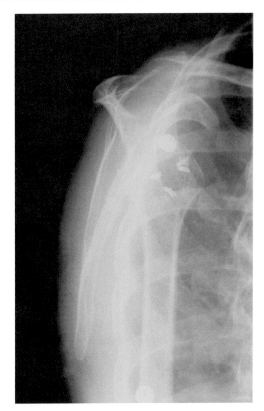

17. (Figure 4-38): _____

_____

_____

CHAPTER 4

STUDY QUESTION ANSWERS

1. A. With the anterior surface up and posterior surface down. Marker is correct.
   B. As if the patient is standing in an upright position. Marker is correct.
   C. As if the patient is standing in an upright position. Marker is reversed.

2. Soft tissue and bony trabecular patterns and cortical outlines of the shoulder structures

3. Table 4-1

Position or Projection	kVp	Grid	AEC Chamber(s)	SID
AP projection, shoulder	65-75	Grid	Center	40-48 inches (100-120 cm)
Inferosuperior (axial) projection, shoulder	65-75			40-48 inches (100-120 cm)
Posterior oblique position (Grashey), shoulder	65-75	Grid	Center	40-48 inches (100-120 cm)
Anterior oblique position, (scapular Y), shoulder	65-75	Grid		40-48 inches (100-120 cm)
AP axial projection (Stryker), shoulder	65-75	Grid		40-48 inches (100-120 cm)
Tangential projection (outlet), shoulder	65-75	Grid		40-48 inches (100-120 cm)
AP and axial projections, clavicle	65-75	Grid		40-48 inches (100-120 cm)
AP projections, AC joint	60-70	Nongrid		72 inches (183 cm)
	65-70	Grid		
AP projection, scapula	65-75	Grid	Center	40-48 inches (100-120 cm)
Lateral position, scapula	70-75	Grid		40-48 inches (100-120 cm)

AC, Acromioclavicular; AEC, automatic exposure control; AP, anteroposterior; kVp, kilovolt peak; SID, source–image receptor distance.

4. Use a compensating filter over the acromion process and lateral clavicular end.

5. When the part thickness measurement is over 5 inches (13 cm)

6. Table 4-2

Position or Projection	IR Size	Placement and Direction
AP projection, shoulder	8 × 10 inches (18 × 24 cm) or 10 × 12 inches (24 × 30 cm)	Crosswise
Inferosuperior (axial) projection, shoulder	8 × 10 inches (18 × 24 cm)	Crosswise
Posterior oblique position (Grashey), shoulder	8 × 10 inches (18 × 24 cm)	Crosswise
Anterior oblique position (scapular Y), shoulder	10 × 12 inches (24 × 30 cm)	Lengthwise
AP axial projection (Stryker), shoulder	8 × 10 inches (18 × 24 cm)	Lengthwise
Tangential projection (outlet), shoulder	8 × 10 inches (18 × 24 cm)	Lengthwise
AP and axial projections, clavicle	10 × 12 inches (24 × 30 cm)	Crosswise
AP projections, AC joint	Unilateral: Two 8 × 10 inches (18 × 24 cm) Bilateral: 14 × 17 inches (35 × 43 cm) or 7 × 17 inches (14 × 43 cm)	Crosswise
AP projection, scapula	10 × 12 inches (24 × 30 cm)	Lengthwise
Lateral position, scapula	10 × 12 inches (24 × 30 cm)	Lengthwise

AC, Acromioclavicular; AP, anteroposterior; IR, image receptor.

Shoulder: AP Projection

1. A. Superior scapular angle
   B. Clavicle
   C. Acromion process
   D. Humeral head
   E. Greater tubercle
   F. Glenoid cavity
   G. Superolateral border of the scapula
   H. Thorax
   I. Coracoid process

2. A. Describes an image that has too much density
   B. Backward movement of the shoulder
   C. Condition that results when the humeral head has been pulled away from the glenoid cavity

3. A. Position the arrow so it is pointing toward the torso.
   B. Position the arrow so it is pointing away from the torso.
4. It should be positioned next to the lateral vertebral column.
5. Position the shoulders at equal distances from the imaging table or IR holder.
6. A. 35 to 40 degrees
   B. Lateral
7. Glenoid cavity
8. Anterior
9. The midcoronal plane should be positioned parallel with the IR.
10. Midclavicle
11. Angle the central ray cephalically until it is perpendicular to the scapular body.
12. A. Laterally
    B. Superiorly
13. A. Greater tubercle
    B. Humeral head
14. A. Position the humeral epicondyles at a 45-degree angle with the IR.
    B. Position the humeral epicondyles perpendicular to the IR.
    C. Position the humeral epicondyles parallel with the IR.
    D. Position the humeral epicondyles parallel with the IR
15. Do not move the patient's arm. The image should be taken with the arm positioned as is.
16. A. Glenohumeral joint
    B. Perpendicular
    C. Inferior to the coracoid process
17. The glenohumeral joint, lateral two thirds of the clavicle, proximal one third of the humerus, and superior scapula
18. The coracoid process is located ¾ inch (2 cm) inferior to the midpoint of the lateral half of the clavicle.
19. The patient was rotated toward the affected shoulder.
20. The patient was rotated toward the unaffected shoulder.
21. The patient's upper midcoronal plane was tilted away from the IR.
22. The patient's humerus was externally rotated until the humeral epicondyles were positioned parallel with the IR.
23. The patient's humerus was rotated internally until the humeral epicondyles were aligned perpendicular to the IR.
24. The superior scapular angle is demonstrated superior to the clavicle, and the lesser tubercle is demonstrated in profile medially. Tilt the upper midcoronal plane posteriorly until it is aligned parallel with the IR, and if a neutral shoulder is

indicated, externally rotate the arm until the humeral epicondyles are at a 45-degree angle to the IR.
25. The superior scapular angle is demonstrated inferior to the clavicle. Tilt the upper midcoronal plane anteriorly until it is aligned parallel with the IR.
26. The medial clavicular end is superimposed over the vertebral column, the superior scapular angle is demonstrated superior to the clavicle, and the lesser tubercle is demonstrated in profile medially. Rotate the patient toward the left shoulder until the shoulders are at equal distances from the IR, and tilt the upper midcoronal plane posteriorly until it is aligned parallel with the IR. If a neutral shoulder is indicated, externally rotate the arm until the humeral epicondyles are at a 45-degree angle to the IR.

Shoulder: Inferosuperior (Axial) Projection

1. A. Greater tubercle
   B. Acromion process
   C. Scapular spine
   D. Glenohumeral joint
   E. Clavicle
   F. Coracoid process
   G. Humeral head
   H. Lesser tubercle
2. A. Inferior
   B. Superior
   C. Aligned
   D. Glenohumeral joint
3. A. Glenohumeral joint
   B. Scapula
4. 30- to 35-degree
5. Align the central ray at a 30- to 35-degree angle with the lateral body surface.
6. A. The angle should be decreased to approximately 20 degrees.
   B. Because the humerus has not been abducted enough to move the glenoid cavity superiorly
7. Position the IR vertically at the top of the affected shoulder so it is aligned perpendicular to the central ray.
8. When it is abducted less than 90 degrees
9. A. Lesser tubercle in profile anteriorly, and the posterolateral aspect of the humeral head in profile posteriorly
   B. Humeral head and neck in profile anteriorly, and the greater tubercle in profile posteriorly
   C. Humeral head and neck in profile posteriorly, and the lesser tubercle in partial profile anteriorly

10. A. Hill-Sachs defect
    B. Arm is externally rotated until humeral epicondyles are at a 45-degree angle with floor
11. Humeral head
12. A. Horizontal
    B. Coracoid process
13. The glenoid cavity, coracoid process, scapular spine, and one third of the proximal humerus
14. Posterior
15. A. Coracoid process
    B. Glenoid cavity
    C. Proximal humerus
16. A. The humeral epicondyles were at a 45-degree angle with the floor.
    B. The humeral epicondyles were perpendicular to the floor.
17. The angle formed between the lateral body surface and the central ray was smaller than needed to align the central ray parallel with the glenohumeral joint space.
18. The angle formed between the lateral body surface and the central ray was larger than needed to align the central ray parallel with the glenohumeral joint.
19. The humerus was externally rotated enough to position the humeral epicondyles perpendicular to the floor.
20. The patient's shoulder was not adequately elevated with a sponge or washcloth.
21. The glenoid fossa is demonstrated lateral to the base of the coracoid process. Increase the angle formed by the lateral body and the central ray.
22. The inferior margin of the glenoid fossa is demonstrated medial to the coracoid process base. Decrease the angle formed by the lateral body and the central ray.
23. The coracoid is not included in the image. Laterally flex the neck toward the right shoulder, and position the IR more medially.

Shoulder: Posterior Oblique Position (Grashey Method)

1. A. Clavicle
   B. Scapular neck
   C. Coracoid process
   D. Humeral head
   E. Glenohumeral joint
2. Forward movement of the shoulder
3. A. Glenoid cavity
   B. Glenohumeral
4. A. Sternoclavicular
   B. Acromioclavicular
5. A. Coracoid process
   B. Acromion angle
6. A. The patient is kyphotic.
   B. The patient is imaged in a recumbent position.

C. The patient leans against the IR while in an upright position.
7. A. The lateral coracoid process will be superimposed over the humeral head by approximately ¼ inch (0.6 cm).
   B. On overrotation, the coracoid process is superimposed over more of the humeral head.
   C. On underrotation, it is superimposed less or is demonstrated superimposing the humeral head.
8. Vertically
9. A. Glenohumeral joint
   B. Perpendicular
   C. Inferior
   D. Medial
   E. Coracoid process
10. The glenoid cavity, humeral head, coracoid process, acromion process, and lateral clavicle
11. The patient was rotated more than needed to obtain an open glenohumeral joint space.
12. The patient was rotated less than needed to obtain an open glenohumeral joint space.
13. The patient was rotated more than needed to obtain an open glenohumeral joint space.
14. The glenohumeral joint space is closed, more than ¼ inch (0.6 cm) of the lateral tip of the coracoid process is superimposed over the humeral head, and the clavicle demonstrates excessive transverse foreshortening. Decrease the degree of patient obliquity.
15. The glenohumeral joint space is closed, the lateral tip of the coracoid process is not superimposed over the humeral head, and the clavicle demonstrates little foreshortening. Increase the degree of patient obliquity.

Shoulder: Anterior Oblique Position (Scapular Y)

1. A. Humeral head
   B. Coracoid
   C. Clavicle
   D. Superior scapular angle
   E. Acromion process
   F. Glenoid cavity
   G. Scapular body
2. A. Least scapular and proximal humerus magnification
   B. Greater scapular and proximal humerus detail sharpness
3. A. Acromion and coracoid processes
   B. Scapular body
   C. Glenoid cavity
4. A. Vertebral (medial)
   B. Lateral
   C. Thoracic cavity

5. Vertebral (medial) border
6. A. Vertebral (medial)
   B. Acromion process angle
   C. Coracoid process
7. A. Shoulder dislocation
   B. Proximal humeral fracture
8. A. Affected
   B. Unaffected
9. The cortical outline of the lateral border is thicker than the cortical outline of the vertebral border.
10. Identify the scapular border that is positioned closest to the thoracic cavity.
11. The humeral head should be superimposed over the glenoid cavity, and the humeral shaft should be superimposed over the scapular body.
12. Yes
13. A. Anteriorly and beneath the coracoid process
    B. Posteriorly and beneath the acromion process
    C. Anterior
14. Position the midcoronal plane vertically so it is parallel with the IR.
15. A. Kyphosis
    B. Angle the central ray caudally until it is perpendicular to the scapular body.
    C. Angle the central ray cephalically until it is perpendicular to the scapular body.
16. A. Midscapular body
    B. Perpendicular
    C. Vertebral (medial)
    D. Inferior scapular angle
    E. Acromion angle
17. The entire scapula and the proximal humerus
18. The patient was rotated more than needed to superimpose the scapular body.
19. The patient was rotated less than needed to superimpose the scapular body.
20. The patient's upper midcoronal plane was leaning toward the IR.
21. The lateral and vertebral borders of the scapula are demonstrated without superimposition. The vertebral scapular border is demonstrated next to the ribs, and the lateral border is demonstrated laterally. Increase the degree of patient obliquity.
22. The lateral and vertebral borders of the scapula are demonstrated without superimposition. The lateral border is demonstrated next to the ribs, and the vertebral border is demonstrated laterally. Decrease the degree of patient rotation.
23. The superior scapular angle is demonstrated superior to the clavicle. Tilt the patient's upper midcoronal plane posteriorly until it is parallel with the IR.
24. The lateral and vertebral borders of the scapula are demonstrated without superimposition. The vertebral scapular border is demonstrated next to the ribs, and the lateral border appears laterally. Increase the degree of patient obliquity.

Shoulder: AP Axial Projection (Stryker "Notch" Method)

1. A. Greater tubercle
   B. Posterolateral humeral head
   C. Conoid tubercle
   D. Coracoid process
   E. Clavicle
   F. Lesser tubercle
2. Lateral
3. A. Hill-Sachs
   B. Posterolateral
4. A. Vertical
   B. On top of the patient's head
5. A. Cephalic
   B. Humeral head
   C. Greater
   D. Lesser
6. A. Coracoid process
   B. Humeral head, coracoid process, lateral clavicle, and glenoid cavity
7. The central ray was angled less than the required 10-degree cephalic angle.
8. The distal humerus is tilted laterally.
9. The humerus was elevated to less than a vertical position
10. The coracoid process is seen inferior to the clavicle, and the humeral shaft demonstrates increased foreshortening. Place a 10-degree cephalic angulation on the central ray.
11. The posterolateral humeral head is obscured, and the humeral shaft demonstrates increased foreshortening and a decrease in density. Elevate the humerus until it is placed at a 90-degree position with the patient's torso.
12. The posterolateral humeral head and lesser tubercle are obscured. The greater tubercle is in profile laterally. Tilt the distal humerus laterally until it is parallel with midsagittal plane.

Shoulder: Tangential Projection (Supraspinatus "Outlet")

1. A. Scapular body
   B. Glenoid cavity
   C. Humeral head
   D. Acromion process
   E. Clavicle
   F. Superior scapular angle
   G. Coracoid process
   H. Thorax
2. Anterior
3. A. Acromion process and coracoid processes
   B. Scapular body
   C. Glenoid cavity
4. A. Vertebral
   B. Lateral

C. Thorax
5. A. Vertebral
   B. 45 degrees
6. The lateral border is thick, with two cortical outlines that are separated by approximately ¼ inch (0.6 cm), whereas the cortical outline of the vertebral border demonstrates a single thin line.
7. Inferior
8. A. ½
   B. Superior
   C. Inferior
   D. Midcoronal
   E. 10 to 15 degrees caudally
9. A. Acromioclavicular joint
   B. Superior aspect of the humeral head
   C. Acromion and coracoid processes, lateral clavicle, superior scapular spine, and half of the scapular body
10. The patient was rotated more than needed to superimpose the scapular body.
11. The upper midcoronal plane was tilted toward the IR, and/or the central ray was not angled 10 to 15 degrees caudally.
12. The lateral and vertebral borders of the scapula are demonstrated without superimposition, and the glenoid cavity is not demonstrated on end but is seen medially. The lateral scapular border is demonstrated next to the ribs, and the vertebral border is demonstrated laterally. Decrease patient obliquity until the scapular borders are superimposed.
13. The lateral clavicle and acromion process are demonstrated less than ½ inch (1.25 cm) superior to the humeral head and supraspinous fossa, and the superior scapular spine appears superior to the clavicle. Tilt the midcoronal plane posteriorly until it is vertical, and place a 10- to 15-degree caudal angle on the central ray.

Clavicle: AP Projection

1. A. Acromion process
   B. Lateral clavicle
   C. Coracoid process
   D. Superior scapular angle
   E. Vertebral border of scapula
   F. Medial clavicle
   G. Vertebral column
2. Over or under the lateral clavicular end
3. A. PA
   B. It results in increased patient discomfort and difficulty in clavicle palpation.
4. It should be adjacent to the lateral edge of the vertebral column.
5. Both shoulders should be placed at equal distances from the table or IR holder.

6. When the midcoronal plane is not positioned parallel with the IR
7. A. Midclavicle
   B. Perpendicular
   C. Medial
   D. Lateral
8. The lateral, middle, and medial thirds of the clavicle and the acromion process
9. The patient was rotated away from the affected shoulder.
10. The patient was rotated toward the affected shoulder.
11. The patient's upper midcoronal plane was leaning away from the IR.
12. The superior scapular angle is demonstrated superior to the clavicle. Tilt the upper midcoronal plane posteriorly until it is aligned parallel with the IR.
13. The medial clavicular end is superimposed over the vertebral column, and the vertebral border of the scapula is positioned away from the thoracic cavity. Rotate the patient toward the affected shoulder.

Clavicle: AP Axial Projection

1. A. Acromion process
   B. Lateral clavicle
   C. Middle clavicle
   D. Superior scapular angle
   E. Medial clavicle
2. Because the anteroposterior measurement of the shoulder thickness varies between the clavicular ends
3. The medial end of the clavicle will be adjacent to the lateral border of the vertebral column.
4. A 15- to 30-degree cephalic angle
5. Middle third of the clavicle
6. A. Middle
   B. Lateral
   C. Thorax and scapula
7. A. Midclavicle
   B. Medial
   C. Lateral
8. The lateral, middle, and medial thirds of the clavicle and the acromion process
9. The patient was rotated toward the affected shoulder.
10. The central ray was not angled enough cephalically.
11. The lateral and medial thirds of the clavicle are superimposed over the scapula, and the medial clavicular end is superimposed over the vertebral column. Increase the degree of cephalic central ray angulation, and rotate the patient toward the right shoulder until the shoulders are at equal distances from the IR.

AC Joint: AP Projection

1. A. Superior scapular angle
   B. Scapular spine
   C. Lateral clavicle
   D. AC joint
   E. Acromial apex
2. A. Act of holding weights or standing to place pressure on the structure
   B. Regarding only one side
   C. Regarding both sides
3. A. To identify the weight-bearing from the non–weight-bearing image
   B. Laterally within the collimated field and pointing downward if it is an arrow
4. A. ⅛
   B. Acromial process apex
5. Both shoulders should be positioned at equal distances from the upright IR holder.
6. To evaluate the AC joint for possible ligament injury
7. Separation between the acromion process and clavicle will be increased when one compares the weight-bearing with the non–weight-bearing images.
8. 5 to 8 lb
9. A. When the upper midcoronal plane is tilted away from the IR and is positioned parallel with the IR
   B. The middle and lateral clavicle are superimposed over the acromion process and scapular spine.
10. A. AC joint
    B. Inferior
    C. Lateral tip of the clavicle
11. The AC joint, lateral clavicle, and acromion process
12. To ensure that the same centering is obtained and the x-ray beam's divergence does not result in a false reading
13. The patient is rotated toward the affected AC joint.
14. The superior scapular angle is demonstrated superior to the clavicle. Tilt the upper midcoronal plane posteriorly until it is parallel with the IR.

Scapula: AP Projection

1. A. Acromion process
   B. Lesser tubercle
   C. Glenoid cavity
   D. Glenoid neck
   E. Lateral border
   F. Inferior angle
   G. Vertebral border
   H. Scapular body
   I. Supraspinous fossa
   J. Scapular spine
   K. Coracoid process
   L. Superior angle
   M. Clavicle
2. A. The amount of darkness demonstrated on an image
   B. The number of atoms in a given area
3. Because the thorax, which is filled with air, has less density than the shoulder soft tissue
4. Expiration
5. A. Longitudinal
   B. Transverse
6. A. 35 to 45 degrees
   B. Transverse
7. A. The arm is abducted to a 90-degree angle with the body, the elbow is flexed, and the hand is supinated by externally rotating the arm.
   B. It forces it to retract.
   C. When the arm is positioned to cause retraction the glenoid cavity is positioned closer to profile.
8. Longitudinal
9. A. Midscapular body
   B. Perpendicular
   C. 2
   D. Inferior
10. The entire scapula, which includes the inferior and superior angles, coracoid and acromion processes, body, and glenoid cavity
11. Place the patient supine to maximize shoulder retraction. If the glenoid cavity area is of interest, roll the patient onto the affected shoulder.
12. Make sure that the arm is abducted to 90 degrees, and externally rotate by flexing the elbow and supinating the hand.
13. A portion of the inferolateral border of the scapula is superimposed by the thoracic cavity, and the superior angle is superimposed by the clavicle. Abduct the humerus to a full 90-degree angle with the body.
14. The inferolateral border of the scapula is superimposed by the thoracic cavity, and the superior angle is superimposed by the clavicle. Abduct the humerus to a 90-degree angle with the body.

Scapula: Lateral Position (Lateromedial or Mediolateral Projection)

1. A. Clavicle
   B. Coracoid process
   C. Thorax
   D. Inferior angle
   E. Scapular body
   F. Acromion process
   G. Glenoid cavity
2. A. Lateral
   B. Vertebral (medial)
   C. Thoracic cavity

3. A. Away from
   B. Toward
4. The elevation of the humerus
5. Lateral
6. The borders of the scapula will not be superimposed.
7. A. Body
   B. Neck
8. Placing the humerus at a 90-degree angle with the body
9. Elevating the humerus higher than a 90-degree angle with the body
10. A. The humerus is not elevated.
    B. Vertebral border
11. A. Less
    B. Because the scapula is drawn laterally around the thorax as the humerus is abducted
12. A. Midscapular body
    B. Perpendicular
    C. Anterior
    D. Inferior scapular
    E. Acromion process

13. The entire scapula, which includes the inferior and superior angles, coracoid and acromion processes, and scapular body
14. The patient was rotated more than needed to superimpose the scapular borders.
15. The patient was rotated less than needed to superimpose the scapular borders.
16. The lateral and vertebral borders of the scapula are demonstrated without superimposition. The vertebral border is visible next to the ribs. Increase the degree of patient rotation.
17. The lateral and vertebral borders of the scapula are demonstrated without superimposition. The lateral border is next to the ribs, and the vertebral border is demonstrated laterally. The patient's arm was not elevated, positioning the vertebral border of the scapula parallel with the IR. Decrease the degree of patient obliquity and elevate the arm to 90 degrees wih the torso.

Image Analysis of the Lower Extremity

LEARNING OBJECTIVES

After completion of this chapter you should be able to:

_____ 1. Identify the required anatomy on toe, foot, calcaneal, ankle, lower leg, knee, and femoral images.

_____ 2. Describe how to properly position the patient, image receptor (IR), and central ray for toe, foot, calcaneal, ankle, lower leg, knee, and femoral images.

_____ 3. State how to properly mark and hang each toe, foot, calcaneal, ankle, lower leg, knee, and femoral image presented.

_____ 4. List the typical artifacts that are found on toe, foot, calcaneal, ankle, lower leg, knee, and femoral images.

_____ 5. List the image requirements for accurate positioning for toe, foot, calcaneal, ankle, lower leg, knee, and femoral images.

_____ 6. State how to properly reposition the patient when toe, foot, calcaneal, ankle, lower leg, knee, or femoral images with poor positioning are produced.

_____ 7. Discuss how to determine the amount of patient or central ray adjustment that is required to improve toe, foot, calcaneal, ankle, lower leg, knee, or femoral images with poor positioning.

_____ 8. State the kilovoltage routinely used for toe, foot, calcaneal, ankle, lower leg, knee, and femoral images, and describe what anatomical structures are visible when the correct technique factors are used.

_____ 9. Describe which aspects of a toe's phalanges are concave and which are convex.

_____ 10. State how the central ray angulation is adjusted for an anteroposterior (AP) toe image when the patient is unable to fully extend the toe.

_____ 11. Discuss how one can locate the metatarsophalangeal (MP), tibiotalar, and femorotibial joints by using palpable anatomical structures.

_____ 12. State why a compensating filter is used when taking an AP foot image, and explain how the filter is positioned on the foot.

_____ 13. Discuss how the degree of central ray angulation is adjusted for an AP foot image and the degree of obliquity is adjusted for an AP oblique foot image in patients with high and low longitudinal arches.

_____ 14. State how one can determine from two different patients' AP oblique foot images which patient's foot has the higher longitudinal arch.

_____ 15. List the soft-tissue structures of interest found on lateral foot and ankle images. State where they are located and why their visualization is important.

_____ 16. State how the height of a patient's longitudinal arch can be evaluated on a lateral foot image.

_____ 17. State what anatomical structures are referred to as the *talar domes* on a lateral foot, calcaneal, or ankle image.

_____ 18. Compare the position of the patient, IR, and central ray for lateromedial and mediolateral projections of the foot.

_____ 19. Describe how the central ray angulation is adjusted when a patient is unable to dorsiflex the foot for an axial calcaneal image.

_____ 20. Describe how routine patient, central ray, and IR relationships and the amount of collimation should be adjusted if an AP, oblique, or lateral ankle image is ordered requesting that more than one fourth of the distal lower leg be included.

_____ 21. State how the medial and lateral talar domes can be identified on a lateral foot, calcaneal, or ankle image with poor positioning.

_____ 22. Describe what effect the anode-heel effect has on lower leg and femoral images.

_____ 23. State how the patient is positioned with respect to the x-ray tube for lower leg and femoral images to take advantage of the anode-heel effect.

_____ 24. Explain why the IR must extend beyond the knee and ankle joints when the lower leg is imaged.

_____ 25. Explain how the patient is positioned if only one of the joints can be in the true position for AP or lateral lower leg images.

_____ 26. Explain how the lower leg might need to be positioned on the IR and the source–image receptor distance (SID) adjusted to include the knee and ankle joints on lower leg images.

_____ 27. Describe the slope of the proximal and distal tibia.

_____ 28. State how the alignment of the central ray with the slope of the proximal and distal tibia will affect the openness of the femorotibial and tibiotalar joints.

_____ 29. Discuss when it is necessary to use a grid for knee images.

_____ 30. Explain how the central ray angulation that is used for AP and oblique knee images is determined by the thickness of the patient's upper thigh and buttocks, and discuss why this adjustment is required.

_____ 31. Describe a valgus and a varus knee deformity.

_____ 32. State how to determine what central ray angulation to use for an AP knee image in a patient who cannot fully extend the knee.

_____ 33. Describe a patella subluxation, and state how it is demonstrated on an AP knee image.

_____ 34. State which anatomical structures are placed in profile on medial and lateral oblique knee images with accurate positioning.

_____ 35. List the soft-tissue structures of interest found on lateral knee images. State where they are located and why their visualization is important.

_____ 36. State how the patient's knee is positioned for a lateral knee image if a patella fracture is suspected.

_____ 37. State the relationship of the medial and lateral femoral condyles, and describe the degree of femoral inclination that is demonstrated in a patient in an erect and a lateral recumbent position.

_____ 38. State the femoral length and pelvic width that demonstrates the least amount of femoral inclination.

_____ 39. Describe two methods that can be used to distinguish the medial and lateral femoral condyles from each other on a lateral knee image with poor positioning.

_____ 40. State two ways that the patient and central ray angle can be aligned to accomplish superimposed femoral condyles for a lateral knee image.

_____ 41. Describe how patellar subluxation is demonstrated on a tangential (axial) projection knee image.

_____ 42. State the importance of securing the legs and instructing the patient to relax the quadriceps femoris muscles for a tangential (axial) projection knee image.

_____ 43. Explain how the positioning setup for a tangential (axial) projection image is adjusted for a patient with large posterior calves.

_____ 44. State why a 72-inch (183 cm) SID is required for a tangential (axial) projection knee image.

_____ 45. Discuss the importance of including the femoral soft tissue on all femoral images.

_____ 46. Explain how a distal and proximal AP and lateral femoral image is obtained in a patient with a suspected fracture.

_____ 47. State why the patient's leg is never rotated when a femoral fracture is suspected.

STUDY QUESTIONS

1. Describe how the following shoulder images should be hung on a view box or displayed on a cathode ray tube (CRT) monitor.

A. AP toe: _____

B. Lateral ankle: _____

C. AP oblique ankle: _____

D. Lateral knee: _____

2. Complete Table 5-1.

TABLE 5-1 **Hip and Pelvic Technical Data**			
Part, Position, and Projection	**kVp**	**Grid**	**SID**
Toe			
Foot			
Plantodorsal (axial) projection, calcaneus			
Lateral position, calcaneus			
Ankle			
Lower leg			
AP projection, knee Lateral position, knee AP oblique position, knee			
PA axial (Holmblad) position, knee			
AP axial (Béclere) projection, knee			
Tangential (axial) projection, knee			
Femur			

AP, Anteroposterior; *kVp,* kilovolt peak; *PA,* posteroanterior; *SID,* source–image receptor distance.

3. Complete Table 5-2.

TABLE 5-2 **IR Size, Placement, and Direction**		
Part, Position, and Projection	**IR Size**	**Placement, Direction, and Number of Images on IR**
AP, oblique, and lateral, toe		
AP and AP oblique, foot		
Lateral, foot		
Plantodorsal (axial) and lateral, calcaneus		
AP and AP oblique, ankle	Screen-film	
	Computed radiography	
Lateral, ankle		
AP, lower leg		
Lateral, lower leg		
AP, oblique, and lateral, knee		
PA axial (Holmblad) position, knee		
AP axial (Béclere) projection, knee		
Tangential (axial) projection, knee		
AP and lateral, femur (proximal and distal)		

AP, Anteroposterior; *IR,* image receptor; *PA,* posteroanterior.

Toe: AP Projection

4. Identify the labeled anatomy in Figure 5-1.

Figure 5–1

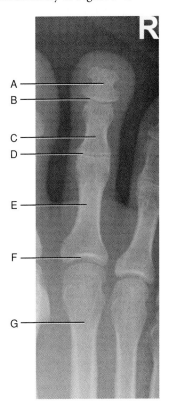

A. _____

B. _____

C. _____

D. _____

E. _____

F. _____

G. _____

5. An AP image of the toe with accurate positioning demonstrates equal
   (A) _____ width and equal (B) _____
   concavity on each side of the phalanges.

6. For an AP toe image, equal pressure is placed on the
   (A) _____ foot surface and the (B) _____,
   (C) _____, and (D) _____ should remain
   aligned.

7. If the toe is medially rotated for a right AP toe image, which side of
   the toe demonstrates the greatest soft-tissue width?

   A. _____ (lateral/medial)

   The greatest phalangeal midshaft concavity?

   B. _____ (lateral/medial)

8. When the toenail is visualized on an AP toe image, it can be used to identify the direction of patient rotation. If the first toenail is rotated medially, in what direction was the patient's foot rotated?

_____

9. To obtain open interphalangeal (IP) and MP joint spaces on an AP toe image, align the central (A) _____ to the joint space and align the joint space (B) _____ to the IR.

10. If the toe is (A) _____ for an AP toe image, the joint spaces will be closed and the phalanges will be (B) _____.

11. State two methods of imaging an AP toe to achieve an image that demonstrates open IP and MP joints and unforeshortened phalanges in a patient who is unable to extend the toe.

   A. _____

   B. _____

12. The long axis of the affected toe is aligned with the long axis of the _____ for toe images to obtain tight collimation.

13. How is the patient positioned for an AP toe image to prevent soft-tissue overlap of adjacent toes onto the affected toe?

   _____

14. On an AP toe image with accurate positioning , the _____ is centered within the collimated field.

15. What anatomical structures are included on an AP toe image with accurate positioning? _____

For the following descriptions of AP toe images with poor positioning, state how the patient would have been mispositioned for such an image to be obtained.

16. The phalanges demonstrate more soft-tissue width on the medial toe surface, and the outline of the toenail is visualized toward the lateral toe surface.

   _____

17. The phalanges demonstrate more midshaft concavity on the lateral surface of the toe than the medial surface.

   _____

18. The IP and MP joint spaces are closed, and the phalanges are foreshortened.

For the following AP toe images with poor positioning, state what anatomical structures are misaligned and how the patient should be repositioned for an optimal image to be obtained.

Figure 5–2

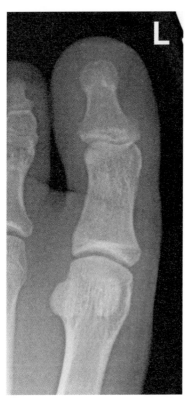

19. (Figure 5-2): _____

_____

_____

_____

Toe: AP Oblique Projection

1. Identify the labeled anatomy in Figure 5-3.

Figure 5–3

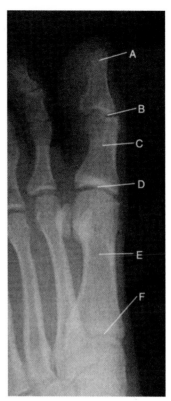

A. _____

B. _____

C. _____

D. _____

E. _____

F. _____

2. What degree of patient toe obliquity is used for an AP oblique toe image?

A. _____

How is the accuracy of the degree of toe obliquity identified on an AP oblique toe image?

B. _____

3. In what direction are the foot and toe rotated for a first through third AP oblique toe image?

A. _____

For a fourth through fifth AP oblique toe image?

B. _____

Why are the patient's foot and toe rotated differently for these examinations?

C. _____

4. The patient was unable to fully extend the toe for an AP oblique toe image. What will the resulting image demonstrate if a perpendicular central ray was used for this patient?

_____

5. The _____ is at the center of the collimated field on an AP oblique toe image with accurate positioning.

6. What anatomical structures are included on an AP oblique toe image with accurate positioning?

_____

7. To ensure that half of the affected toe's metatarsal is included on an AP oblique toe image, the longitudinally collimated field should extend 2 inches (5 cm) proximal to the _____.

For the following descriptions of AP oblique toe images with poor positioning, state how the patient would have been mispositioned for such an image to be obtained.

8. The soft-tissue width demonstrated on each side of the phalanges is nearly equal.

_____

9. The proximal phalanx demonstrates more concavity on the posterior aspect than on the anterior aspect.

_____

10. The IP and MP joint spaces are obscured and the phalanges foreshortened.

_____

For the following AP oblique toe images with poor positioning, state what anatomical structures are misaligned and how the patient should be repositioned for such an image to be obtained.

Figure 5–4

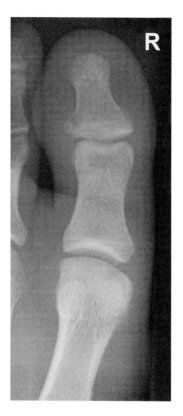

11. (Figure 5-4): _____

_____

_____

_____

Figure 5–5

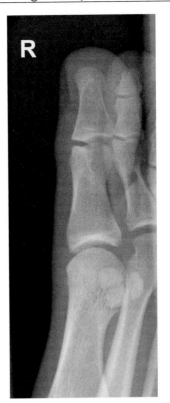

12. (Figure 5-5): _____

_____

_____

_____

Figure 5–6

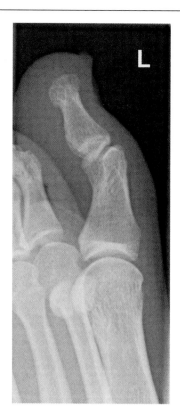

13. (Figure 5-6): _____

_____

_____

_____

Toe: Lateral Position

1. Identify the labeled anatomy in Figure 5-7.

Figure 5–7

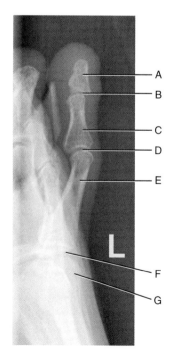

A. _____

B. _____

C. _____

D. _____

E. _____

F. _____

G. _____

2. To image the toe in a lateral position, the foot is rotated
   (A) _____ (medially/laterally) when the first, second, and
   third toes are imaged and (B) _____ (medially/laterally)
   when the fourth and fifth toes are imaged.

3. In a lateral position, the (A) _____ (anterior/posterior)
   surface of the proximal phalanx demonstrates more concavity than
   the (B) _____ (anterior/posterior) surface, and the distal
   phalanx demonstrates more concavity on the (C) _____
   (anterior/posterior) surface.

4. Where is the toenail demonstrated on a lateral toe image with accurate
   positioning? _____

5. The (A) _____ joint is centered within the collimated
   field on a lateral toe image with accurate positioning. This is
   accomplished by centering a (B) _____ central ray to the
   (C) _____.

6. What anatomical structures are included on a lateral toe image with
   accurate positioning?

   _____

**For the following descriptions of lateral toe images with poor position-
ing, state how the patient would have been mispositioned for such an
image to be obtained.**

7. The proximal phalanx demonstrates nearly equal midshaft concavity,
   the condyles appear without superimposition, and the metatarsal
   heads appear without superimposition.

   _____

8. The proximal phalanx demonstrates nearly equal midshaft concavity,
   the condyles are shown without superimposition, and the metatarsal
   heads are slightly superimposed.

   _____

9. Soft-tissue and bony overlap of unaffected digits onto the affected
   digit is present.

   _____

For the following lateral toe images with poor positioning, state what anatomical structures are misaligned and how the patient should be repositioned for an optimal image to be obtained.

Figure 5-8

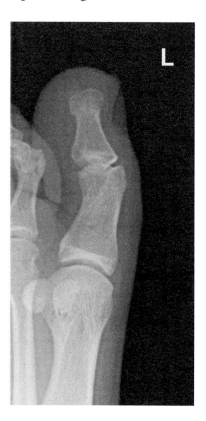

10. (Figure 5-8): _____

_____

_____

_____

Figure 5-9

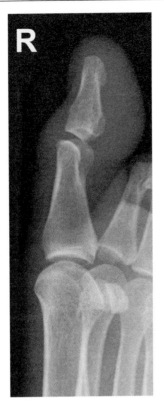

11. (Figure 5-9): _____

_____

_____

Foot: AP Projection (Dorsoplantar Projection)

1. Identify the labeled anatomy in Figure 5-10.

Figure 5–10

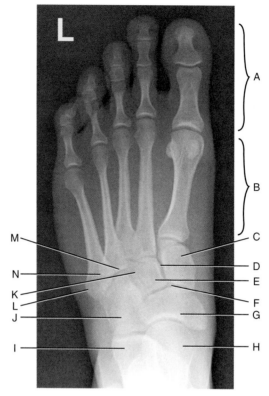

A. _____

B. _____

C. _____

D. _____

E. _____

F. _____

G. _____

H. _____

I. _____

J. _____

K. _____

L. _____

M. _____

N. _____

2. When an exposure is set that adequately demonstrates the proximal metatarsals and tarsals, the distal metatarsals and phalanges are overexposed. Why does this density variation exist?

A. _____

How can the positioning setup be adjusted to obtain uniform image density over the entire foot?

B. _____

3. The MP joints of the foot are located (A) _____ inch
   (B) _____ to the toe interconnecting tissue.

4. An AP foot image with accurate positioning demonstrates an open
   joint space between the (A) _____ and (B)
   _____ cuneiforms and approximately ¾ inch (2 cm) of the
   calcaneus without (C) _____ superimposition.

5. For an AP foot image, equal pressure is placed on the
   (A) _____ foot surface and the (B) _____,
   (C) _____, and (D) _____ should remain
   aligned.

6. Should the navicular bone be demonstrated on an AP foot image with
   accurate positioning? _____ (Yes/No)

7. Will medial or lateral foot rotation result in the talus moving away
   from the calcaneus? _____

8. Will medial or lateral foot rotation result in increased superimposition
   of the metatarsal bases? _____

9. A 10- to 15-degree proximal angulation is required
   for an AP foot image to demonstrate open
   (A) _____ and
   (B) _____ joint spaces. Is a higher
   degree of central ray angulation needed in a patient with a low
   longitudinal arch or a high longitudinal arch?
   (C) _____

10. On an AP foot image with accurate positioning, the proximal
    (A) _____ are centered within
    the collimated field when the central ray is centered to the
    midline of the foot at a level (B) _____ inch distal to the
    (C) _____.

11. What anatomical structures are included on an AP foot image with
    accurate positioning?

**For the following descriptions of AP foot images with poor positioning,
state how the patient or central ray would have been mispositioned for
such an image to be obtained.**

12. The joint space between the medial and intermediate cuneiforms is
    closed, the navicular bone is demonstrated in profile, and less than ¾
    inch (2 cm) of the calcaneus is demonstrated without talar
    superimposition.

---

13. The joint space between the medial and intermediate cuneiforms is
    closed, the calcaneus is demonstrated without talar superimposition,
    and the metatarsal bases demonstrate decreased superimposition.

---

14. The tarsometatarsal and navicular-cuneiform joint spaces are
    obscured.

For the following AP foot images with poor positioning, state what anatomical structures are misaligned and how the patient should be repositioned for an optimal image to be obtained.

Figure 5–11

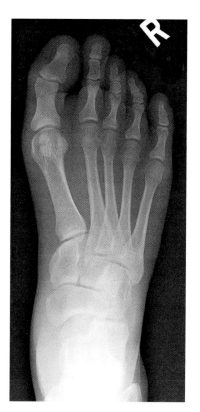

15. (Figure 5-11): _____

_____

_____

_____

Figure 5–12

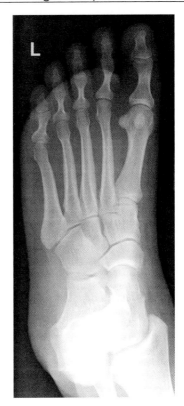

16. (Figure 5-12): _____

_____

_____

_____

Foot: AP Oblique Projection (Medial Rotation)

1. Identify the labeled anatomy in Figure 5-13.

Figure 5–13

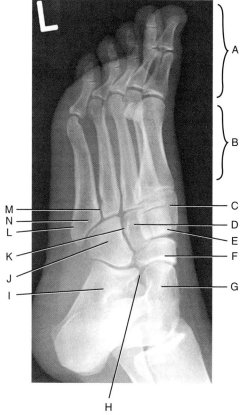

A. _____

B. _____

C. _____

D. _____

E. _____

F. _____

G. _____

H. _____

I. _____

J. _____

K. _____

L. _____

M. _____

N. _____

2. What joint spaces are open on an AP oblique foot image with accurate positioning?

A. _____

B. _____

3. Which of the joint spaces that surround the cuboid is the first to close if the patient's foot is not adequately rotated? _____

4. An AP oblique foot image is obtained by rotating the patient 30 to 60 degrees _____ (medially/laterally).

5. The degree of foot obliquity needed for an AP oblique foot image varies according to the height of the patient's longitudinal arch. What degree of obliquity is used in a patient with a high longitudinal arch?

   A. _____

   In a patient with a low longitudinal arch?

   B. _____

   On a patient with an average longitudinal arch?

   C. _____

6. View the AP oblique foot image in Figure 5-13. State whether the patient has a high or low longitudinal arch.

   A. _____

   How did you determine this?

   B. _____

   _____

7. View the lateral foot images in Figures 5-15 and 5-17. State which image was obtained from the patient with the higher longitudinal arch.

   A. _____

   How did you determine this difference?

   B. _____

   _____

8. As a patient's foot is rotated medially from an AP projection, the (A) _____ metatarsal base rotates beneath the (B) _____ metatarsal base and the second through third metatarsal heads move (C) _____ (closer to/farther away from) one another.

9. Is the fourth metatarsal tubercle or the fifth metatarsal located more posteriorly when the patient's foot is overrotated for an AP oblique foot image?

   A. _____

   When the foot is medially rotated more than needed for an AP oblique foot image with accurate positioning, will the fourth metatarsal tubercle be superimposed over the fifth metatarsal or will the fifth metatarsal be superimposed over the fourth metatarsal?

   B. _____

   _____

10. On an AP oblique foot image with accurate positioning, the (A) _____ is centered within the collimated field. This is accomplished by centering a (B) _____ central ray to the (C) _____ of the foot at the level of the (D) _____.

11. What anatomical structures are demonstrated within the collimated field on an AP oblique foot image with accurate positioning? _____

For the following descriptions of AP oblique foot images with poor positioning, state how the patient would have been mispositioned for such an image to be obtained.

12. The lateral cuneiform-cuboid, navicular-cuboid, and third through fifth intermetatarsal spaces are closed, and the fourth metatarsal tubercle is demonstrated without fifth metatarsal superimposition.

13. The lateral cuneiform-cuboid, navicular-cuboid, and intermetatarsal joint spaces are closed, and the fifth metatarsal is superimposed over the fourth metatarsal tubercle.

For the following AP oblique foot image with poor positioning, state what anatomical structures are misaligned and how the patient should be repositioned for an optimal image to be obtained.

Figure 5–14

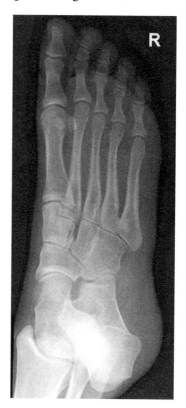

14. (Figure 5-14): _____

_____

_____

_____

Foot: Lateral Position (Mediolateral and Lateromedial Projections)

1. Identify the labeled anatomy in Figure 5-15.

Figure 5–15

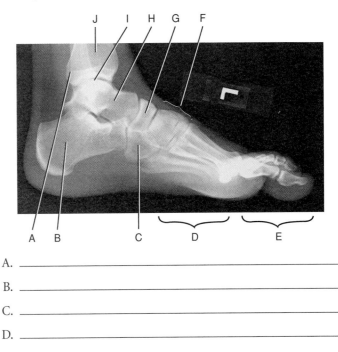

A. _____

B. _____

C. _____

D. _____

E. _____

F. _____

G. _____

H. _____

I. _____

J. _____

2. Define the following terms.

   A. Joint effusion: _____

   B. Dorsiflex foot: _____

   C. Plantar foot surface: _____

   D. Plantar foot flexion: _____

3. Which surface of the foot is positioned against the IR for a mediolateral projection of the foot? _____

4. List the two soft-tissue fat pads that should be demonstrated on a lateral foot image, and describe their locations.

   A. _____

   B. _____

5. A lateral foot image demonstrates (A) _____ talar domes, an open (B) _____ joint, and the (C) _____ superimposed by the posterior half of the tibia.

6. How is the patient's lower leg placed to obtain a lateral foot image with accurate positioning?

_____

7. How is the patient's foot positioned with the lower leg and IR to obtain a lateral foot image with accurate positioning?

A. Lower leg: _____

B. IR: _____

8. A lateral foot image was requested for a patient with a large upper thigh that prevented the lower leg from aligning parallel with the imaging table when the patient was positioned. If the image was obtained with the patient positioned in this manner, how would this poor positioning be identified on the resulting image?

A. _____

How is the positioning setup adjusted in this situation before the image is obtained?

B. _____

9. The height of the longitudinal arch can be determined on a lateral foot image with accurate positioning by measuring the amount of cuboid that appears (A) _____ to the (B) _____.

10. The average foot image demonstrates approximately _____ inch of the cuboid distal to the navicular bone.

11. In a patient with a low foot arch, (A) _____ (more/less) of the cuboid will be demonstrated distal to the navicular bone, and in a patient with a high foot arch, (B) _____ (more/less) will be demonstrated.

12. The actual height of the foot arch on a lateral foot image is accurate only when the _____ are superimposed.

13. What anatomical structures form the talar domes?

_____

14. Misalignment of the talar domes can be caused by poor (A) _____ and/or (B) _____ positioning.

15. If the distal tibia is positioned farther from the imaging table than the proximal tibia for a lateral foot image, the (A) _____ (lateral/medial) dome is demonstrated (B) _____ to the (C) _____ (lateral/medial) talar dome and the longitudinal foot arch appears (D) _____ (higher/lower) on the resulting image.

16. If the proximal tibia is positioned farther from the imaging table than the distal tibia for a lateral foot image, the (A) _____ dome is demonstrated (B) _____ to the (C) _____ talar dome and the longitudinal foot arch appears (D) _____ (higher/lower) on the resulting image.

17. If a lateral foot image with poor positioning demonstrates an obscured tibiotalar joint space, one talar dome proximal to the other, and the navicular bone superimposed over most of the cuboid, which dome is proximal? _____

18. If the calcaneus is positioned too close to the IR and the forefoot is raised off the IR for a lateral foot image, the (A) _____ talar dome is demonstrated (B) _____ to the (C) _____ talar dome and the fibula is demonstrated too far (D) _____ on the tibia.

19. If the forefoot is positioned too close to the IR and the calcaneus is elevated off the IR for a lateral foot image, the (A) _____ talar dome is demonstrated (B) _____ to the (C) _____ talar dome and the fibula is demonstrated too far (D) _____ on the tibia.

20. Why is it important to dorsiflex the foot to a 90-degree angle with the lower leg?

    A. _____

    B. _____

    C. _____

21. Against what aspect of the foot is the IR placed for a standing lateromedial projection of the foot?

    A. _____

    What surface (medial/lateral) of the foot is aligned parallel with the IR for a lateromedial projection of the foot with accurate positioning?

    B. _____

22. If a standing lateromedial projection of the foot with poor positioning demonstrates one talar dome posterior to the other talar dome and the fibula is situated too far posterior on the tibia, how should the patient's position be adjusted for an optimal image to be obtained?

    _____

23. On a lateral foot image with accurate positioning, the (A) _____ are centered to the collimated field. This is accomplished by centering a (B) _____ central ray halfway between the distal toes and the (C) _____.

24. What anatomical structures are included on a lateral foot image with accurate positioning? _____

    _____

For the following descriptions of mediolateral foot images with poor positioning, state how the patient would have been mispositioned for such an image to be obtained.

25. The tibiotalar joint space is obscured, one talar dome is demonstrated proximal to the other dome, and the navicular bone is superimposed over most of the cuboid.

    _____

26. The tibiotalar joint space is obscured, one talar dome is demonstrated proximal to the other dome, and more than ½ inch (1.25 cm) of the cuboid appears distal to the navicular bone.

    _____

27. The tibiotalar joint is obscured, one talar dome is demonstrated anterior to the other dome, and the fibula is demonstrated too posterior on the tibia.

    _____

28. The tibiotalar joint is obscured, one talar dome is demonstrated anterior to the other dome, and the fibula is demonstrated too anterior on the tibia.

For the following lateral foot images with poor positioning, state what anatomical structures are misaligned and how the patient should be repositioned for an optimal image to be obtained.

Figure 5–16

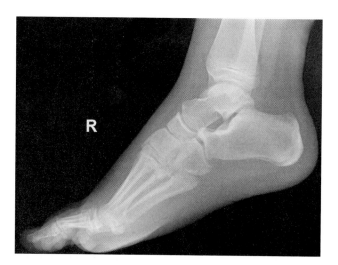

29. (Figure 5-16): _____ , _____

_____

_____

_____

Figure 5–17

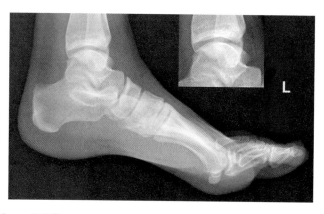

30. (Figure 5-17): _____

_____

_____

_____

Calcaneus: Plantodorsal (Axial) Projection

1. Identify the labeled anatomy in Figure 5-18.

Figure 5–18

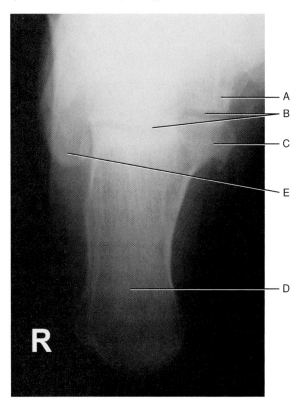

A. _____

B. _____

C. _____

D. _____

E. _____

2. An axial calcaneal image with accurate positioning demonstrates an open (A) _____ joint space and demonstrates the (B) _____ without distortion.

3. To obtain an axial calcaneal image with accurate positioning, position the foot (A) _____ and direct a (B) _____-degree central ray angulation toward the (C) _____ foot surface.

4. When the central ray and foot are accurately aligned, the central ray is aligned (A) _____ to the talocalcaneal joint space and (B) _____ to the calcaneal tuberosity.

5. If an axial calcaneal image is requested for a patient who is unable to dorsiflex the foot to a vertical position, how is the positioning setup adjusted before the image is obtained?

A. _____

How is the setup changed if the patient dorsiflexed the foot beyond the vertical position?

B. _____

6. What anatomical structures can be used to estimate the central ray angulation needed when the patient is unable to dorsiflex the foot into a vertical position?

   _____

7. Describe where to palpate to locate the fifth metatarsal base.

   _____

8. How is the patient positioned to prevent calcaneal tilting?

   A. _____

   How is calcaneal tilting identified on an axial calcaneal image with poor positioning?

   B. _____

9. On an axial calcaneal image with accurate positioning, the
   (A) _____
   is centered within the collimated field. This is accomplished by centering the central ray to the midline of the foot at the level of the
   (B) _____.

10. What anatomical structures are included on an axial calcaneal image with accurate positioning?

    _____

11. List three practices that should be followed to produce optimal digital extremity images.

    A. _____

    B. _____

    C. _____

For the following descriptions of axial calcaneal images with poor positioning, state how the patient would have been mispositioned for such an image to be obtained.

12. The talocalcaneal joint space is obscured, and the calcaneal tuberosity is elongated. The standard 40-degree angulation was used.

    _____

13. The talocalcaneal joint space is obscured, and the calcaneal tuberosity is foreshortened. The standard 40-degree angulation was used.

    _____

14. The first metatarsal is demonstrated medially.

_____

15. The fourth and fifth metatarsals are demonstrated laterally.

_____

For the following axial calcaneal image with poor positioning, state what anatomical structures are misaligned and how the patient should be repositioned for an optimal image to be obtained.

Figure 5–19

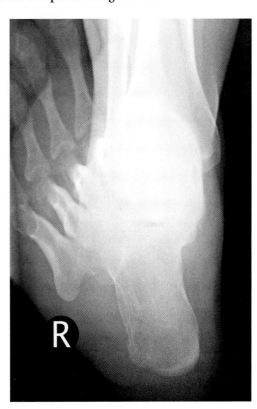

16. (Figure 5-19): _____

_____

_____

_____

Figure 5–20

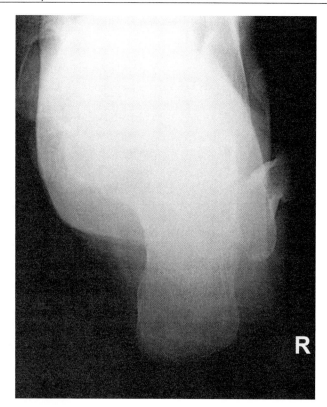

17. (Figure 5-20): _____

_____

_____

_____

Figure 5–21

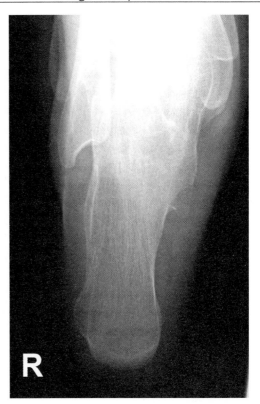

18. (Figure 5-21): _____

_____

_____

_____

Calcaneus: Lateral Position (Mediolateral Projection)

1. Identify the labeled anatomy in Figure 5-22.

Figure 5-22

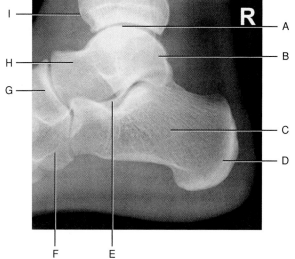

A. _____

B. _____

C. _____

D. _____

E. _____

F. _____

G. _____

H. _____

I. _____

2. A lateral calcaneal image demonstrates (A) _____ talar domes, an open (B) _____ joint, and the distal fibula superimposed by the (C) _____ (posterior/anterior) half of the (D) _____.

3. How is the patient's lower leg positioned to obtain a lateral calcaneal image with accurate positioning? _____

4. How is the patient's foot positioned with the lower leg and IR to obtain a lateral calcaneal image with accurate positioning?

   A. Lower leg: _____

   B. IR: _____

5. A calcaneal foot image was requested for a patient with a large upper thigh that prevented the lower leg from aligning parallel with the imaging table when the patient was positioned. If the image was obtained with the patient positioned in this manner, how would this poor positioning be identified on the resulting image? _____

   _____

6. The height of the longitudinal arch is determined on a lateral calcaneal image with accurate positioning by measuring the amount of cuboid that appears (A) _____ to the (B) _____.

7. The average calcaneal image demonstrates approximately _____ inch of the cuboid distal to the navicular bone.

8. An image from a patient with a low foot arch shows (A) _____ (more/ less) of the cuboid distal to the navicular bone, and an image from a patient with a high foot arch shows (B) _____ (more/less).

9. The actual height of the foot arch on a lateral calcaneal image is accurate only when the _____ are superimposed.

10. What anatomical structures form the talar domes on a lateral calcaneal image?

_____

11. Misalignment of the talar domes can be caused by poor (A) _____ and/or (B) _____ positioning.

12. If the distal tibia is positioned farther from the imaging table than the proximal tibia for a lateral calcaneal image, the (A) _____ dome is demonstrated (B) _____ to the (C) _____ talar dome and the longitudinal foot arch appears (D) _____ (higher/lower) on the resulting image.

13. If the proximal tibia is positioned farther from the imaging table than the distal tibia for a lateral calcaneal image, the (A) _____ dome is demonstrated (B) _____ to the (C) _____ talar dome and the longitudinal foot arch appears (D) _____ (higher/lower) on the resulting image.

14. If the calcaneus is positioned too close to the IR and the forefoot is raised off the IR for a lateral calcaneal image, the (A) _____ talar dome is demonstrated (B) _____ to the (C) _____ talar dome and the fibula is demonstrated too far (D) _____ on the tibia.

15. If the forefoot is positioned too close to the IR and the calcaneus is raised off the IR for a lateral calcaneal image, the (A) _____ talar dome is demonstrated (B) _____ to the (C) _____ talar dome and the fibula is demonstrated too far (D) _____ on the tibia.

16. Positioning the long axis of the foot at a 90-degree angle with the lower leg prevents _____ rotation.

17. On a lateral calcaneal image with accurate positioning, the (A) _____ is centered within the collimated field. This is accomplished by centering a (B) _____ central ray 1 inch (2.5 cm) (C) _____ to the (D) _____.

18. What anatomical structures are included on a lateral calcaneal image with accurate positioning?

_____

19. To ensure that the needed joint spaces are included on a lateral calcaneal image, the longitudinal collimation is open to the level of the (A) _____ and transverse collimation extends 2 inches (5 cm) anterior to the (B) _____.

For the following descriptions of lateral calcaneal images with poor positioning, state how the patient would have been mispositioned for such an image to be obtained.

20. The tibiotalar joint space is obscured, one talar dome is demonstrated proximal to the other, and the navicular bone is superimposed over most of the cuboid.

_____

21. The tibiotalar joint space is obscured, one talar dome is demonstrated proximal to the other, and more than ½ inch (1.25 cm) of cuboid appears distal to the navicular bone.

_____

22. The tibiotalar joint is obscured, one talar dome is demonstrated anterior to the other dome, and the fibula is demonstrated too posterior on the tibia.

_____

23. The tibiotalar joint is obscured, one talar dome is demonstrated anterior to the other dome, and the fibula is demonstrated too anterior on the tibia.

_____

For the following axial calcaneal images with poor positioning, state what anatomical structures are misaligned and how the patient should be repositioned for an optimal image to be obtained.

Figure 5–23

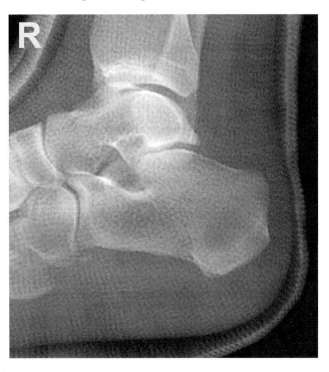

24. (Figure 5-23): _____

_____

_____

_____

Figure 5–24

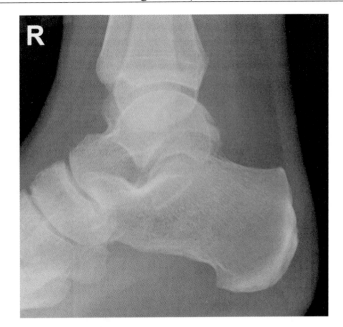

25. (Figure 5-24): _____

_____

_____

_____

Figure 5–25

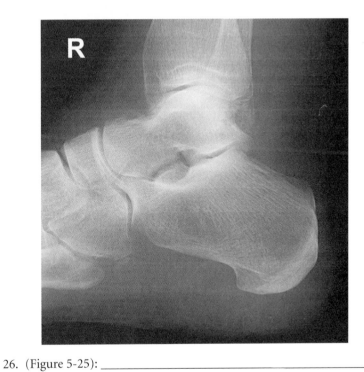

26. (Figure 5-25): _____

_____

_____

_____

Ankle: AP Projection

1. Identify the labeled anatomy in figure 5-26.

Figure 5–26

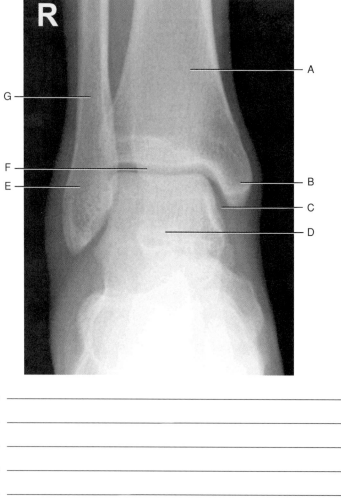

A. _____

B. _____

C. _____

D. _____

E. _____

F. _____

G. _____

2. Define the following terms.

A. Intermalleolar line: _____

B. Medial mortise: _____

C. Lateral mortise: _____

3. An AP ankle image with accurate positioning demonstrates what open joint spaces?

A. _____

B. _____

4. The ankle joint is located at the same level as what palpable anatomical structure? _____

5. Is the distal fibula superimposed by the tibia or is the tibia superimposed by the distal fibula on an AP ankle image?

   _____

6. The intermalleolar line is at what angle with the IR when the patient is accurately positioned for an AP ankle image? _____

7. The patient's leg was laterally rotated for an AP ankle image. How can this mispositioning be identified on an AP ankle image?

   _____

   _____

8. How is the patient positioned for an AP ankle image to obtain an open tibiotalar joint space?

   _____

9. The central ray was centered proximal to the ankle joint space for an AP ankle image. How is this mispositioning identified on an AP ankle image? _____

   _____

10. On an AP ankle image with accurate positioning, the
    (A) _____ is centered to the collimated field.
    This is accomplished by centering a (B) _____
    central ray to the ankle midline at the level of the
    (C) _____.

11. What anatomical structures are included on an AP ankle image with accurate positioning?

    _____

For the following descriptions of AP ankle images with poor positioning, state how the patient would have been mispositioned for such an image to be obtained.

12. The medial mortise is obscured, the tibia and talus demonstrate increased superimposition of the fibula, and the posterior aspect of the medial malleolus is situated lateral to the anterior aspect.

    _____

13. The medial mortise is closed, and the fibula demonstrates no talar superimposition.

    _____

14. The tibiotalar joint is closed, and the anterior tibial margin has been projected into the joint space.

    _____

For the following AP ankle image with poor positioning, state what anatomical structures are misaligned and how the patient should be repositioned for an optimal image to be obtained.

Figure 5–27

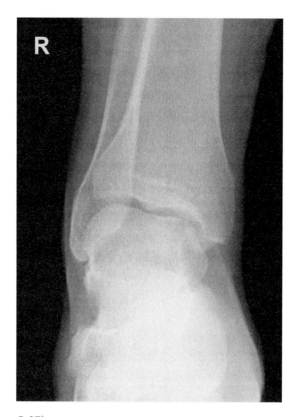

15. (Figure 5-27): _____

_____

_____

_____

Figure 5–28

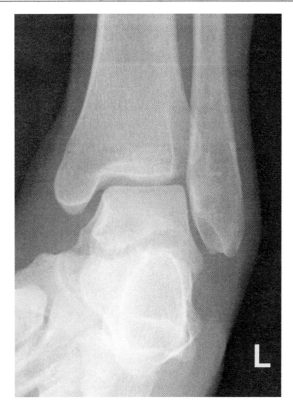

16. (Figure 5-28): _____

_____

_____

_____

Ankle: AP Oblique Projection (Internal Rotation: 15- to 20-Degree Mortise and 45-Degree Oblique)

1. Identify the labeled anatomy in Figure 5-29.

Figure 5–29

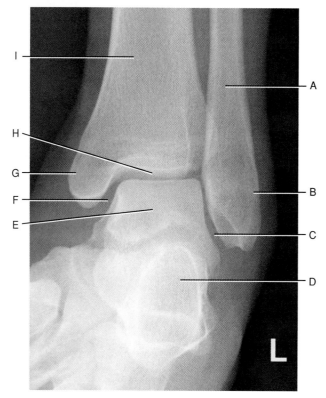

A. _____

B. _____

C. _____

D. _____

E. _____

F. _____

G. _____

H. _____

I. _____

2. Define *tarsal sinus*. _____

3. On a mortise AP oblique ankle image with accurate positioning, the distal fibula is demonstrated without (A) _____ superimposition and the (B) _____ joint space is open. This joint space is also referred to as the (C) _____ (medial/lateral) mortise.

4. Approximately how much ankle obliquity is needed for a mortise AP oblique ankle image with accurate positioning?

   A. _____

   In which direction is the patient's leg rotated?

   B. _____

5. On a 45-degree AP oblique ankle image with accurate positioning the medial mortise is (A) _____ and the fibula is demonstrated (B) _____ (with/without) tibial superimposition.

6. How is the patient positioned to obtain an open tibiotalar joint space on an AP oblique ankle image with accurate positioning?

   _____

7. The central ray was centered distal to the ankle joint for an AP oblique ankle image. How can this mispositioning be identified on an AP oblique ankle image? _____

   _____

8. How is the patient positioned to demonstrate the calcaneus distal to the lateral mortise and fibula on an AP oblique ankle image?

   _____

   _____

9. On an AP oblique ankle image with accurate positioning, the (A) _____ is centered within the collimated field. This is accomplished by centering a (B) _____ central ray to the ankle midline at the level of the (C) _____.

10. What anatomical structures are included on an AP ankle image with accurate positioning?

    _____

For the following descriptions of AP oblique ankle images with poor positioning, state how the patient would have been mispositioned for such an image to be obtained.

11. Mortise oblique: The lateral mortise is closed, and the medial mortise is demonstrated as an open space. The tarsal sinus is not shown.

_____

12. Mortise oblique: The lateral and medial mortises are closed, and the tarsal sinus is demonstrated.

_____

13. 45-degree oblique: the lateral and medial mortises and closed, the fibula is demonstrated without tibial superimposition, and the tarsal sinus is demonstrated.

_____

14. Mortise oblique: The tibiotalar joint space is expanded, the anterior tibial margin is projected superior to the posterior margin, and the tibial articulating surface is demonstrated.

_____

15. 45 degree oblique: The calcaneus is obscuring the distal aspect of the lateral mortise and the distal fibula.

_____

For the following AP oblique ankle images with poor positioning, state what anatomical structures are misaligned and how the patient should be repositioned for an optimal image to be obtained.

Figure 5–30

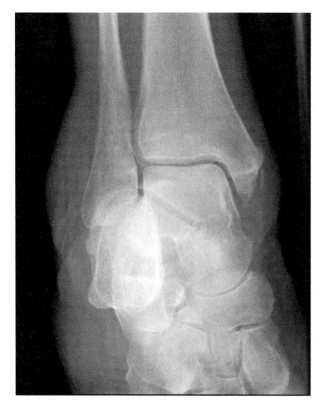

16. (Figure 5-30, mortise oblique): _____

_____

_____

_____

_____

_____

Figure 5–31

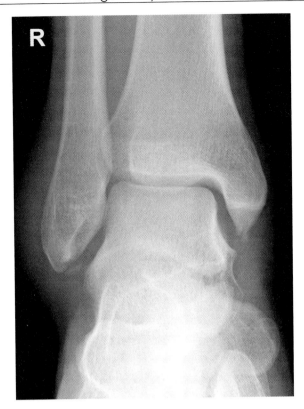

17. (Figure 5-31, mortise oblique): _____

_____

_____

_____

Figure 5–32

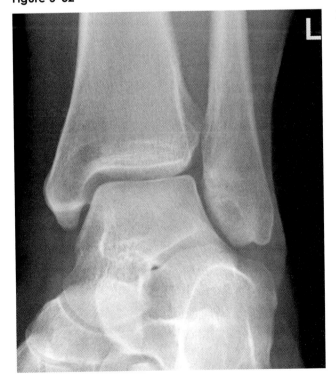

18. (Figure 5-32, mortise oblique): _____

_____

_____

_____

_____

_____

Figure 5–33

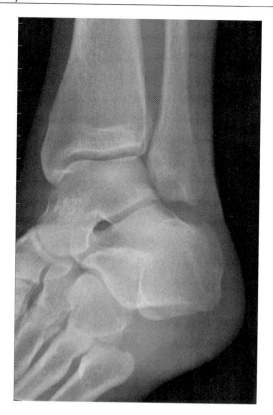

19. (Figure 5-33, 45-degree oblique): _____

_____

_____

_____

Figure 5–34

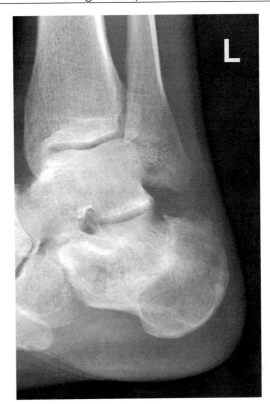

20. (Figure 5-34, 45-degree oblique): _____

_____

_____

_____

Ankle: Lateral Position (Mediolateral Projection)

1. Identify the labeled anatomy in Figure 5-35.

Figure 5–35

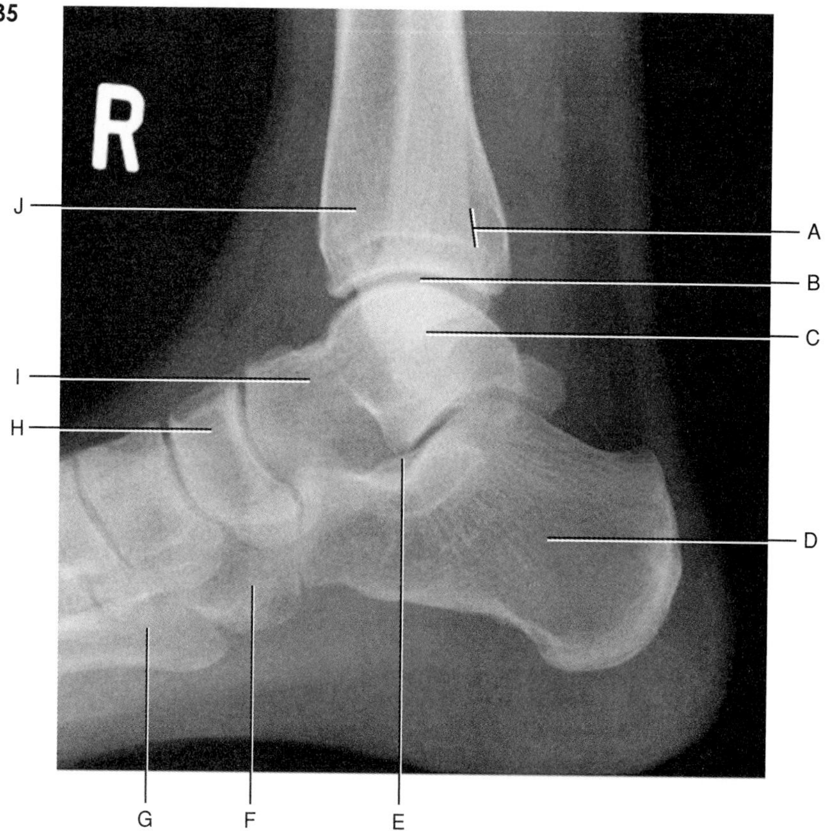

A. _____

B. _____

C. _____

D. _____

E. _____

F. _____

G. _____

H. _____

I. _____

2. Describe the location of the anterior pretalar and posterior pericapsular fat pads on a lateral ankle image.

   A. Anterior pretalar: _____

   B. Posterior pericapsular: _____

3. Why is the visualization of the anterior pretalar and posterior pericapsular fat pads important on a lateral ankle image? _____

_____

4. A lateral ankle image demonstrates (A) _____ talar domes, an open (B) _____ joint, and the distal fibula superimposed by the (C) _____ half of the (D) _____.

5. To obtain a lateral ankle image with accurate positioning, the patient's leg is extended with the lower leg positioned (A) _____ to the imaging table and the foot dorsiflexed with its (B) _____ surface aligned parallel to the IR.

6. The height of the longitudinal arch can be determined on a lateral ankle image with accurate positioning by measuring the amount of cuboid that appears (A) _____ to the (B) _____. The average ankle image demonstrates approximately (C) _____ inch of the cuboid, while a high-arched patient demonstrates approximately (D) _____ inch and a low arched patient demonstrates approximately (E) _____ inch.

7. What anatomical structures form the structures referred to as the *talar domes* on a lateral foot image?

   _____

   _____

8. Accurate lower leg positioning for a lateral ankle image ensures accurate _____ alignment of the talar domes.

9. If the distal tibia is positioned farther from the imaging table than the proximal tibia for a lateral ankle image, the (A) _____ dome is demonstrated (B) _____ to the (C) _____ talar dome and the longitudinal foot arch appears (D) _____ on the resulting image.

10. If the proximal tibia is positioned farther from the imaging table than the distal tibia for a lateral ankle image, the (A) _____ dome is demonstrated (B) _____ to the (C) _____ talar dome and the longitudinal foot arch appears (D) _____ on the resulting image.

11. Accurate lateral foot surface positioning for a lateral ankle image ensures proper _____ alignment of the talar domes.

12. If the calcaneus is positioned too close to the IR and the toes are raised off the IR for a lateral ankle image, the (A) _____ talar dome is demonstrated (B) _____ to the (C) _____ talar dome and the fibula is demonstrated too far (D) _____ on the tibia.

13. If the toes are positioned too close to the IR and the calcaneus is raised off the IR for a lateral ankle image, the (A) _____ talar domes are demonstrated (B) _____ to the (C) _____ talar dome and the fibula is demonstrated too far (D) _____ on the tibia.

14. Why is it important to dorsiflex the foot to a 90-degree angle with the lower leg?

   A. _____

   B. _____

   C. _____

15. On a lateral ankle image with accurate positioning, the (A) _____ is centered within the collimated field. This is accomplished by centering a (B) _____ central ray to the (C) _____.

16. What anatomical structures are included on a lateral ankle image with accurate positioning? _____

_____

17. What is a Jones fracture? _____

18. Why should the transversely collimated field remain open to include 3 inches (7.5 cm) of the proximal forefoot? _____

_____

For the following descriptions of lateral ankle images with poor positioning, state how the patient would have been mispositioned for such an image to be obtained.

19. The tibiotalar joint space is obscured, one talar dome is demonstrated proximal to the other dome, and the navicular bone is superimposed over most of the cuboid.

_____

20. Average longitudenial arch: The tibiotalar joint space is obscured, one talar dome is demonstrated proximal to the other dome, and more than ½ inch (1.25 cm) of the cuboid appears distal to the navicular bone.

_____

21. The tibiotalar joint is obscured, one talar dome is demonstrated anterior to the other dome, and the fibula is demonstrated too posterior on the tibia.

_____

22. The tibiotalar joint is obscured, one talar dome is demonstrated anterior to the other dome, and the fibula is demonstrated too anterior on the tibia.

_____

For the following lateral ankle images with poor positioning, state what anatomical structures are misaligned and how the patient should be repositioned for an optimal image to be obtained.

Figure 5–36

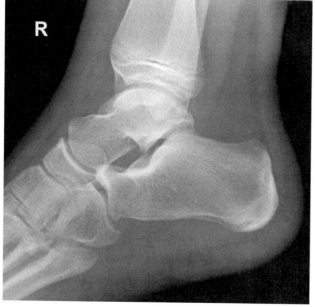

23. (Figure 5-36): _____

_____

_____

_____

_____

_____

Figure 5–37

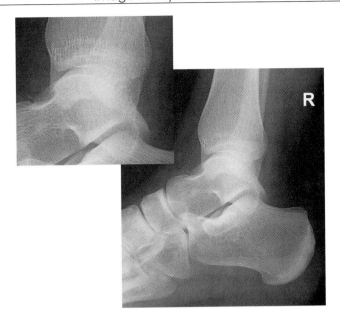

24. (Figure 5-37): _____

_____

_____

_____

Figure 5–38

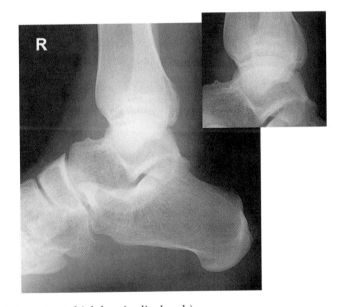

25. (Figure 5-38, high longitudinal arch): _____

_____

_____

_____

Figure 5–39

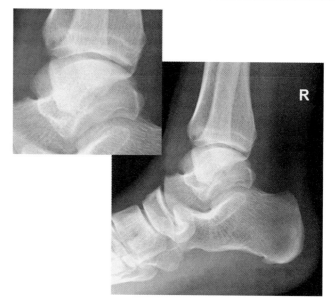

26. (Figure 5-39, average longitudinal arch): _____

_____

_____

_____

Figure 5–40

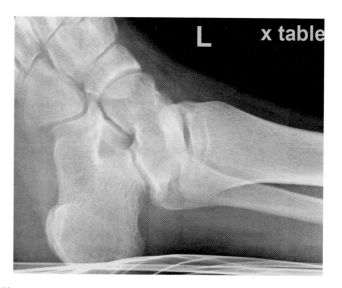

27. (Figure 5-40, trauma, lateromedial projection): _____

_____

_____

_____

Figure 5–41

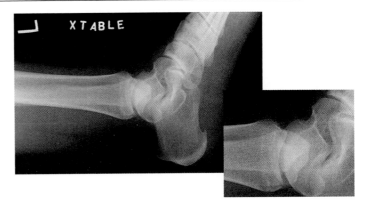

28. (Figure 5-41, trauma, lateromedial projection):_____

_____

_____

_____

Lower Leg: AP Projection

Figure 5–42

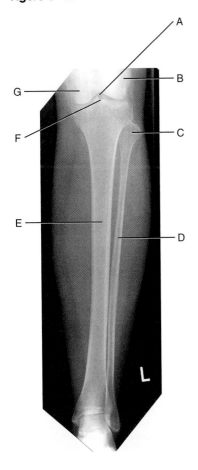

1. Identify the labeled anatomy in Figure 5-42.

A. _____

B. _____

C. _____

D. _____

E. _____

F. _____

G. _____

2. How should the lower leg be positioned with respect to the x-ray tube to take advantage of the anode-heel effect? _____

_____

3. An AP projection of the lower leg is obtained by (A) _____ the patient's knee and (B) _____ rotating the leg until the medial and lateral (C) _____ are positioned at equal distances from the IR.

4. An AP projection of the distal lower leg is demonstrated when the _____ mortise is open.

5. Describe the relationship of the tibia and fibula at the knee, midshaft, and ankle on an AP lower leg image with accurate positioning.

   A. Knee: _____

   B. Midshaft: _____

   C. Ankle: _____

6. Describe how the tibia and fibula on an AP lower leg image are misaligned at the knee and ankle if the leg is internally rotated.

   A. Knee: _____

   B. Ankle: _____

7. A patient from the emergency room is unable to position the ankle and knee in a true AP projection simultaneously for an AP lower leg image. If the area of interest is closer to the knee joint, how should the leg be positioned for the image?

   _____

8. Are the femorotibial and tibiotalar joint spaces closed on an AP lower leg image with accurate positioning?

   A. _____ (Yes/No)

   Explain how the divergence of the x-ray beam used to record these two joints affects their openness.

   B. _____

9. Why is it necessary for the IR to extend at least 1 inch (2.5 cm) beyond the ankle and knee joints when the lower leg is imaged in an AP projection?

   _____

10. The ankle joint is located at the level of the palpable
    (A) _____, and the knee joint is located ¾ inch
    (2 cm) (B) _____ to the palpable
    (C) _____.

11. The _____ is centered to the collimated field on an AP lower leg image with accurate positioning.

12. What anatomical structures are included on an AP lower leg image with accurate positioning?

_____

For the following descriptions of AP lower leg images with poor positioning, state how the patient would have been mispositioned for such an image to be obtained.

13. The medial mortise is closed, and the tibia and talus demonstrate excessive fibular superimposition.

_____

14. The distal fibula is free of talar superimposition, and the proximal fibula is free of tibial superimposition.

_____

For the following AP lower leg image with poor positioning, state what anatomical structures are misaligned and how the patient should be repositioned for an optimal image to be obtained.

Figure 5–43

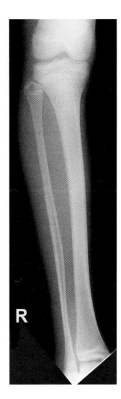

15. (Figure 5-43): _____

_____

_____

_____

Lower Leg: Lateral Position (Mediolateral Projection)

1. Identify the labeled anatomy in Figure 5-44.

Figure 5–44

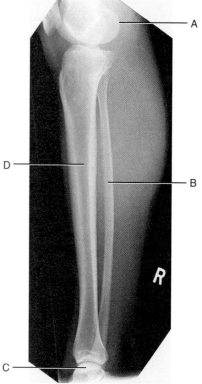

A. _____

B. _____

C. _____

D. _____

2. State how the lower leg is positioned with respect to the x-ray tube to take advantage of the anode-heel effect. _____

_____

3. What aspect of the patient's leg is positioned against the IR for a lateral lower leg image with accurate positioning? _____ (Medial/Lateral)

4. Describe the anatomical relationship of the tibia and fibula at the knee, midshaft, and ankle on a lateral lower leg image with accurate positioning.

A. Knee: _____

B. Midshaft: _____

C. Ankle: _____

5. How does the relationship between the tibia and fibula at the knee and ankle described in question 4 change if the patient's medial femoral epicondyle is rotated anterior to the lateral epicondyle for the image?

   A. Knee: _____

   B. Ankle: _____

6. The degree of knee flexion determines how superimposed the femoral condyles will be on a lateral lower leg image. Will the femoral condyles be superimposed if the image is obtained with the knee extended?

   A. _____ (Yes/No)

   If the image is obtained with the knee flexed 30 degrees?

   B. _____ (Yes/No)

7. A patient from the emergency room is unable to position the knee and ankle in a true lateral position simultaneously for a lateral lower leg image. If the area of interest is closest to the ankle joint, how should the leg be positioned for this image?

   _____

8. To ensure that both joints are included on a lateral lower leg image, how far should the IR and longitudinally collimated field extend beyond the knee and ankle joints?

   _____

9. The _____ is centered to the collimated field on a lateral lower leg image with accurate positioning.

10. What anatomical structures are included on a lateral lower leg image with accurate positioning?

    _____

For the following descriptions of lateral lower leg images with poor positioning, state how the patient would have been mispositioned for such an image to be obtained.

11. The distal fibula is situated too far posterior on the tibia, the medial talar dome is anterior to the lateral dome, and the fibular head is free of tibial superimposition.

    _____

12. The distal fibula is situated too far anterior on the tibia, the medial talar dome is posterior to the lateral dome, and the fibular head and midshaft are superimposed by the tibia.

    _____

For the following lateral lower leg images with poor positioning, state what anatomical structures are misaligned and how the patient should be repositioned for an optimal image to be obtained.

Figure 5–45

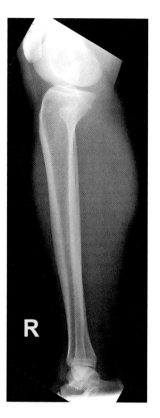

13. (Figure 5-45): _____

_____

_____

_____

Figure 5–46

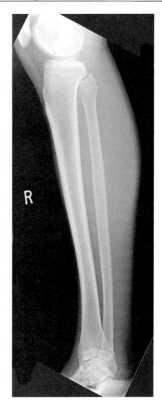

14. (Figure 5-46): _____

_____

_____

_____

Knee: AP Projection

1. Identify the labeled anatomy in Figure 5-47.

Figure 5–47

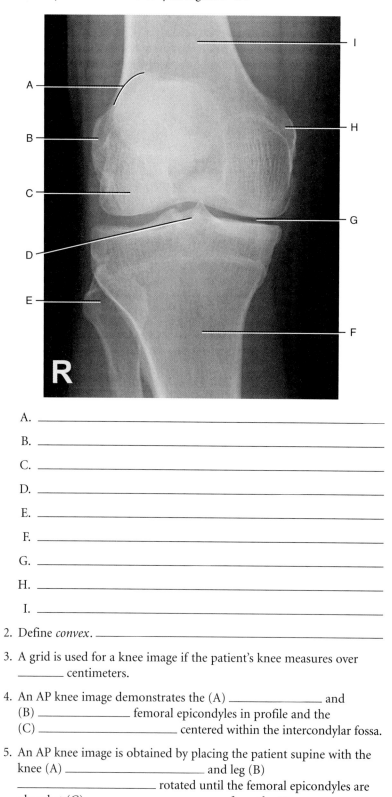

A. _____

B. _____

C. _____

D. _____

E. _____

F. _____

G. _____

H. _____

I. _____

2. Define *convex*. _____

3. A grid is used for a knee image if the patient's knee measures over _____ centimeters.

4. An AP knee image demonstrates the (A) _____ and (B) _____ femoral epicondyles in profile and the (C) _____ centered within the intercondylar fossa.

5. An AP knee image is obtained by placing the patient supine with the knee (A) _____ and leg (B) _____ rotated until the femoral epicondyles are placed at (C) _____ from the IR.

6. Is the proximal tibia superimposed over the proximal fibula or is the proximal fibula superimposed over the proximal tibia when the knee is in an AP projection?

_____

7. If the knee is rotated from an AP projection, will the femoral condyle positioned closer to or farther away from the IR appear larger on the resulting image? _____

8. If the patient's leg is not internally rotated to accurately position the femoral epicondyles, how will the appearances of the femoral condyles and the alignment of the tibia and fibula change? _____

_____

9. When the central ray and proximal tibia are accurately aligned for an AP knee image, the (A) _____ joint space is open, the anterior and posterior condylar margins of the tibia are (B) _____, and the fibular head is demonstrated approximately (C) _____ inch distal to the tibial plateau.

10. How does the central ray have to be aligned with the femorotibial joint space and tibial plateau to demonstrate them as open spaces on an AP knee image? _____

11. Describe the slope of the tibial plateau. _____

_____

12. Why is it necessary to vary the degree of central ray angulation for AP knee images in patients with different upper thigh and buttock thicknesses? _____

_____

13. Should the patient's abdominal thickness be included in the anterior superior iliac spine (ASIS)-to-imaging table measurement obtained for a patient undergoing AP knee imaging? _____ (Yes/No)

14. What central ray angulation is used when obtaining an AP knee image in a patient with a large (greater than 24 cm) ASIS-to-imaging table measurement?

A. _____

When imaging a patient with a small (less than 18 cm) ASIS-to-imaging table measurement?

B. _____

15. If the wrong central ray angle is used for an AP knee image, the shape of the fibular head and its proximity to the tibial plateau change from that demonstrated on an AP knee image in which an accurate central ray angle was used. For each situation that follows, state the change that occurs.

A. Central ray angled too cephalically: _____

_____

B. Central ray angled too caudally: _____

_____

16. Which knee compartment on an AP knee image is the narrower when a valgus deformity is present?

    A. _____

    When a varus deformity is present?

    B. _____

17. What deformity is demonstrated in Figure 5-48? _____

Figure 5–48

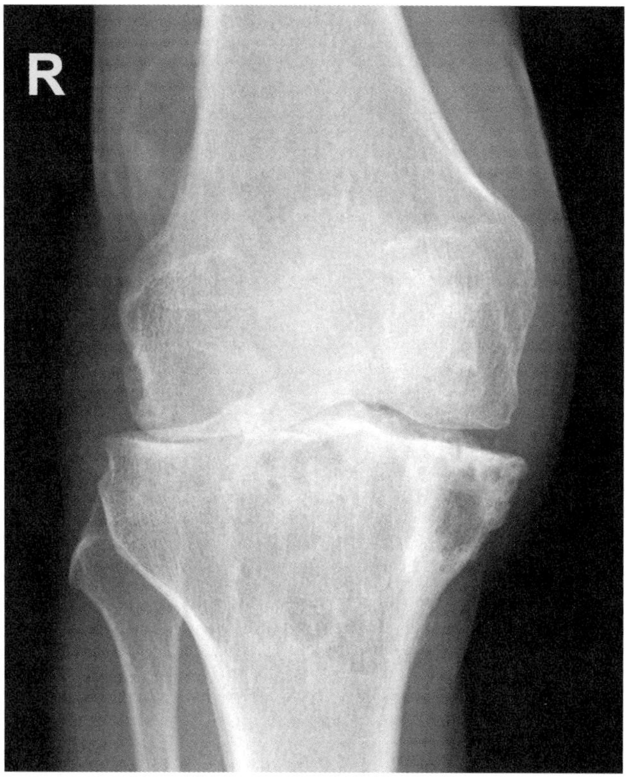

18. An AP knee image is requested for a patient who is unable to fully extend the knee. The technologist angled the central ray until it was perpendicular to the anterior surface of the lower leg and obtained a 10-degree cephalic angle. How is this angle adjusted to align the central ray parallel with the tibial plateau and obtain an open femorotibial joint? _____

    _____

19. State the location of the patella on an AP knee image with accurate positioning and without pathology. _____

    _____

20. When the knee is flexed, the patella shifts (A) _____ (proximally/distally) and (B) _____ (medially/laterally) onto the patellar surface of the femur and then (C) _____ (medially/laterally) onto the intercondylar fossa.

21. State the location of the patella for each of the following degrees of knee flexion.

    A. 10 degrees: _____

    B. 20 degrees: _____

    C. 60 degrees: _____

22. Where is the patella demonstrated on an AP knee image with accurate positioning in a patient with a subluxed patella?

    A. _____

    _____

    What type of knee rotation situates the patella in the same location?

    B. _____

    How can one distinguish patellar subluxation from knee rotation on an AP knee image?

    C. _____

23. On an AP knee image with accurate positioning, the
    (A) _____ is centered within the
    collimated field. This is accomplished by centering the central ray
    (B) _____ inch (C) _____ to the palpable
    (D) _____.

24. What anatomical structures are included on an AP knee image with accurate positioning? _____

    _____

For the following descriptions of AP knee images with poor positioning, state how the patient or central ray would have been mispositioned for such an image to be obtained.

25. The medial femoral condyle appears larger than the lateral condyle, and the head, neck, and shaft of the fibula are almost entirely superimposed by the tibia.

    _____

26. The lateral femoral condyle appears larger than the medial condyle, and the tibia demonstrates very little superimposition of the fibular head.

    _____

27. The femorotibial joint space is obscured, the tibial plateau is demonstrated, the proximal ridges of the femoral condyles are concave, and the fibular head is foreshortened and demonstrated more than ½ inch (1.25 cm) distal to the tibial plateau.

    _____

28. The medial femorotibial joint space is closed, the proximal ridges of the femoral condyles are convex, and the fibular head is elongated and demonstrated less than ½ inch (1.25 cm) distal to the tibial plateau.

    _____

For the following AP knee images with poor positioning, state what anatomical structures are misaligned and how the patient should be repositioned for an optimal image to be obtained.

Figure 5–49

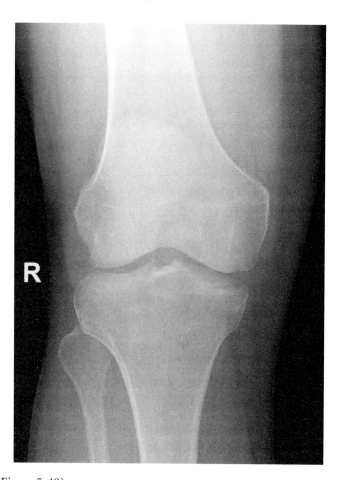

29. (Figure 5-49): _____

_____

_____

_____

Figure 5–50

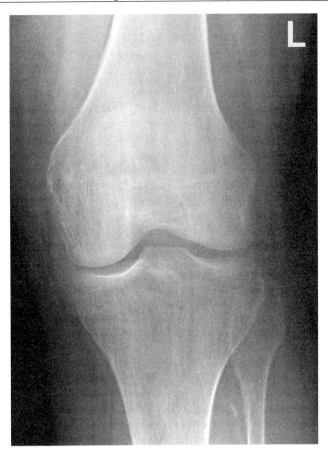

30. (Figure 5-50): _____

_____

_____

_____

Figure 5–51

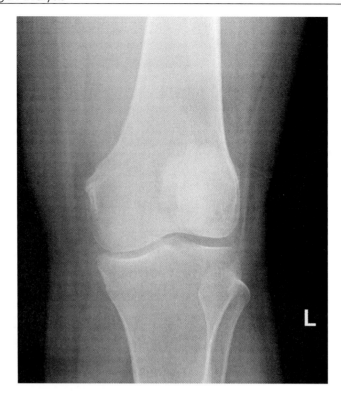

31. (Figure 5-51): _____

_____

_____

_____

Figure 5–52

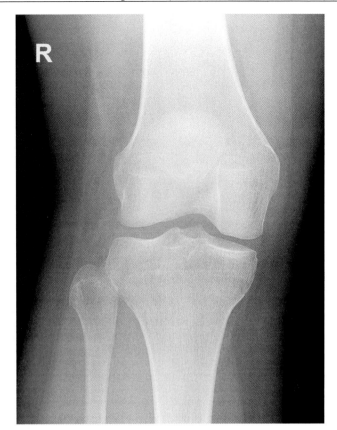

32. (Figure 5-52): _____

_____

_____

_____

Figure 5–53

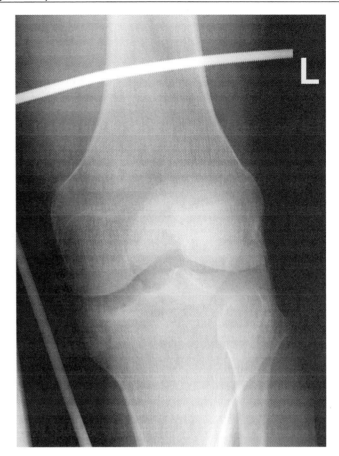

33. (Figure 5-53, trauma): _____

_____

_____

_____

Knee: AP Oblique Projection (Internal and External Rotation)

1. Identify the labeled anatomy in Figure 5-54.

Figure 5–54

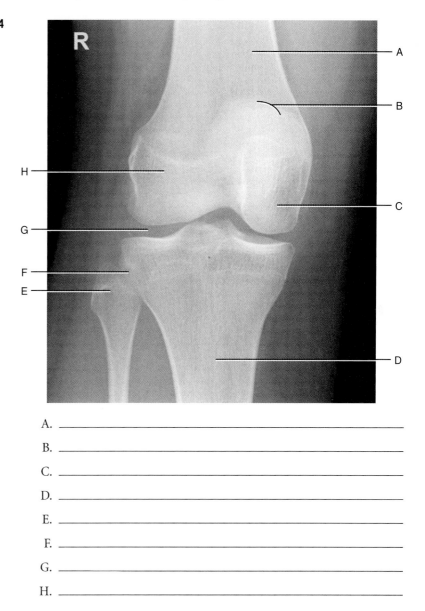

A. _____

B. _____

C. _____

D. _____

E. _____

F. _____

G. _____

H. _____

2. Identify the labeled anatomy in Figure 5-55.

Figure 5–55

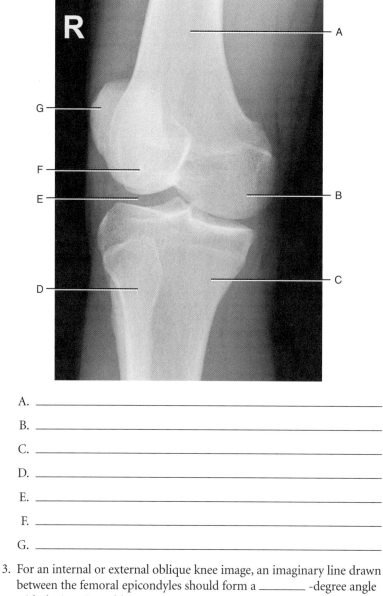

A. _____

B. _____

C. _____

D. _____

E. _____

F. _____

G. _____

3. For an internal or external oblique knee image, an imaginary line drawn between the femoral epicondyles should form a _____ -degree angle with the imaging table.

4. What is the relationship of the fibular head and tibia on an accurately rotated medial knee image?

A. _____

_____

Which femoral condyle is demonstrated in profile?

B. _____

5. How can one determine from a knee image with internal rotation that the patient was overrotated? _____

_____

6. What is the relationship of the tibia and fibular head on a knee image with accurate external rotation?

   A. _____

   _____

   Which femoral condyle is demonstrated in profile?

   B. _____

7. How can one determine from a knee image with external rotation that the patient was overrotated?

   _____

8. When the central ray and tibial plateau are accurately aligned for oblique knee images, the (A) _____ joint is open, the anterior and posterior condylar margins of the tibia are (B) _____, and the fibular head is demonstrated approximately (C) _____ inch (D) _____ to the tibial plateau.

9. What degree of central ray angulation is used for a knee image with lateral rotation in a patient whose ASIS-to-imaging table measurement is 12 cm?

   A. _____.

   Why is it not uncommon to need a cephalic angle for the medially (internally) oblique knee image?

   B. _____

   To need a caudal angle for the lateral (externally) oblique image?

   C. _____

10. On a knee image with accurate rotation, the (A) _____ is centered within the collimated field. This centering is obtained by centering the central ray to the (B) _____ at the level of the (C) _____

11. What anatomical structures are included on an oblique knee image with accurate positioning?

    _____

For the following descriptions of AP oblique knee images with poor positioning, state how the patient or central ray would have been mispositioned for such an image to be obtained.

12. On an internally rotated knee image, the tibia is partially superimposed over the fibular head.

    _____

13. On an externally rotated knee image, the lateral femoral condyle is superimposed over the medial condyle, and the fibula is located in the center of the tibia.

    _____

14. On an externally rotated knee image, the fibula is not entirely superimposed by the tibia.

    _____

15. On an internally rotated knee image, the femorotibial joint space is obscured, the proximal ridges of the femoral condyles are concave, and the fibular head is foreshortened and demonstrated more than ½ inch (1.25 cm) distal to the tibial plateau.

For the following AP oblique knee images with poor positioning, state what anatomical structures are misaligned and how the patient should be repositioned for an optimal image to be obtained.

Figure 5–56

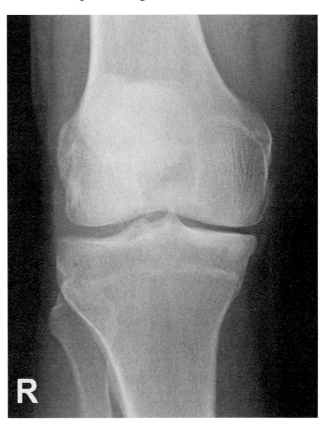

16. (Figure 5-56, internal oblique): _____

_____

_____

_____

Figure 5–57

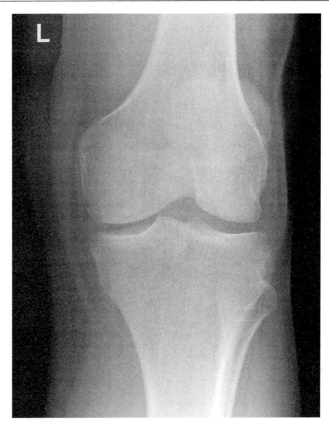

17. (Figure 5-57, external oblique): _____

_____

_____

Figure 5–58

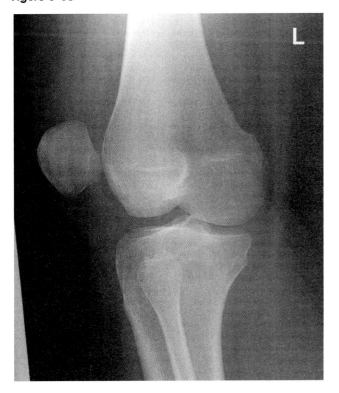

18. (Figure 5-58, external oblique): _____

_____

_____

_____

_____

_____

Knee: Lateral Position (Mediolateral Projection)

1. Identify the labeled anatomy in Figure 5-59.

Figure 5–59

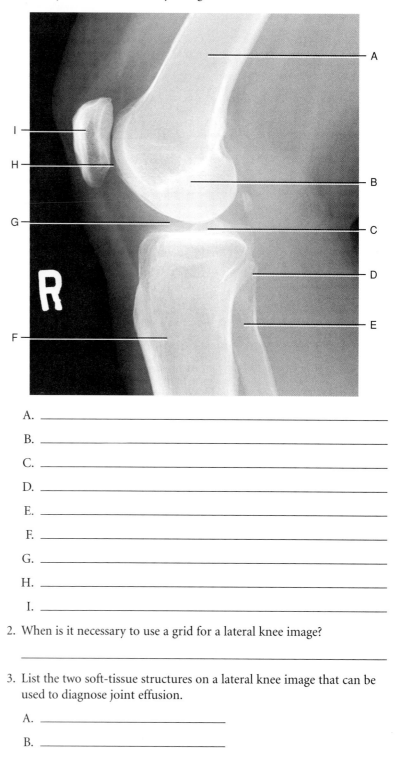

A. _____

B. _____

C. _____

D. _____

E. _____

F. _____

G. _____

H. _____

I. _____

2. When is it necessary to use a grid for a lateral knee image?

_____

3. List the two soft-tissue structures on a lateral knee image that can be used to diagnose joint effusion.

A. _____

B. _____

4. Why can a joint effusion diagnosis be made when evaluating a lateral knee image if the knee is flexed less than 20 degrees but become difficult to make when the knee is flexed more than 20 degrees?

_____

_____

5. When a patient is erect, the distal femoral condylar surfaces are aligned (A) _____ to the floor and the femoral shaft inclines (B) _____ approximately (C) _____ degrees. A patient that demonstrates the greatest femoral inclination will have a (D) _____ (wide/narrow) pelvis and (E) _____ (long/short) femoral shaft length.

6. When the average patient is placed in a recumbent lateral position for a lateral knee image, the femoral shaft inclination displayed in the erect position is reduced, causing the (A) _____ condyle to be projected (B) _____ to the (C) _____ condyle.

7. To obtain superimposed distal femoral condylar surfaces when imaging the average patient for a lateral knee image, a (A) _____-degree cephalic central ray angulation is used to shift the (B) _____ condyle anteriorly and proximally. The central ray angulation is (C) _____ (increased/reduced) when imaging a patient with a narrow pelvis and long femora.

8. State two methods of distinguishing the medial femoral condyle from the lateral femoral condyle on a lateral knee image with poor positioning.

   A. _____

   B. _____

9. When is it necessary to use a cephalic central ray angulation for a lateral knee image in a patient in a supine position?

_____

_____

10. What is the relationship between the tibia and the fibular head on a lateral knee image with accurate positioning if superimposed condyles were obtained by aligning the femoral epicondyles perpendicular to the IR and directing the central ray across the femur to project the medial condyle anteriorly and proximally?

   A. _____

   How will this relationship change if superimposed condyles are obtained by rolling the patient's patella approximately ¼ inch (0.6 cm) closer to the IR and directing the central ray toward the femur so it only moves the medial condyle proximally?

   B. _____

11. Why is the medial condyle shifted more than the lateral condyle when the degree of central ray angulation is adjusted?

_____

12. If the distal surfaces of the femoral condyles are demonstrated without superimposition, how does one determine the degree of central ray adjustment that would be required to superimpose them?

_____

_____

13. The abductor tubercle is located (A) _____ (anteriorly/posteriorly) on the (B) _____ condyle.

14. Is the proximal fibula superimposed over the tibia or is the tibia superimposed over the proximal fibula on a mediolateral knee projection with accurate positioning?

_____

15. If the medial condyle is demonstrated anterior to the lateral condyle on a lateral knee image with poor positioning, what will the tibia and fibular relationship be?

_____

16. If the lateral condyle is demonstrated anterior to the medial condyle on a lateral knee image with poor positioning, what will the tibia and fibular relationship be?

_____

17. On a lateral knee image with accurate positioning, the (A) _____ is centered within the collimated field. This is accomplished by centering the central ray to the midline of the knee at a level (B) _____ inch (C) _____ to the palpable (D) _____.

18. What anatomical structures are included on a lateral knee image with accurate positioning?

_____

For the following descriptions of lateral knee images with poor positioning, state how the patient or central ray would have been mispositioned for such an image to be obtained.

19. The patient's patella is in contact with the patellar surface of the femur, and the suprapatellar fat pads are obscured.

_____

20. The distal articulating surfaces of the femoral condyles are demonstrated without superimposition. The condyle that has the adductor tubercle attached to it is demonstrated approximately ¼ inch (0.6 cm) distal to the other condyle.

_____

21. The distal articulating surfaces of the femoral condyles are demonstrated without superimposition. The condyle that has the flattest distal surface is demonstrated approximately ½ inch (1.25 cm) distal to the other condyle.

_____

22. The anterior and posterior aspects of the femoral condyles are demonstrated without superimposition. The medial condyle is demonstrated posteriorly.

23. The anterior and posterior aspects of the femoral condyles are demonstrated without superimposition. The medial condyle is demonstrated anteriorly.

For the following lateral knee images with poor positioning, state what anatomical structures are misaligned and how the patient should be repositioned for an optimal image to be obtained.

Figure 5–60

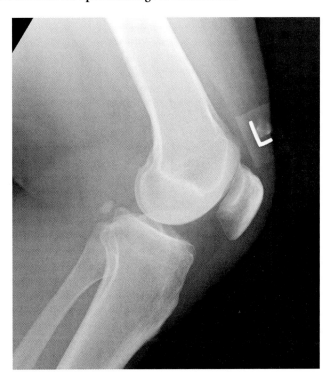

24. (Figure 5-60): _____

_____

_____

_____

Figure 5–61

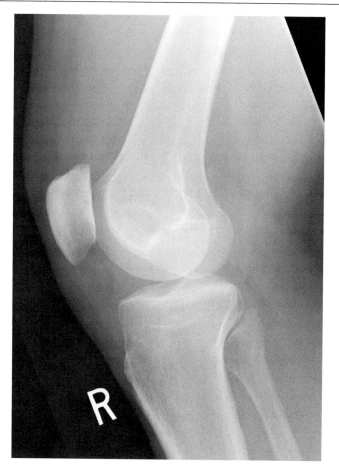

25. (Figure 5-61): _____

_____

_____

_____

Figure 5–62

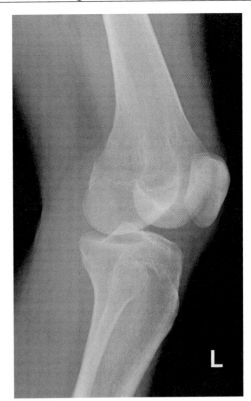

26. (Figure 5-62): _____

_____

_____

_____

Figure 5–63

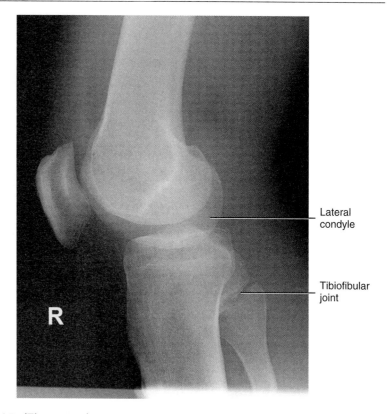

Lateral condyle

Tibiofibular joint

R

27. (Figure 5-63): _____

_____

_____

_____

Figure 5–64

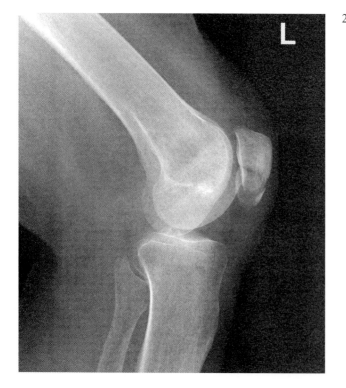

L

28. (Figure 5-64, trauma, mediolateral projection):

_____

_____

_____

_____

_____

Figure 5–65

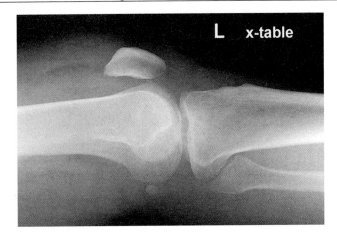

29. (Figure 5-65, trauma, lateromedial): _____

_____

_____

_____

Figure 5–66

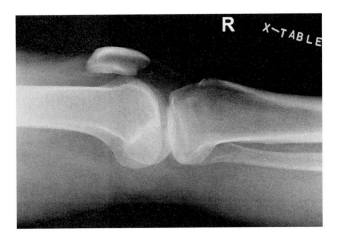

30. (Figure 5-66, trauma, lateromedial projection): _____

_____

_____

_____

Knee: Intercondylar Fossa—PA Axial Projection (Holmblad Method)

1. Identify the labeled anatomy in Figure 5-67.

Figure 5–67

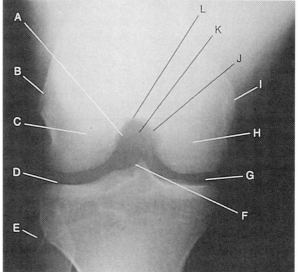

A. _____

B. _____

C. _____

D. _____

E. _____

F. _____

G. _____

H. _____

I. _____

J. _____

K. _____

L. _____

2. A PA axial (Holmblad) knee image with accurate positioning demonstrates the (A) _____, (B) _____, and (C) _____ surfaces of the intercondylar fossa and the femoral epicondyles in profile.

3. How are the femur and foot positioned to demonstrate superimposed medial and lateral intercondylar fossa surfaces on a PA axial knee image?

   A. Femur: _____

   B. Foot: _____

4. Which direction does the patella move when the patient is positioned for a PA axial knee image and the heel is rotated as indicated below?

   A. Internally: _____

   B. Externally: _____

5. To superimpose the proximal surfaces of the intercondylar fossa in the PA axial knee position, position the patient's femur at
   (A) _____ degrees from vertical or
   (B) _____ degrees from the imaging table.

6. What direction does the patella move when the knee is flexed? _____ (Proximally/Distally)

7. If the knee is flexed more than needed to superimpose the proximal surfaces of the intercondylar fossa, is the patella demonstrated proximally or distally to where it is demonstrated on an AP axial knee image with accurate positioning? _____

8. What is the relationship of the tibial plateau to the imaging table in a patient whose foot is plantar-flexed?

   A. _____

   How is the patient positioned for the anterior and posterior condylar margins of the tibia to be superimposed on a Holmblad knee image?

   B. _____

   This positioning also demonstrates an open (C) _____ joint space and the (D) _____ and (E) _____ without foreshortening.

9. On a PA axial knee image with accurate positioning, the
   (A) _____ is centered within the collimated field. This is accomplished by centering a
   (B) _____ central ray to the midline of the knee at a level (C) _____ inch distal to the palpable
   (D) _____.

10. What anatomical structures are included on a Holmblad knee image with accurate positioning?

For the following descriptions of PA axial (Holmblad) knee images with poor positioning, state how the patient would have been mispositioned for such an image to be obtained.

11. The medial and lateral aspects of the intercondylar fossa are demonstrated without superimposition, and the patella is situated laterally.

---

12. The medial and lateral aspects of the intercondylar fossa are demonstrated without superimposition, the patella is situated medially, and the tibia is demonstrated without fibular head superimposition.

---

13. The proximal surfaces of the intercondylar fossa are demonstrated without superimposition, and the patella is positioned within the intercondylar fossa.

---

14. The proximal surfaces of the intercondylar fossa are demonstrated without superimposition, and the patella is positioned too far proximal to the intercondylar fossa.

---

15. The femorotibial joint is obscured, and the tibial plateau is demonstrated.

For the following PA axial (Holmblad) knee images with poor positioning, state what anatomical structures are misaligned and how the patient should be repositioned for an optimal image to be obtained.

Figure 5–68

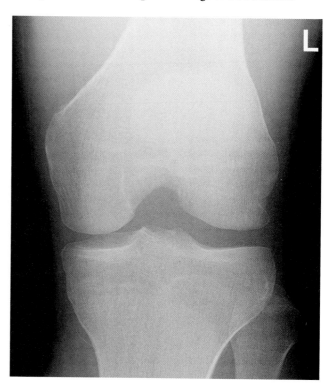

16. (Figure 5-68): _____

_____

_____

_____

Figure 5–69

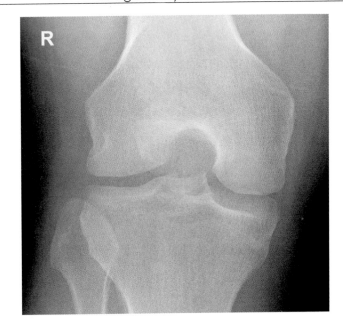

17. (Figure 5-69): _____

_____

_____

_____

Figure 5–70

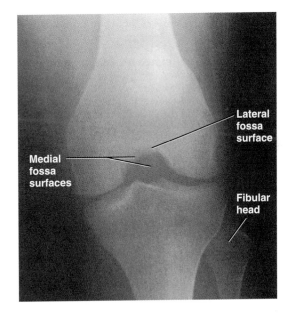

18. (Figure 5-70): _____

_____

_____

_____

Knee: Intercondylar Fossa—AP Axial Projection (Béclere Method)

1. Identify the labeled anatomy in Figure 5-71.

Figure 5–71

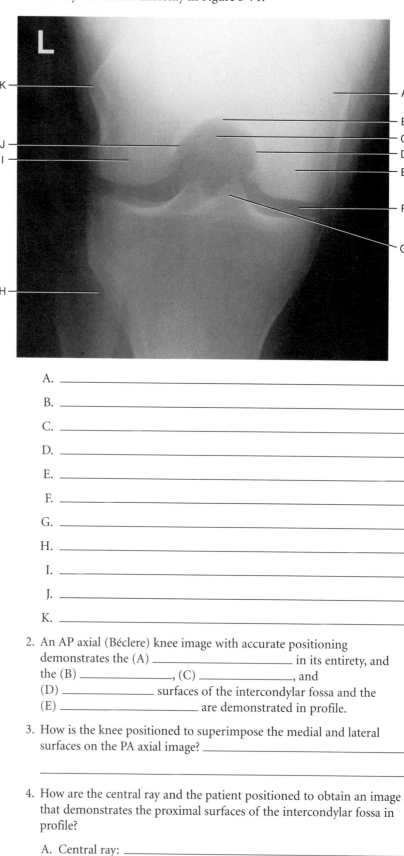

A. _____

B. _____

C. _____

D. _____

E. _____

F. _____

G. _____

H. _____

I. _____

J. _____

K. _____

2. An AP axial (Béclere) knee image with accurate positioning demonstrates the (A) _____ in its entirety, and the (B) _____, (C) _____, and (D) _____ surfaces of the intercondylar fossa and the (E) _____ are demonstrated in profile.

3. How is the knee positioned to superimpose the medial and lateral surfaces on the PA axial image? _____ _____

4. How are the central ray and the patient positioned to obtain an image that demonstrates the proximal surfaces of the intercondylar fossa in profile?

   A. Central ray: _____

   B. Patient: _____

5. As the knee is flexed, the patella shifts (A) _____ onto the patellar surface of the femur and then into the (B) _____ with increased flexion.

6. For an open knee joint space and demonstration of the intercondylar eminence and tubercles in profile, the (A) _____ and (B) _____ must be aligned parallel with each other.

7. On an AP axial (Béclere) image with accurate positioning, the (A) _____ is centered within the collimated field. This is accomplished by first positioning the central ray (B) _____ with the anterior lower leg surface, then (C) _____ the obtained angulation by 5 degrees and centering the central ray 1 inch (2.5 cm) distal to the (D) _____.

8. What anatomical structures are included on an AP axial knee image with accurate positioning?

_____

For the following descriptions of AP axial (Béclere) knee images with poor positioning, state how the patient would have been mispositioned for such an image to be obtained.

9. The medial and lateral aspects of the intercondylar fossa are not superimposed, the lateral femoral condyle is wider than the lateral condyle, and the fibular head demonstrates decreased tibial superimposition.

_____

10. The medial and lateral aspects of the intercondylar fossa are not superimposed, the medial femoral condyle is wider than the medial condyle, and the fibular head demonstrates increased tibial superimposition.

_____

11. The proximal surfaces of the intercondylar fossa are not superimposed, and the patellar apex is demonstrated within the intercondylar fossa.

_____

12. The proximal surfaces of the intercondylar fossa are not superimposed, and the patellar apex is demonstrated proximal to the intercondylar fossa.

_____

13. The knee joint space is closed, and the fibular head is shown less than ½ inch (1.25 cm) distal to the tibial plateau.

_____

14. The knee joint space is closed, and the fibular head is shown more than ½ inch (1.25 cm) distal to the tibial plateau.

_____

For the following AP axial (Béclere) knee images with poor positioning, state what anatomical structures are misaligned and how the patient should be repositioned for an optimal image to be obtained.

Figure 5–72

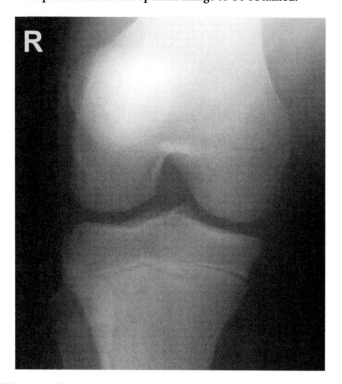

15. (Figure 5-72): _____

_____

_____

_____

Figure 5–73

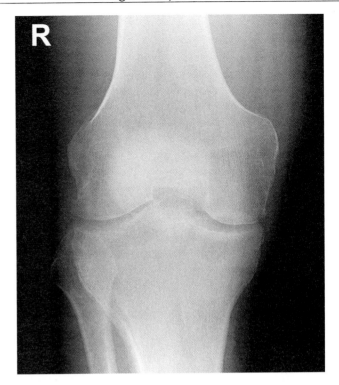

16. (Figure 5-73): _____

_____

_____

_____

Patella: Tangential (Axial) Projection (Merchant Method)

1. Identify the labeled anatomy in Figure 5-74.

Figure 5–74

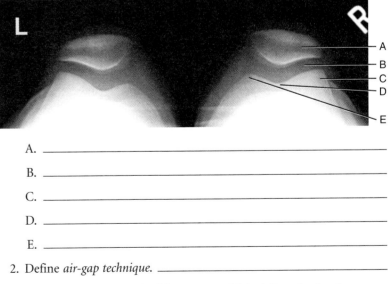

A. _____

B. _____

C. _____

D. _____

E. _____

2. Define *air-gap technique.* _____

3. Why is a grid not required for a tangential (axial) projection knee image? _____

4. What open joint spaces are demonstrated on a tangential (axial) projection knee image? _____

5. A nonrotated tangential (axial) projection knee image will demonstrate the patellae, anterior femoral condyles, and intercondylar sulci positioned (A) _____ (superiorly/laterally/medially) and the (B) _____ femoral condyle with more height than the (C) _____ condyle.

6. How are the patient's legs positioned to prevent rotation on a tangential (axial) projection knee image?

_____

7. How do the positions of the patellae and femoral condyles change when the knees are in external rotation for a tangential (axial) projection knee image?

   A. Patellae: _____

   B. Femoral condyles: _____

8. The tangential (axial) projection knee image is most often obtained to demonstrate what patient condition?

   A. _____

   How is this condition demonstrated on a tangential (axial) projection knee image with accurate positioning?

   B. _____

   How can one distinguish this condition from rotation on a tangential (axial) projection knee image?

   C. _____

9. Why is it important for the patient to relax the quadriceps femoris muscles for the tangential (axial) projection knee position?

_____

10. How are the long axes of the patient's femurs positioned to obtain a tangential (axial) projection knee image with accurate positioning?

_____

11. Where are the long axes of the long axes of the patient's posterior knee curves positioned with respect to the axial viewer for a tangential (axial) projection knee image with accurate positioning?

_____

12. How is the positioning setup for a tangential (axial) projection knee image adjusted when imaging a patient with large posterior calves?

   A. _____

_____

If this positioning setup is not changed, what anatomical misalignment appears on the resulting image?

B. _____

_____

13. What are the standard direction and degree of central ray angulation used for the tangential (axial) projection position?

_____

14. What is the sum of the central ray angle and the angle of the axial viewer for all tangential (axial) projection positions?

_____

15. Why is a 72-inch (183 cm) SID used for the tangential (axial) projection position?

_____

16. On a tangential (axial) projection knee image with accurate positioning, the _____ are centered along the longitudinal axis of the collimated field.

17. What anatomical structures are included on a tangential (axial) projection knee image with accurate positioning?

_____

For the following descriptions of tangential (axial) projection knee images with poor positioning, state how the patient would have been mispositioned for such an image to be obtained.

18. The patellae are demonstrated directly above the intercondylar sulci and rotated laterally. The medial femoral condyles demonstrate more height than the lateral condyles.

_____

19. Soft tissue from the patient's anterior thighs has been projected onto the patellae and patellofemoral joint spaces.

_____

20. The patellae are resting against the intercondylar sulci, obscuring the patellofemoral joint spaces.

_____

21. The tibial tuberosities are demonstrated within the patellofemoral joint spaces. The patient's calves were not large.

_____

For the following tangential (axial) projection knee images with poor positioning, state what anatomical structures are misaligned and how the patient should be repositioned for an optimal image to be obtained.

Figure 5–75

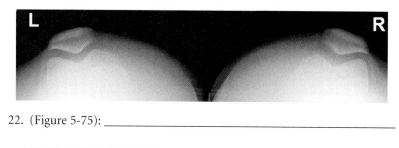

22. (Figure 5-75): _____

_____

_____

_____

Figure 5–76

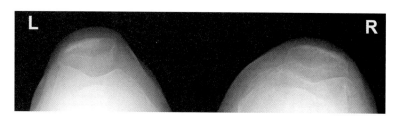

23. (Figure 5-76): _____

_____

_____

_____

Figure 5–77

24. (Figure 5-77): _____

_____

_____

_____

Figure 5–78

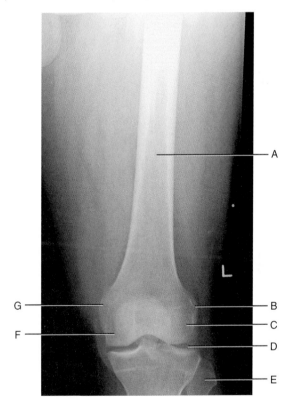

25. (Figure 5-78): _____

_____

_____

_____

Femur: AP Projection

1. Identify the labeled anatomy in Figure 5-79.

Figure 5–79

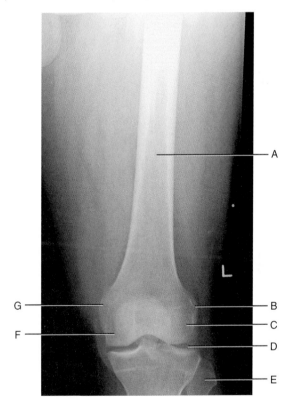

A. _____

B. _____

C. _____

D. _____

E. _____

F. _____

G. _____

2. Identify the labeled anatomy in Figure 5-80.

Figure 5–80

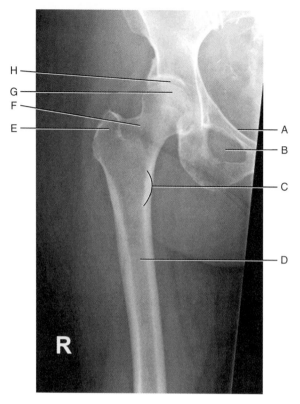

A. _____

B. _____

C. _____

D. _____

E. _____

F. _____

G. _____

H. _____

3. How is the femur positioned with respect to the x-ray tube for an AP femoral image to take advantage of the anode-heel effect? _____

_____

4. Why is it necessary to include all the femoral soft tissue when imaging the femur?

_____

5. An AP image of the distal femur demonstrates the
(A) _____ and (B) _____ femoral epicondyles in profile, symmetrical femoral condyles, and the
(C) _____ centered within the intercondylar fossa.

6. An AP distal femur is obtained by placing the patient in a
(A) _____ position with the knee (B) _____ and leg
(C) _____ rotated until the femoral epicondyles are at equal distances from the IR.

7. Should the technologist rotate a patient with a suspected fractured femur in an attempt to position the leg in an AP projection?

A. _____ (Yes/No)

Justify your answer.

B. _____

8. Why is the femorotibial joint space narrowed on an AP femoral image?

_____

9. On a distal femoral image with accurate positioning, the (A) _____ is centered within the collimated field. This centering is accomplished by positioning the lower IR edge approximately (B) _____ inches below the (C) _____ joint.

10. What anatomical structures are included on an AP distal femur image with accurate positioning?

_____

11. How can the patient be positioned to prevent pelvic rotation on an AP proximal femur image?

_____

12. How are the femoral epicondyles positioned for an AP proximal femur image?

A. _____

How will this positioning demonstrate the femoral neck and greater trochanter on the resulting image?

B. _____

13. On an AP proximal femur image with accurate positioning, the (A) _____ is centered within the collimated field. This is accomplished by placing the upper IR edge at the level of the (B) _____.

14. Why should the surrounding soft tissue be included on femoral images?

_____

15. What anatomical structures are included on an AP proximal femur image with accurate positioning?

_____

For the following descriptions of AP femoral images with poor positioning, state how the patient would have been mispositioned for such an image to be obtained.

16. The medial femoral condyle appears larger than the lateral condyle, and the intercondylar eminence is not centered within the intercondylar fossa.

_____

17. The lateral femoral condyle appears larger than the medial condyle, and the intercondylar eminence is not centered within the intercondylar fossa.

_____

18. The affected side's obturator foramen is narrowed, and the iliac spine is demonstrated without pelvic brim superimposition.

_____

19. The affected side's obturator foramen is open, and the ischial spine is not aligned with the pelvic brim but is demonstrated closer to the acetabulum.

_____

20. The femoral neck is partially foreshortened, and the lesser trochanter is demonstrated in profile.

_____

For the following AP femoral images with poor positioning, state what anatomical structures are misaligned and how the patient should be repositioned for an optimal image to be obtained.

Figure 5–81

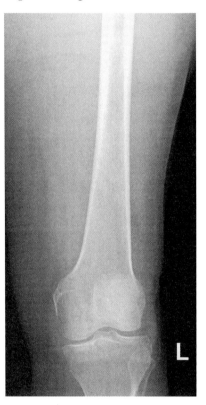

21. (Figure 5-81, distal femur): _____

_____

_____

_____

Figure 5–82

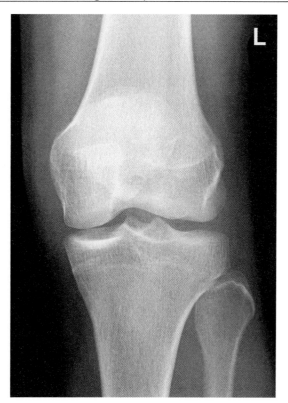

22. (Figure 5-82, distal femur): _____

_____

_____

_____

Figure 5–83

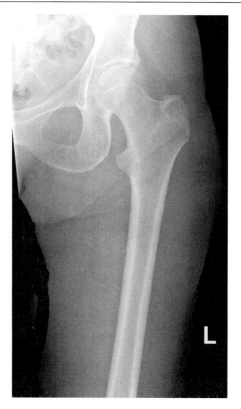

23. (Figure 5-83, proximal femur): _____

_____

_____

_____

Femur: Lateral Position (Mediolateral Projection)

1. Identify the labeled anatomy in Figure 5-84.

Figure 5–84

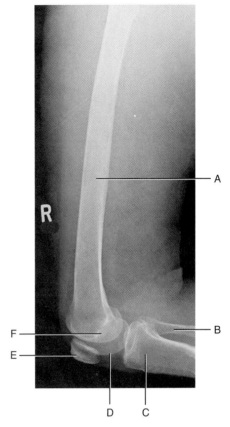

A. _____

B. _____

C. _____

D. _____

E. _____

F. _____

2. Identify the labeled anatomy in Figure 5-85.

Figure 5–85

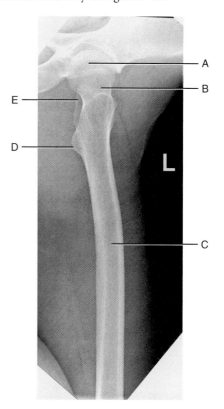

A. _____

B. _____

C. _____

D. _____

E. _____

3. Identify the labeled anatomy in Figure 5-86.

Figure 5–86

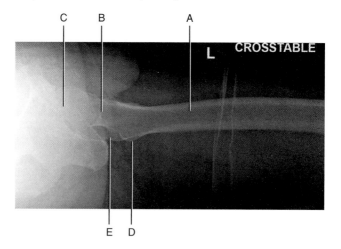

A. _____

B. _____

C. _____

D. _____

E. _____

4. To take advantage of the anode-heel effect, how is the femur positioned with respect to the x-ray tube for a lateral femur image?

_____

_____

5. A lateral distal femur image is obtained by rotating the patient onto the (A) _____ (medial/lateral) aspect of the affected femur until an imaginary line connecting the femoral epicondyles is aligned (B) _____ to the IR.

6. A distal femur image with accurate positioning demonstrates alignment of the (A) _____ and (B) _____ surfaces of the femoral condyles and demonstrates the (C) _____ with partial superimposition of the tibia.

7. Which of the femoral condyles is positioned distally on a lateral distal femur image with accurate positioning?

A. _____

What causes this distal positioning?

B. _____

C. _____

8. How is a lateral distal femur image obtained in a patient with a known or suspected femur fracture? _____

_____

9. What advantage is gained by aligning the long axis of the femoral shaft with the long axis of the collimated field? _____

10. On a lateral distal femur image with accurate positioning, the (A) _____ is centered within the collimated field. This centering is accomplished by placing the lower IR edge approximately (B) _____ inches below the (C) _____.

11. What anatomical structures are included on a lateral distal femur image with accurate positioning? _____

_____

12. How is the patient positioned to place the lesser trochanter in profile and the greater trochanter beneath the femoral neck on a lateral proximal femur image? _____

_____

13. How is the patient positioned for a lateral proximal femur image to demonstrate the femoral shaft without foreshortening and the femoral neck on end? _____

_____

14. What position is performed to demonstrate a lateral proximal femur when a fracture is suspected or known to be present? _____

_____

15. On a lateral proximal femoral image with accurate positioning, the (A) _____ is centered within the collimated field. This is accomplished by positioning the upper IR edge at the level of the (B) _____.

16. What anatomical structures are included on a lateral proximal femoral image with accurate positioning? _____

For the following descriptions of lateral femoral images with poor positioning, state how the patient would have been mispositioned for such an image to be obtained.

17. The anterior and posterior surfaces of the medial and lateral femoral condyles are demonstrated without alignment. The medial condyle is posterior to the lateral condyle.

   _____

18. The anterior and posterior surfaces of the medial and lateral femoral condyles are demonstrated without alignment. The medial condyle is anterior to the lateral condyle.

   _____

19. The greater trochanter is demonstrated medially (next to the ischial tuberosity), and the lesser trochanter is obscured.

   _____

20. The greater trochanter is demonstrated laterally, and the lesser trochanter is obscured.

   _____

For the following lateral femoral images with poor positioning, state what anatomical structures are misaligned and how the patient should be repositioned for an optimal image to be obtained.

Figure 5–87

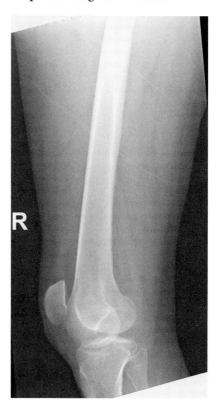

21. (Figure 5-87, distal femur): _____

_____

_____

_____

Figure 5–88

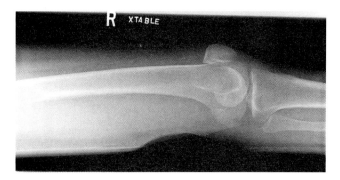

22. (Figure 5-88, trauma lateromedial distal femur): _____

_____

_____

_____

Figure 5–89

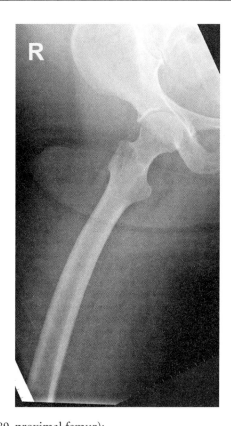

23. (Figure 5-89, proximal femur): _____

_____

_____

_____

Figure 5–90

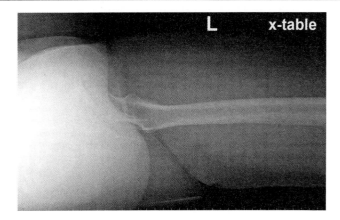

24. (Figure 5-90, proximal femur): _____

_____

_____

_____

Figure 5–91

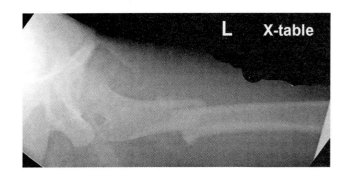

25. (Figure 5-91, trauma proximal femur): _____

_____

_____

_____

CHAPTER 5
STUDY QUESTION ANSWERS

1. A. As if the patient is hanging from the toes. The marker is correct.
   B. As if hung by the patient's hip or in an upright position. The marker is correct.
   C. As if hung by the patient's hip or in an upright position. The marker is correct.
   D. As if hung by the patient's hip or in an upright position. The marker is correct.

2. Table 5-1

Part, Position, and Projection	kVp	Grid	SID
Toe	55-65		40-48 inches (100-120 cm)
Foot	55-65		40-48 inches (100-120 cm)
Plantodorsal (axial) projection, calcaneus	65-75		40-48 inches (100-120 cm)
Lateral position, calcaneus	55-65		40-48 inches (100-120 cm)
Ankle	55-65		40-48 inches (100-120 cm)
Lower leg	65-75		40-48 inches (100-120 cm)
AP projection, knee Lateral position, knee AP oblique position, knee	Nongrid: 60-70 Grid: 65-75	If measures over 13 cm	40-48 inches (100-120 cm)
PA axial (Holmblad) position, knee	60-70		40-48 inches (100-120 cm)
AP axial (Béclere) projection, knee	60-70		40-48 inches (100-120 cm)
Tangential (axial) projection, knee	60-70		48-72 inches (120-180 cm)
Femur	70-80	Grid	40-48 inches (100-120 cm)

AP, Anteroposterior; *kVp,* kilovolt peak; *PA,* posteroanterior; *SID,* source–image receptor distance.

3. Table 5-2

Part, Position, and Projection	IR Size	Placement, Direction, and Number of Images on IR
AP, oblique, and lateral, toe	8 × 10 inches (18 × 24 cm)	Crosswise
AP and AP oblique, foot	10 × 12 inches (24 × 30 cm)	Lengthwise
Lateral, foot	8 × 10 inches (18 × 24 cm) or 10 × 12 inches (24 × 30 cm)	Diagonally or crosswise
Plantodorsal (axial) and lateral, calcaneus	8 × 10 inches (24 × 30 cm)	Crosswise
AP and AP oblique, ankle	Screen-film 10 × 12 (24 × 30 cm) Computed radiography 8 × 10 inches (18 × 24 cm)	Crosswise—two images on IR Lengthwise—one image on IR
Lateral, ankle	8 × 10 inches (18 × 24 cm) or 10 × 12 inches (24 × 30 cm)	Lengthwise
AP, lower leg	14 × 17 inches (35 × 43 cm)	Lengthwise
Lateral, lower leg	14 × 17 inches (35 × 43 cm)	Lengthwise
AP, oblique, and lateral, knee	8 × 10 inches (18 × 24 cm) or 10 × 12 inches (24 × 30 cm)	Lengthwise—one image on IR
PA axial (Holmblad) position, knee	8 × 10 inches (18 × 24 cm)	Lengthwise

Part, Position, and Projection	IR Size	Placement, Direction, and Number of Images on IR
AP axial (Béclere) projection, knee	8 × 10 inches (18 × 24 cm)	Crosswise or curved cassette
Tangential (axial) projection, knee	10 × 12 inches (24 × 30 cm) or 11 × 14 inches (28 × 35 cm)	Crosswise
AP and lateral, femur (proximal and distal)	14 × 17 inches (35 × 43 cm)	Lengthwise

AP, Anteroposterior; *IR*, image receptor; *PA*, posteroanterior.

Toe: AP Projection

4. A. Distal phalanx
   B. Distal interphalangeal joint
   C. Middle phalanx
   D. Proximal interphalangeal joint
   E. Proximal phalanx
   F. Metatarsophalangeal joint
   G. Metatarsal
5. A. Soft-tissue
   B. Midshaft
6. A. Plantar
   B. Foot
   C. Ankle
   D. Lower leg
7. A. Lateral
   B. Lateral
8. Medially
9. A. Parallel
   B. Perpendicular
10. A. Closed
    B. Foreshortened
11. A. Elevate the toe on a radiolucent sponge to bring the phalanges parallel with the IR.
    B. Angle the central ray until it is perpendicular to the phalanx of interest or parallel with the joint space of interest.
12. Collimated field
13. The toes are spread.
14. MP joint
15. The distal and proximal phalanges and half of the metatarsal
16. The foot and toe were laterally rotated.
17. The foot and toe were medially rotated.
18. The patient's toe was flexed.
19. The proximal phalanx demonstrates greater soft-tissue width and midshaft concavity on the lateral surface. The toenail is facing medially. Laterally rotate the foot and toe until they are placed flat against the IR. The IP joint space is closed, and the distal phalanx is foreshortened. Angle the central ray proximally until it is aligned perpendicular to the distal phalanx.

Toe: AP Oblique Projection

1. A. Distal phalanx
   B. Interphalangeal joint
   C. Proximal phalanx
   D. Metatarsophalangeal joint
   E. Metatarsal
   F. Tarsometatarsal joint
2. A. 45 degrees
   B. Twice as much soft-tissue width is present on the side of the digit rotated away from the IR when accurate.
3. A. Medially
   B. Laterally
   C. To obtain an oblique using the least amount of OID
4. Closed joint spaces and foreshortened phalanges
5. MP joint
6. The distal and proximal phalanges and half of the metatarsal
7. Connecting tissue between the toes
8. The patient's toe and foot were close to an AP projection.
9. The patient's toe was close to a lateral position.
10. The patient's toe was flexed, and the central ray was not aligned perpendicular to the phalanges or parallel with the joint spaces.
11. Nearly equal soft-tissue width and midshaft concavity are demonstrated on each side of the phalanges. Increase the degree of toe and foot obliquity until the affected toe is at a 45-degree angle with the IR.
12. Soft-tissue and bony overlap of the adjacent digit onto the affected digit is present. Draw the unaffected toes away from the affected toe.
13. The proximal phalanx demonstrates more concavity on the lateral aspect of the toe than the medial aspect, and more than twice as much soft tissue is shown on one side of the toe as on the other. Decrease the degree of toe and foot obliquity until the toe is at a 45-degree angle with the IR.

Toe: Lateral Position

1. A. Distal phalanx
   B. Distal interphalangeal joint
   C. Middle phalanx
   D. Proximal interphalangeal joint
   E. Proximal phalanx
   F. Metatarsophalangeal joint
   G. Metatarsal
2. A. Medially
   B. Laterally
3. A. Posterior
   B. Anterior
   C. Anterior
4. Anteriorly
5. A. PIP joint
   B. Perpendicular
   C. PIP joint
6. The distal and proximal phalanges and the MP joint space
7. The foot and toe were not rotated enough to place the toe in a lateral position.
8. The foot and toe were rotated too much to place the toe in a lateral position.
9. The adjacent unaffected digits were not drawn away from the affected digit.
10. The proximal and distal phalanges demonstrate nearly equal midshaft concavity, the condyles of the proximal phalanx are demonstrated without superimposition, and the first and second metacarpal heads are not superimposed. Increase the patient's toe and foot obliquity until the affected toe is in a lateral position.
11. The proximal phalange's condyles are not superimposed, and the metacarpal heads demonstrate slight superimposition. Decrease the patient's toe and foot obliquity until the affected toe is in a lateral position.

Foot: AP Projection (Dorsoplantar Projection)

1. A. Phalanges
   B. Metatarsals
   C. Medial cuneiform
   D. Medial-intermediate cuneiform joint
   E. Intermediate cuneiform
   F. Navicular-cuneiform joint
   G. Navicular bone
   H. Talus
   I. Calcaneus
   J. Cuboid
   K. Lateral cuneiform
   L. Fifth metatarsal tuberosity
   M. Fourth tarsometatarsal joint
   N. Fifth metatarsal base

2. A. Because of the anteroposterior thickness difference that exists between the distal and proximal foot
   B. Position a compensating filter over the phalanges and distal metatarsals.
3. A. 1
   B. Proximal
4. A. Medial
   B. Intermediate
   C. Talar
5. A. Plantar
   B. Lower leg
   C. Ankle
   D. Foot
6. No
7. Medial
8. Lateral
9. A. Tarsometatarsal
   B. Navicular-cuneiform
   C. High arch requires more angulation.
10. A. Second and third metatarsal bases
    B. ½ (1.25 cm)
    C. Fifth metatarsal tuberosity
11. Proximal calcaneus, talar neck, tarsals, metatarsals, phalanges, and surrounding soft tissue
12. The foot was laterally rotated.
13. The foot was medially rotated.
14. The central ray was not angled enough proximally.
15. The joint space between the medial and intermediate cuneiforms is closed, the navicular bone is demonstrated in profile, and less than ¾ inch (2 cm) of the calcaneus is demonstrated without talar superimposition. Rotate the foot medially until the pressure is equal over the entire plantar surface.
16. The joint space between the medial and intermediate cuneiforms is closed, the distal calcaneus is demonstrated without talar superimposition, and the metatarsal bases demonstrate decreased superimposition. Rotate the foot laterally until the pressure is equal over the entire plantar surface.

Foot: AP Oblique Projection (Medial Rotation)

1. A. Phalanges
   B. Metatarsals
   C. Medial cuneiform
   D. Lateral cuneiform
   E. Intermediate cuneiform
   F. Navicular bone
   G. Talus
   H. Tarsal sinus
   I. Calcaneus
   J. Cuboid

K. Cuboid-cuneiform joint
L. Fifth metatarsal tuberosity
M. Intermetatarsal joint
N. Fourth metatarsal base
2. A. Spaces surrounding the cuboid
   B. Second through fifth intermetatarsal joint spaces
3. Cuneiform-cuboid
4. Medially
5. A. 60 degrees
   B. 30 degrees
   C. 45 degrees
6. A. Figure 5-15
   B. The first metatarsal base is superimposed by the second and part of the third metatarsal bases.
7. A. Figure 5-15
   B. More of the cuboid is demonstrated posterior to the navicular bone in Figure 5-15 than in Figure 5-17.
8. A. First
   B. Second
   C. Closer to
9. A. Fourth metatarsal tubercle
   B. The fifth metatarsal will be superimposed over the fourth metatarsal tubercle.
10. A. Third metatarsal base
    B. Perpendicular
    C. Midline
    D. Fifth tuberosity
11. The phalanges, metatarsals, tarsals, calcaneus, and surrounding soft tissue
12. The patient's foot was positioned too close to an AP projection.
13. The patient's foot was positioned too close to a lateral position.
14. The lateral cuneiform-cuboid, navicular-cuboid, and third through fifth intermetatarsal joint spaces are closed. The fifth metatarsal is not superimposed over the fourth metatarsal tubercle. Increase the degree of medial foot obliquity.

Foot: Lateral Position (Mediolateral and Lateromedial Projections)

1. A. Fibula
   B. Calcaneus
   C. Cuboid
   D. Metatarsals
   E. Phalanges
   F. Cuneiforms
   G. Navicular bone
   H. Talus
   I. Tibiotalar joint
   J. Tibia

2. A. Evasion of fluid into a joint
   B. Act of moving the forefoot superiorly
   C. Sole of the foot
   D. Act of moving the forefoot inferiorly
3. Lateral
4. A. Posterior pericapsular located within indention formed by the articulation of the posterior tibia and talar bone
   B. Anterior pretalar located anterior to the ankle joint, next to the talus
5. A. Superimposed
   B. Tibiotalar
   C. Distal fibula
6. Position the lower leg parallel with the imaging table.
7. A. Position the long axis of the foot at a 90-degree angle with the lower leg.
   B. Position the lateral foot surface parallel with the IR.
8. A. The medial talar dome would be demonstrated distal to the lateral talar dome.
   B. Elevate the distal lower leg and ankle until the lower leg is parallel with the imaging table.
9. A. Posterior
   B. Navicular bone
10. ½ (1.25 cm)
11. A. Less
    B. More
12. Talar domes
13. The most medial and lateral aspects of the talar's trochlear surface
14. A. Leg
    B. Foot
15. This question can be answered two different ways:
    A. Medial   A. Lateral
    B. Proximal   B. Distal
    C. Lateral   C. Medial
    D. Higher   D. Higher
16. This question can be answered two different ways:
    A. Medial   A. Lateral
    B. Distal   B. Proximal
    C. Lateral   C. Medial
    D. Lower   D. Lower
17. Lateral
18. This question can be answered two different ways:
    A. Medial   A. Lateral
    B. Posterior   B. Anterior
    C. Lateral   C. Medial
    D. Anterior   D. Anterior
19. This question can be answered two different ways:
    A. Medial   A. Lateral
    B. Anterior   B. Posterior
    C. Lateral   C. Medial
    D. Posterior   D. Posterior
20. A. It demonstrates the anterior pretalar fat pad without forced flattening.
    B. It places the tibiotalar joint in a neutral position.
    C. It prevents anterior foot rotation.

21. A. Medial
    B. Lateral
22. Move the patient's heel away from the IR.
23. A. Proximal metatarsals
    B. Perpendicular
    C. Heel
24. The phalanges, metatarsals, tarsals, talus, calcaneus, 1 inch (2.5 cm) of the distal lower leg, and the surrounding foot soft tissue
25. The proximal lower leg was elevated higher than the distal lower leg.
26. The distal lower leg was elevated higher than the proximal lower leg.
27. The heel was elevated, and the forefoot was depressed.
28. The heel was depressed, and the forefoot was elevated.
29. The lower leg and long axis of the foot do not form a 90-degree angle. The patient's foot was in plantar flexion. Dorsiflex the foot until the lower leg and long axis of the foot form a 90-degree angle.
30. The medial talar dome is positioned posterior to the lateral dome, and the distal fibula is anterior on the tibia. Depress the patient's forefoot and elevate the heel (external leg rotation) until the lateral foot surface is parallel with the IR.

Calcaneus: Plantodorsal (Axial) Projection

1. A. Talus
   B. Talocalcaneal joint
   C. Sustentaculum tali
   D. Tuberosity
   E. Fifth metatarsal base
2. A. Talocalcaneal
   B. Calcaneal tuberosity
3. A. Vertical
   B. 40
   C. Plantar
4. A. Parallel
   B. Perpendicular
5. A. Increase the degree of central ray angulation.
   B. Decrease the degree of central ray angulation.
6. Base of the fifth metatarsal and distal point of the fibula.
7. Along the lateral foot surface approximately halfway between the ball of the foot and the heel
8. A. Place the ankle in an AP projection without medial or lateral rotation.
   B. The first metatarsal will be demonstrated medially, or the fourth and fifth metatarsals will be demonstrated laterally.
9. A. Proximal calcaneal tuberosity
   B. Fifth metatarsal base
10. The calcaneal tuberosity and talocalcaneal joint

11. A. Tight collimation
    B. Lead masking
    C. No overlap of individual exposures
12. Foot was dorsiflexed beyond the vertical position.
13. The foot was in plantar flexion.
14. The leg and ankle were medially rotated.
15. The leg and ankle were laterally rotated.
16. The second through fifth metatarsals are demonstrated laterally. Internally rotate the leg until the ankle is in an AP projection.
17. The talocalcaneal joint space is obscured and the calcaneal tuberosity is foreshortened. If the patient's condition allows, dorsiflex the foot to a vertical, neutral position. If the patient cannot dorsiflex the foot, increase the central ray angulation, aligning the central ray with the fifth metatarsal base and the distal point of the fibula.
18. The talocalcaneal joint space is obscured, and the calcaneal tuberosity is elongated. The foot was dorsiflexed beyond the vertical position, and a 40-degree central angulation was used. Plantar-flex the foot to a vertical position, and use a 40-degree angulation.

Calcaneus: Lateral Position (Mediolateral Projection)

1. A. Tibiotalar joint
   B. Talar domes
   C. Calcaneus
   D. Tuberosity
   E. Talocalcaneal joint
   F. Cuboid
   G. Navicular bone
   H. Talus
   I. Tibia
2. A. Superimposed
   B. Tibiotalar
   C. Posterior
   D. Tibia
3. Parallel with the imaging table
4. A. Position the long axis of the foot at a 90-degree angle with the lower leg.
   B. Position the lateral foot surface parallel with the IR.
5. The medial talar dome would be demonstrated distal to the lateral talar dome.
6. A. Posterior
   B. Navicular bone
7. ½ (1.25 cm)
8. A. Less
   B. More
9. Talar domes
10. The most medial and lateral aspects of the talar's trochlear surface

11. A. Leg
    B. Foot
12. This question can be answered two different ways:
    A. Medial   A. Lateral
    B. Proximal   B. Distal
    C. Lateral   C. Medial
    D. Higher   D. Higher
13. This question can be answered two different ways:
    A. Medial   A. Lateral
    B. Distal   B. Proximal
    C. Lateral   C. Medial
    D. Lower   D. Lower
14. This question can be answered two different ways:
    A. Medial   A. Lateral
    B. Posterior   B. Anterior
    C. Lateral   C. Medial
    D. Anterior   D. Anterior
15. This question can be answered two different ways:
    A. Medial   A. Lateral
    B. Anterior   B. Posterior
    C. Lateral   C. Medial
    D. Posterior   D. Posterior
16. Anterior
17. A. Midcalcaneus
    B. Perpendicular
    C. Distal
    D. Medial malleolus
18. The tibiotalar joint, talus, calcaneus, and calcaneal articulating tarsal bones
19. A. Medial malleolus
    B. Medial malleolus
20. The proximal tibia was elevated.
21. The distal tibia was elevated.
22. The forefoot was depressed, and the heel was elevated (leg externally rotated).
23. The forefoot was elevated, and the heel was depressed (leg internally rotated).
24. The medial talar dome is anterior to the lateral talar dome, and the fibula is too posterior on the tibia. Elevate the forefoot and depress the heel until the lateral foot surface is parallel with the IR.
25. The foot is plantar-flexed, the medial talar dome is posterior and distal to the lateral talar dome, the fibula is too anterior on the tibia, and less than ½ inch (1.25 cm) of the cuboid is demonstrated posterior to the navicular bone. Dorsiflex the foot to a 90-degree angle with the lower leg, depress the forefoot and elevate the heel (externally rotate leg) until the lateral foot surface is parallel with the IR, and depress the proximal lower leg until it is parallel with the imaging table.
26. The lateral talar dome is posterior and proximal to the medial talar dome, the fibula is too far posterior on the tibia, and more than ½ inch (1.25 cm) of the cuboid is demonstrated posterior to the navicular bone. Internally rotate the leg until the lateral foot surface is parallel with the IR

and elevate the proximal lower leg until it is parallel with the IR.

Ankle: AP Projection

1. A. Tibia
   B. Medial malleolus
   C. Medial mortise
   D. Talus
   E. Lateral malleolus
   F. Tibiotalar joint
   G. Fibula
2. A. Imaginary line drawn between the medial and lateral malleoli
   B. Joint space formed between the fibula and talus
   C. Joint space formed between the lateral tibia and talus
3. A. Tibiotalar
   B. Medial mortise
4. Medial malleolus
5. The tibia is superimposed over the fibula.
6. 15 to 20 degrees
7. The tibia and talus will demonstrate increased superimposition of the fibula, and the medial mortise will be closed.
8. The lower leg should be positioned parallel with the IR.
9. The tibiotalar joint space will be closed or narrowed, and the anterior tibial margin will be projected distally.
10. A. Tibiotalar joint
    B. Perpendicular
    C. Medial malleolus
11. The distal one fourth of the tibia and fibula, talus, and surrounding ankle soft tissue
12. The ankle was laterally rotated.
13. The ankle was medially rotated.
14. The proximal tibia was elevated, or the central ray was centered too proximally.
15. The medial mortise is obscured, the tibia and talus demonstrate increased superimposition of the fibula, and the posterior aspect of the medial malleolus is situated medial to the anterior aspect. Rotate the leg internally, placing the long axis of the foot in a vertical position.
16. The talus is demonstrated without fibular superimposition. Externally rotate the leg until the long axis of the foot is vertical.

Ankle: AP Oblique Projection (Internal Rotation: 15- to 20-Degree Mortise and 45-Degree Oblique)

1. A. Fibula
   B. Lateral malleolus
   C. Lateral mortise
   D. Calcaneus

E. Talus

F. Medial mortise

G. Medial malleolus

H. Tibiotalar joint

I. Tibia

2. Opening between the calcaneus and talus

3. A. Tibial

B. Talofibular

C. Lateral

4. A. 15 to 20 degrees

B. Medially (internally)

5. A. Closed

B. Without

6. Position the lower leg parallel with the imaging table.

7. The anterior tibial margin will be projected too far superior to the posterior margin, expanding the tibiotalar joint space.

8. Dorsiflex the foot to a 90-degree angle with the lower leg.

9. A. Tibiotalar joint

B. Perpendicular

C. Medial malleolus

10. The distal one fourth of the fibula and tibia, talus, and surrounding ankle soft tissue

11. The patient's leg and ankle were underrotated.

12. The patient's leg and ankle were overrotated.

13. The patient's leg and ankle were internally rotated more than 45 degrees.

14. The distal tibia was elevated, or the central ray was positioned distal to the joint space.

15. The foot was in plantar flexion.

16. The calcaneus is obscuring the distal aspect of the lateral mortise and the distal fibula. Dorsiflex the foot until its long axis forms a 90-degree angle with the lower leg.

17. The lateral mortise is closed, the medial mortise is open, and the tarsal sinus is not demonstrated. Increase the degree of internal (medial) leg rotation until the most prominent aspects of the malleoli are positioned at equal distances from the IR.

18. The medial mortise is partially closed, the fibula is demonstrated without tibial superimposition, and the tarsal sinus is partially shown. Decrease the degree of internal (medial) leg rotation until the malleoli are positioned at equal distances from the IR.

19. The lateral and medial mortises are closed, and the tarsal sinus is demonstrated. Rotate the leg laterally until the long axis of the foot is at a 45-degree angle with the IR.

20. The lateral and medial mortises are closed, and the tarsal sinus is demonstrated. Rotate the leg laterally until the long axis of the foot is at a 45-degree angle with the IR.

Ankle: Lateral Position (Mediolateral Projection)

1. A. Fibula

B. Tibiotalar joint

C. Talar domes

D. Calcaneus

E. Talocancaneal joint

F. Cuboid

G. Fifth metatarsal tuberosity

H. Navicular bone

I. Talus

J. Tibia

2. A. Anterior to the ankle joint

B. Within the indention formed by the joint of the posterior tibia and talar bone

3. Displacement of these pads may indicate underlying injuries and joint effusion.

4. A. Superimposed

B. Tibiotalar

C. Posterior

D. Tibia

5. A. Parallel

B. Lateral

6. A. Posterior

B. Navicular

C. ½ (1.25 cm)

D. ¾ (2 cm)

E. ¼ (0.6 cm)

7. The most medial and lateral aspects of the talar's trochlear surface

8. Proximal-distal

9. This question can be answered two different ways:

A. Medial	A. Lateral
B. Proximal	B. Distal
C. Lateral	C. Medial
D. Higher	D. Higher

10. This question can be answered two different ways:

A. Medial	A. Lateral
B. Distal	B. Proximal
C. Lateral	C. Medial
D. Lower	D. Lower

11. Anteroposterior

12. This question can be answered two different ways:

A. Medial	A. Lateral
B. Posterior	B. Anterior
C. Lateral	C. Medial
D. Anterior	D. Anterior

13. This question can be answered two different ways:

A. Medial	A. Lateral
B. Anterior	B. Posterior
C. Lateral	C. Medial
D. Posterior	D. Posterior

14. A. It allows the anterior pretalar fat pad to be used to detect joint effusion.

B. It places the ankle joint in a neutral position.

C. It prevents the patient from rotating anteriorly.

15. A. Tibiotalar joint
     B. Perpendicular
     C. Medial malleolus
16. The talus, 1 inch (2.5 cm) of the fifth metatarsal base, surrounding ankle soft tissue, and distal one fourth of the fibula and tibia
17. A fracture of the fifth metatarsal base that results from inversion of the foot
18. So the fifth metatarsal base will be included on the image to rule out a Jones fracture
19. The proximal lower leg was elevated.
20. The distal lower leg was elevated.
21. The heel was elevated, and the forefoot was depressed.
22. The heel was depressed, and the forefoot was elevated.
23. The foot is plantar-flexed. Dorsiflex the foot until the long axis of the foot forms a 90-degree angle with the lower leg.
24. The lateral talar dome is demonstrated distal to the medial dome, more than ½ inch (1.25 cm) of the cuboid is demonstrated posterior to the navicular bone, and the talocalcaneal joint is widened. Depress the distal lower leg until the lower leg is aligned parallel with the IR.
25. The lateral talar dome is proximal to the medial dome. Less than ¾ inch (2 cm) of the cuboid is demonstrated posterior to the navicular bone, and the talocalcaneal joint is narrowed. Elevate the distal lower leg until the lower leg is parallel with the IR.
26. The lateral talar dome is demonstrated anterior to the medial dome and the fibula is too far anterior on the tibia. Depress the forefoot (externally rotate leg) until the lateral surface of the foot is aligned parallel with the IR.
27. The lateral talar dome is posterior to the medial dome, and the fibula is posterior on the tibia. Adjust the central ray anteriorly until it is aligned perpendicular to the lateral aspect of the foot or 10 degrees (the domes are physically approximately 1 inch (2.5 cm) apart and are off by ¼ (0.6 cm) inch on image, with a needed 5-degree angulation adjustment for every ⅛ inch (0.3 cm) that the domes are off).
28. The lateral talar dome is proximal and anterior to the medial talar dome.
     Patient: Adjust the distal lower leg ⅛ inch (0.3 cm) away from to the IR (need to move half the distance the talar domes are off), and externally rotate the ankle and leg ⅛ inch (0.3 cm) or until the lateral foot surface is parallel with the IR.
     Central ray: Adjust the central ray distally and posteriorly 5 degrees for every ⅛ inch (0.3 cm) the domes are off anterior-posteriorly and proximal-distally, respectively (10 degrees proximally and anteriorly).

Lower Leg: AP Projection

1. A. Intercondylar fossa
    B. Lateral femoral condyle
    C. Fibular head
    D. Fibula
    E. Tibia
    F. Intercondylar eminence
    G. Medial femoral condyle
2. Position the ankle toward the anode end of the tube and the knee toward the cathode end.
3. A. Extending
    B. Internally
    C. Femoral epicondyles
4. Medial
5. A. The tibia is partially superimposed over the fibular head.
    B. The tibia and fibula are demonstrated without superimposition.
    C. The distal tibia and talus are partially superimposed over the fibula.
6. A. The fibula will be demonstrated with reduced or without tibial superimposition.
    B. The fibula will be demonstrated with reduced or without tibial and talar superimposition.
7. Place the knee in an AP projection and allow the ankle to be positioned as is.
8. A. Yes
    B. The proximal tibia slopes in the opposite direction as the diverged x-rays, and the distal tibia does not slope at the same degree as the diverged x-rays. If the x-ray divergence and joints are not parallel, the joints will be closed.
9. To ensure that the diverged beams used to record the ankle and knee will be included on the image
10. A. Medial malleolus
    B. Distal
    C. Femoral epicondyles
11. Tibial midshaft
12. The tibia, fibula, ankle and knee joints, and surrounding lower leg soft tissue
13. The patient's leg was externally rotated.
14. The patient's leg was internally rotated.
15. The distal lower leg has been clipped and the distal and proximal fibula are free of talar superimposition. Move the central ray and IR 1 inch (2.5 cm) distally and laterally rotate the patient's leg until the femoral epicondyles are positioned at equal distances from the IR.

Lower Leg: Lateral Position (Mediolateral Projection)

1. A. Medial femoral condyle
    B. Fibula
    C. Talar domes
    D. Tibia

2. Position the distal lower leg at the anode end of the tube and the proximal lower leg at the cathode end.
3. Lateral
4. A. The tibia is partially superimposed over the fibular head.
   B. The tibia and fibula are free of superimposition.
   C. The distal fibula is superimposed by the posterior half of the distal tibia.
5. A. The fibula will be demonstrated with reduced or without tibial superimposition.
   B. The fibula will be demonstrated with reduced or without tibial superimposition.
6. A. No
   B. Yes
7. Place the ankle in a lateral position, and allow the knee to be positioned as is.
8. At least 1 inch
9. Tibial midshaft
10. The tibia, fibula, ankle and knee joints, and surrounding lower leg soft tissue
11. The patient's leg was rotated too far anteriorly.
12. The patient's leg was rotated too far posteriorly.
13. The fibula is superimposed by the tibia. Rotate the patient's leg externally.
14. The fibular head is demonstrated without tibia superimposition, and the fibula is demonstrated too posterior on the tibia. Rotate the patient's leg internally.

Knee: AP Projection

1. A. Patella
   B. Lateral epicondyle
   C. Lateral condyle
   D. Intercondylar eminence
   E. Fibular head
   F. Femur
   G. Femorotibial joint
   H. Medial epicondyles
   I. Femur
2. Structure that is curved or rounded outward
3. 13
4. A. Medial
   B. Lateral
   C. Intercondylar eminence
5. A. Extended
   B. Internally
   C. Equal distances
6. The proximal tibia is superimposed over the proximal fibula.
7. Farther away
8. The medial condyle will appear larger than the lateral condyle, and the head, neck, and possibly the shaft of the fibula will be superimposed by the tibia.

9. A. Femorotibial
   B. Superimposed
   C. ½ (1.25 cm)
10. Parallel with it
11. The tibial plateau slopes approximately 5 degrees anterior to posterior.
12. The thicker the upper thigh, the more the leg slopes down toward the IR and the more distal the anterior tibial margin and proximal the posterior tibial margin will move.
13. No
14. A. 5 degrees cephalic
    B. 5 degrees caudal
15. A. The fibular head will be foreshortened and demonstrated more than ½ inch (1.25 cm) distal to the tibial plateau.
    B. The fibular head will be elongated and demonstrated less than ½ inch (1.25 cm) distal to the tibial plateau.
16. A. Lateral compartment
    B. Medial compartment
17. Valgus
18. Decrease the angulation approximately 5 degrees to align it with the tibial plateau.
19. The patella lies just superior to the patellar surface of the femur and is situated slightly lateral to the knee midline.
20. A. Distally
    B. Medially
    C. Laterally
21. A. It is demonstrated superior to the patellar surface.
    B. It is demonstrated on the patellar surface.
    C. It is demonstrated between the patellar surface and intercondylar fossa.
22. A. It is demonstrated farther laterally than it would be demonstrated on a nonsubluxed knee image.
    B. Lateral (external)
    C. When the patella is subluxed, the condyles will remain symmetrical and the tibia will be superimposed over the fibular head. Rotation will alter these two relationships.
23. A. Femorotibial joint
    B. 1 (2.5 cm)
    C. Distal
    D. Medial epicondyle
24. One fourth of the distal femur and proximal lower leg and surrounding knee soft tissue
25. The patient's leg was externally (laterally) rotated.
26. The patient's leg was internally (medially) rotated.
27. The central ray was angled too cephalically.
28. The central ray was angled too caudally.
29. The femorotibial joint space is obscured, the fibular head is more than ½ inch (1.25 cm) distal to the tibial plateau, and the fibular head is foreshortened. Adjust the central ray angulation 5 degrees caudally.

30. The femorotibial joint space is obscured, the fibular head is less than ½ inch (1.25 cm) distal to the tibial plateau, and the fibular head is elongated. Adjust the central ray angulation 5 degrees cephalically.
31. The medial femoral condyle appears larger than the lateral condyle, and the head, neck, and shaft of the fibula are almost entirely superimposed by the tibia. Internally rotate the patient's leg until the femoral epicondyles are at equal distances from the IR. The femorotibial joint space is obscured, and the fibular head is less than ½ inch (1.25 cm) distal to the tibial plateau. Adjust the central ray angulation 5 degrees cephalically.
32. The lateral femoral condyle appears larger than the medial condyle, and the tibia demonstrates very little superimposition of the fibular head. Externally rotate the patient's leg until the femoral epicondyles are at equal distances from the IR.
33. Angle the central ray until it is perpendicular to the anterior surface of the lower leg, then adjust the angle 5 degrees distally, aligning the central ray with the tibial plateau.

Knee: AP Oblique Projection (Internal and External Rotation)

1. A. Femur
   B. Patella
   C. Medial condyle
   D. Tibia
   E. Fibular head
   F. Tibiofibular joint
   G. Femorotibial joint
   H. Lateral condyle
2. A. Femur
   B. Medial condyle
   C. Tibia
   D. Fibula
   E. Femorotibial joint
   F. Lateral condyle
   G. Patella
3. 45
4. A. The fibular head should be demonstrated without tibial superimposition.
   B. Lateral
5. The femoral condyles will be nearly superimposed.
6. A. The fibula is superimposed by the tibia, and the fibular head is aligned with the anterior edge of the tibia.
   B. Medial
7. The fibular head will be aligned with the anterior edge of the tibia, but will be positioned posterior to this placement.
8. A. Femorotibial
   B. Superimposed
C. ½
D. Distal
9. A. Angle 5 degrees caudally
   B. The patient's hip is often elevated to accomplish the degree of needed internal obliquity.
   C. The patient's hip is placed closer to the imaging table to obtain the needed external obliquity.
10. A. Femorotibial joint
    B. Midline of the knee
    C. Knee joint
11. One fourth of the distal femur and proximal lower leg and surrounding knee soft tissue
12. The patient's knee was rotated less than 45 degrees.
13. The patient's knee was rotated more than 45 degrees.
14. The patient's knee was rotated less than 45 degrees.
15. The central ray was angled too cephalically.
16. The tibia is partially superimposed over the fibular head. Increase the degree of internal knee obliquity until an imaginary line connecting the femoral epicondyles is aligned at a 45-degree angle with the IR.
17. The fibular head, neck, and shaft are not entirely superimposed by the tibia. Increase the degree of external knee obliquity until an imaginary line connecting the femoral epicondyles is aligned at a 45-degree angle with the IR.
19. The fibular head is not aligned with the anterior edge of the tibia but is situated posterior to this placement. Decrease the degree of external knee rotation until the femoral epicondyles are aligned at a 45-degree angle with the IR.

Knee: Lateral Position (Mediolateral Projection)

1. A. Femur
   B. Femoral condyles
   C. Intercondylar eminence
   D. Fibular head
   E. Fibular neck
   F. Tibia
   G. Femorotibial joint
   H. Patellofemoral joint
   I. Patella
2. When the knee measures over 5 inches (13 cm)
3. A. Anterior suprapatellar fat pad
   B. Posterior suprapatellar fat pad
4. When the knee is flexed more than 20 degrees, the muscles and tendons tighten, forcing the patella to come in contact with the patellar surface of the femur and obscuring the fat pads.

5. A. Parallel
   B. Medially
   C. 10 to 15
   D. Wide
   E. Short
6. A. Medial
   B. Distal
   C. Lateral
7. A. 5 to 7
   B. Medial
   C. Reduced
8. A. Locate the adductor tubercle on the posterior aspect of the medial condyle.
   B. Locate the distal articulating surface that is the flattest. It is the lateral condyle.
9. When the leg is laterally abducted
10. A. The tibia will be partially superimposed over the fibular head.
    B. The fibula will be demonstrated free of tibial superimposition.
11. Because it is situated farthest from the IR
12. Adjust the angle approximately 5 degrees for every ¼ inch (0.6 cm) of distance demonstrated between the distal surfaces of the condyles.
13. A. Posteriorly
    B. Medial
14. The proximal tibia is superimposed over the proximal fibula.
15. The fibula will be demonstrated with decreased or without tibial superimposition.
16. The fibula will be demonstrated with increased or complete tibial superimposition.
17. A. Femorotibial joint
    B. 1 (2.5 cm)
    C. Distal
    D. Medial epicondyle
18. One fourth of the distal femur and proximal lower leg and surrounding knee soft tissue
19. The patient's knee was overflexed.
20. The central ray was angled too caudally.
21. The central ray was angled too cephalically.
22. The patient's patella was situated too far away from the IR (leg internally rotated).
23. The patient's patella was situated too close to the IR (leg externally rotated).
24. The patient's knee is overflexed; the patella is in contact with the patellar surface of the femur. The marker is superimposed over the soft-tissue structures. Decrease the degree of knee flexion to meet your facility's requirements. Move the marker off of the soft-tissue structures.
25. The medial femoral condyle is anterior to the lateral condyle. Rotate the patella farther away from the IR (internal leg rotation).
26. The medial femoral condyle is posterior to the lateral condyle. Rotate the patella closer to the IR (external leg rotation).
27. The medial femoral condyle is proximal to the lateral condyle and the tibiofibular joint is visualized. Adjust the central ray angle 5 to 7 degrees caudally.
28. The knee is overflexed; the patella demonstrates a fracture. If a patellar or other knee fracture is suspected, the knee should remain extended to prevent displacement of bony fragments or vascular injury.
29. The medial femoral condyle is anterior to the lateral condyle. Rotate the knee internally until the femoral epicondyles are parallel with the imaging table or the cart on which the patient is lying, or adjust the central ray anteriorly until it is aligned parallel with the femoral epicondyles.
30. The medial femoral condyle is distal to the lateral condyle. Adduct the patient's leg until the epicondyles are perpendicular to the IR, or rotate the x-ray tube toward the patient's feet, adjusting the central ray caudally (moves the lateral condyle toward the medial condyle).

Knee: Intercondylar Fossa—PA Axial Projection (Holmblad Method)

1. A. Lateral fossa surfaces
   B. Lateral epicondyle
   C. Lateral condyle
   D. Tibial condylar margin
   E. Fibular head
   F. Intercondylar eminence
   G. Femorotibial joint
   H. Medial condyle
   I. Medial epicondyle
   J. Medial fossa surfaces
   K. Intercondylar fossa
   L. Proximal fossa surfaces
2. A. Proximal
   B. Medial
   C. Lateral
3. A. Allow the femur to incline medially approximately 10 to 15 degrees.
   B. Position the long axis of the foot perpendicular to the imaging table.
4. A. The patella rotates laterally.
   B. The patella rotates medially.
5. A. 20 to 30
   B. 60 to 70
6. Distally
7. Distally
8. A. The posterior tibial margin is distal to the anterior tibial margin.
   B. Dorsiflex the foot until its long axis is aligned perpendicular to the imaging table.
   C. Femorotibial
   D. Intercondylar eminence
   E. Tubercles

9. A. Intercondylar fossa
   B. Perpendicular
   C. 1
   D. Medial femoral epicondyle
10. The distal femur, proximal tibia and intercondylar fossa, eminence, and tubercles
11. The femur was too vertical, or the heel was rotated medially.
12. The patient's heel was laterally rotated.
13. The patient's knee was overflexed; the femur was too close to vertical.
14. The patient's knee was underflexed; the femur was more than 20 to 30 degrees from vertical.
15. The foot was in plantar-flexion.
16. The proximal surfaces of the intercondylar fossa are demonstrated without superimposition, and the patellar apex is positioned at the intercondylar fossa. Unflex the knee, positioning the proximal femur closer to the imaging table. The femorotibial joint is closed, and the fibular head is slightly more than ½ inch (1.25 cm) from the tibial plateau. Increase the degree of foot dorsiflexion, elevating the distal lower leg.
17. The femorotibial joint is obscured, the tibial plateau is demonstrated, and the fibular head is less than ½ inch (1.25 cm) from the tibial plateau. Plantar-flex the foot, lowering the distal lower leg.
18. The medial and the lateral aspects of the intercondylar fossa are not superimposed, the patella is situated medially, and the tibia is demonstrated without fibular head superimposition. The knee joint is obscured, the tibial plateau is demonstrated, and the fibula is positioned closer than ½ inch (1.25 cm) closer to the tibial plateau. Rotate the heel medially until the foot's long axis is aligned perpendicular to the imaging table, and depress the distal lower leg by decreasing the amount of foot dorsiflexion.

Knee: Intercondylar Fossa—AP Axial Projection (Béclere Method)

1. A. Medial epicondyle
   B. Proximal intercondylar fossa surfaces
   C. Intercondylar fossa
   D. Medial intercondylar fossa surfaces
   E. Medial Femoral condyle
   F. Femorotibial joint space
   G. Intercondylar eminence
   H. Fibular head
   I. Lateral condyle
   J. Lateral intercondylar fossa surfaces
   K. Lateral epicondyle
2. A. Intercondylar Fossa
   B. Medial

C. Lateral
D. Proximal
E. Femoral epicondyles
3. Internally rotated to AP projection, with femoral epicondyles parallel with the imaging table
4. A. Femur position at a 60-degree angle with the imaging table
   B. Central ray aligned with tibial plateau
5. A. Distally
   B. Intercondylar fossa
6. A. Central ray
   B. Tibial plateau
7. A. Intercondylar fossa
   B. Perpendicular
   C. Decreasing
   D. Medial femoral condyle
8. Distal femur, proximal tibia, and intercondylar fossa, eminences, and tubercles
9. The patient's leg was internally rotated.
10. The patient's leg was externally rotated.
11. The femur was angled more than 60 degrees with the imaging table.
12. The femur was angled less than 60 degrees with the imaging table.
13. The distal lower leg was depressed, or the central ray was angled too caudally.
14. The distal lower leg was elevated too high, or the central ray was angled too cephalically.
15. The medial and the lateral aspects of the intercondylar fossa are not superimposed, the medial femoral condyle is wider than the lateral condyle, and the fibular head demonstrates increased tibial superimposition. Internally rotate the leg until an imaginary line connecting the femoral epicondyles is aligned parallel with the imaging table.
16. The proximal surfaces of the intercondylar fossa are not superimposed, and the patellar apex is demonstrated within the intercondylar fossa. Decrease the degree of hip and knee flexion until the long axis of the femur is aligned 60 degrees with the imaging table. The femorotibial joint is closed, and the fibular head is demonstrated less than ½ inch (1.25 cm) distal to the tibial plateau. Elevate the distal lower leg until the knee is flexed 45 degrees, or adjust the central ray cephalically.

Patella: Tangential (Axial) Projection (Merchant Method)

1. A. Patella
   B. Patellofemoral joint
   C. Anterolateral femoral condyle
   D. Intercondylar sulcus
   E. Anteromedial femoral condyle
2. Technique in which a large OID is used and scatter radiation misses the IR

3. Because a long OID is used
4. Patellofemoral joint spaces
5. A. Superiorly
   B. Lateral
   C. Medial
6. Internally rotate the legs, and secure them by wrapping the Velcro straps of the axial viewer around the patient's calves.
7. A. They will be situated laterally.
   B. The condyles will demonstrate equal heights, or the medial condyle will demonstrate more height than the lateral condyle.
8. A. Patellar subluxation
   B. The patella will be demonstrated laterally.
   C. The intercondylar sulci will remain facing superiorly on a subluxed patella but not on a rotated one.
9. Because tightening of the quadriceps muscles will prevent patella subluxation from being demonstrated
10. Parallel with the imaging table
11. Directly above the bend of the axial viewer until the knees are flexed 45 degrees
12. A. Decrease the angulation set on the axial viewer, or increase the central ray angulation 5 to 10 degrees.
    B. The tibial tuberosities will be demonstrated within the patellofemoral joint spaces.
13. 60 degrees caudally
14. 105 degrees
15. To offset the magnification caused by the large OID
16. Patellofemoral joints
17. The patellae, anterior femoral condyles, and intercondylar sulci
18. The patient's legs were externally rotated.
19. The height of the axial viewer was not set high enough to position the long axes of the femurs parallel with the imaging table.
20. The posterior knee curve was positioned at or below the bend of the axial viewer.
21. The posterior knee curve was positioned too far above the bend of the axial viewer.
22. The patellae are demonstrated directly above the intercondylar sulci and rotated laterally, and the heights of the lateral and medial condyles are nearly equal. Internally rotate the patient's legs until the patellae are situated superiorly, and restrain the legs with the Velcro straps of the axial viewer.
23. The patellae are resting against the intercondylar sulci, obscuring the patellofemoral joint spaces. Slide the patient's knees away from the axial viewer until the patient's posterior knee curvatures are positioned just superior to the bend of the axial viewer.
24. The tibial tuberosities are demonstrated within the patellofemoral joint spaces. Slide the patient's

knees toward the axial viewer until the posterior knee curvatures are just superior to the bend of the axial viewer.
25. The patellae, anterior femoral condyles, and intercondylar sulci are demonstrated superiorly, the lateral femoral condyle demonstrates more height than the medial condyle, the patellofemoral joint space is open, and the patellae are laterally located. Positioning is accurate; the patient's patellae are subluxed.

Femur: AP Projection

1. A. Femoral shaft
   B. Lateral epicondyle
   C. Lateral condyle
   D. Femorotibial joint
   E. Fibular head
   F. Medial condyle
   G. Medial epicondyle
2. A. Pelvic brim
   B. Obturator foramen
   C. Lesser trochanter
   D. Femoral shaft
   E. Greater trochanter
   F. Femoral neck
   G. Femoral head
   H. Acetabulum
3. Position the knee toward the anode end of the tube and the hip toward the cathode end.
4. It can be used to detect subcutaneous air or hematomas.
5. A. Medial
   B. Lateral
   C. Intercondylar eminence
6. A. Supine
   B. Extended
   C. Internally
7. A. No
   B. Forced internal rotation of a fractured femur may cause injury to the blood supply and nerves that surround the injured area.
8. The diverged x-rays used to record the femorotibial joint are angled against the joint.
9. A. Distal femoral shaft
   B. 2
   C. Femorotibial
10. The distal femoral shaft, surrounding femoral soft tissue, femorotibial joint, and 1 inch (2.5 cm) of the lower leg
11. Position the anterior superior iliac spines at equal distances from the imaging table.
12. A. Parallel with the imaging table
    B. It will demonstrate the femoral neck without foreshortening and the greater trochanter in profile.

13. A. Proximal femoral shaft
    B. ASIS
14. To allow the reviewer to detect subcutaneous air or hematomas
15. The proximal femoral shaft, hip joint, and surrounding femoral soft tissue
16. The patient's leg was externally rotated.
17. The patient's leg was internally rotated.
18. The patient's pelvis was rotated toward the affected femur.
19. The patient was rotated away from the affected femur.
20. The patient's leg was externally rotated.
21. The femoral epicondyles are not in profile, the medial condyle appears larger than the lateral condyle, and the tibia superimposes the fibular head. Internally rotate the leg until the femoral epicondyles are at equal distances from the IR.
22. The femoral epicondyles are not in profile, the lateral condyle appears larger than the medial condyle, the fibular head is demonstrated without tibial superimposition and not enough of the femur has been included. Externally rotate the leg until the femoral epicondyles are at equal distances from the IR, increase the IR size, and enter the central ray proximally, including more of the proximal femurs.
23. The femoral neck is partially foreshortened, and the lesser trochanter is demonstrated in profile medially. Internally rotate the patient's leg until the femoral epicondyles are positioned at equal distances from the imaging table.

Femur: Lateral Position (Mediolateral Projection)

1. A. Femoral shaft
   B. Fibula
   C. Tibia
   D. Medial femoral condyle
   E. Patella
   F. Lateral femoral condyle
2. A. Femoral head
   B. Femoral neck
   C. Femoral shaft
   D. Lesser trochanter
   E. Greater trochanter
3. A. Femoral shaft
   B. Femoral neck
   C. Femoral head
   D. Lesser trochanter
   E. Greater trochanter
4. Position the knee toward the anode end of the tube and the hip toward the cathode end.
5. A. Lateral
   B. Perpendicular
6. A. Anterior
   B. Posterior
   C. Fibula

7. A. Medial
   B. The reduction in medial femoral inclination that results when the patient is in a lateral recumbent position
   C. The x-rays used to record the condyles are caudally diverged and project the medial condyle, which is situated farther from the IR distally.
8. The femur should not be moved or the patient rotated. The image is obtained using a cross-table (horizontal) beam.
9. It allows the technologist to collimate tightly.
10. A. Distal femoral shaft
    B. 2
    C. Femorotibial joint
11. The distal femoral shaft, surrounding femoral soft tissue, femorotibial joint, and 1 inch (2.5 cm) of the lower leg
12. The pelvis is rotated until the femoral epicondyles are aligned perpendicular to the imaging table.
13. Lateral surface of femur is placed next to the imaging table.
14. The patient's leg should not be moved, nor the body rotated. Take the image with the patient in an axiolateral position.
15. A. Proximal femoral shaft
    B. ASIS
16. The proximal femoral shaft, hip joint, and surrounding femoral soft tissue
17. The patient's patella was positioned too far away from the IR.
18. The patient's patella was positioned too close to the IR.
19. The pelvis is overrotated, and the femoral epicondyles are not aligned perpendicular to the imaging table; the medial epicondyle is anterior to the lateral epicondyle.
20. The pelvis is underrotated, and the femoral epicondyles are not aligned perpendicular to the imaging table; the medial epicondyle is posterior to the lateral epicondyle.
21. The medial femoral condyle is anterior to the lateral epicondyle. Internally rotate the leg (moving the patella away from the IR).
22. The medial femoral condyle is anterior to the lateral epicondyle. Internally rotate the femur until the femoral epicondyles are aligned perpendicular to the IR, or angle the central ray anteriorly until it is aligned parallel with the femoral epicondyles.
23. The greater trochanter is positioned laterally, the femoral neck is demonstrated with only partial foreshortening, and the femoral shaft is foreshortened. Rotate the pelvis, increase the degree of external leg rotation, and abduct the leg as needed to place the femur against the imaging table, with the femoral epicondyles aligned perpendicular to the IR.

24. The soft tissue from the unaffected thigh is superimposed over the acetabulum and femoral head of the affected femur. Flex and abduct the unaffected leg, drawing it away from the affected acetabulum and femoral head.

25. The greater trochanter is demonstrated posteriorly, and the lesser trochanter is superimposed over the femoral shaft. A proximal femoral shaft fracture is present. The patient's affected leg was in external rotation. Do not attempt to adjust the patient's leg position if a fracture of the proximal femur is suspected. No corrective movement is needed.

Image Analysis of the Hip and Pelvis

LEARNING OBJECTIVES

After completion of this chapter you should be able to:

_____ 1. Identify the required anatomy on images of the hip, pelvis, and sacroiliac joints.

_____ 2. Describe how to properly position the patient, image receptor (IR), and central ray for hip, pelvic, and sacroiliac joint images.

_____ 3. State how to properly mark and hang hip, pelvic, and sacroiliac joint images.

_____ 4. List the typical artifacts that are found on hip, pelvic, and sacroiliac joint images.

_____ 5. List the requirements for accurate positioning for hip, pelvic, and sacroiliac joint images.

_____ 6. State how to properly reposition the patient when hip, pelvic, and sacroiliac joint images with poor positioning are produced.

_____ 7. Discuss how to determine the amount of patient or central ray adjustment that is required to improve hip, pelvic, and sacroiliac joint images with poor positioning.

_____ 8. State the kilovoltage (kVp) routinely used for hip, pelvic, and sacroiliac joint images, and describe what anatomical structures are visible when the correct technique factors are used.

_____ 9. List the soft-tissue fat planes that are demonstrated on anteroposterior (AP) hip and pelvic images, and describe their locations.

_____ 10. Discuss the importance of using a technique that adequately demonstrates the soft-tissue fat planes on AP hip and pelvic images.

_____ 11. Explain how leg rotation affects which anatomical structures of the proximal femur are demonstrated.

_____ 12. Discuss why the leg of a patient with a proximal femoral fracture should never be rotated to obtain AP and lateral images, and state how these images should be taken.

_____ 13. Define the differences demonstrated between the pelvic bones of female and those of male patients.

_____ 14. Explain when gonadal shielding is used for hip and pelvic images.

_____ 15. Describe how the anatomical structures of the proximal femur are demonstrated differently for frog-leg hip and pelvic images when the distal femur is elevated at different angles to the imaging table.

_____ 16. Describe how the anatomical structures of the proximal femur are demonstrated differently for frog-leg hip and pelvic images when the distal femur is abducted at different angles to the imaging table.

_____ 17. Explain how to position a compensating filter for an axiolateral hip image to obtain uniform density of the hip joint and proximal femur.

_____ 18. Describe how to localize the femoral neck for an axiolateral hip image.

_____ 19. State which sacroiliac joint is of interest when the patient is rotated for oblique sacroiliac joint images.

STUDY QUESTIONS

1. Describe how the following hip and pelvic images should be hung on a view box or displayed on a cathode ray tube (CRT) monitor.

    A. Left axial lateral hip: _____

    _____

    B. AP pelvis: _____

    _____

    C. Left oblique sacroiliac joints: _____

    _____

2. What anatomical artifact is common on AP hip and pelvic images?

    _____

3. Sharply defined bony trabecular patterns and cortical outlines of the proximal femur and pelvic girdle are obtained when:

    A. _____

    B. _____

    C. _____

4. To provide optimal spatial resolution when using computed radiography to image the pelvic girdle and proximal femur, the _____ IR size should be chosen.

5. List the four soft-tissue structures that are demonstrated on accurately exposed AP hip and pelvis images, and describe their locations.

    A. _____

    B. _____

    C. _____

    D. _____

    Why is it important that these soft-tissue structures are visualized?

    E. _____

6. Complete Table 6-1.

TABLE 6-1   Hip and Pelvic Technical Data

Position or Projection	kVp	Grid	AEC Chamber(s)	SID
AP projection, hip				
Mediolateral (frog-leg) projection, hip				
Axiolateral (inferosuperior) projection, hip				
AP projection, pelvis				
AP oblique (frog-leg) projection, pelvis				
AP axial projection, sacroiliac joints				
AP oblique projection, sacroiliac joints				

AEC, Automatic exposure control; *AP,* anteroposterior; *kVp,* kilovolt peak; *SID,* source–image receptor distance.

7. Complete Table 6-2.

TABLE 6-2   IR Size, Placement, and Direction

Position or Projection	IR Size	Placement or Direction
AP projection, hip		
Mediolateral (frog-leg) projection, hip		
Axiolateral (inferosuperior) projection, hip		
AP projection, pelvis		
AP oblique (frog-leg) projection, pelvis		
AP axial projection, sacroiliac joints		
AP oblique projection, sacroiliac joints		

AP, Anteroposterior; *IR,* image receptor.

Hip: AP Projection

1. Identify the labeled anatomy in Figure 6-1.

Figure 6–1

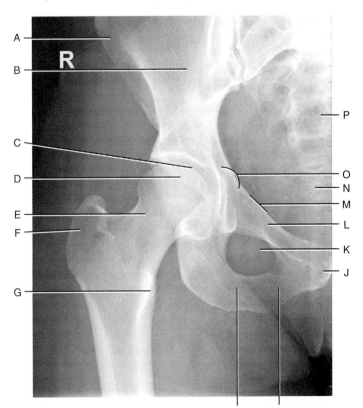

A. _____

B. _____

C. _____

D. _____

E. _____

F. _____

G. _____

H. _____

I. _____

J. _____

K. _____

L. _____

M. _____

N. _____

O. _____

P. _____

2. On an AP hip image with accurate positioning, the ischial spine is aligned with the (A) _____ and the sacrum and coccyx are aligned with the (B) _____.

3. How can patient positioning be evaluated to ensure that pelvic rotation is not present on an AP hip image?

_____

4. Describe the relationship that would result between the following anatomical structures on an AP hip image if the affected side was rotated away from the IR.

   A. Sacrum and symphysis pubis: _____

   B. Iliac spine and pelvic brim: _____

5. If the affected hip is rotated toward the IR for an AP hip image, how will the obturator foramen appear in comparison with a nonrotated AP hip image? _____

6. When the patient's leg is adequately rotated for an AP hip image, the femoral neck is demonstrated without (A) _____, the (B) _____ trochanter is demonstrated in profile (C) _____ (medially/laterally), and the (D) _____ trochanter is superimposed by the femoral neck.

7. The demonstration of the femoral neck and lesser trochanter on an AP hip image depends on the position of the femoral epicondyles. For each epicondyle position in the following list, describe how the femoral neck and lesser trochanter are demonstrated on an AP hip image.

   A. Leg is externally rotated, with the foot at a 45-degree angle and an imaginary line connecting the femoral epicondyles at a 60- to 65-degree angle with the imaging table:

   _____

B. Leg is internally rotated, with the foot vertical and an imaginary line connecting the femoral epicondyles at a 15- to 20-degree angle with imaging table:

_____

C. Leg is internally rotated, with the foot 15 to 20 degrees from vertical and an imaginary line connecting the femoral epicondyles aligned parallel with imaging table:

_____

8. How are the patient's foot and femoral epicondyles positioned to obtain an AP hip image with accurate positioning? _____

_____

9. Should the technologist attempt to rotate the leg of a patient with a suspected fracture or dislocated hip?

   A. _____ (Yes/No)

   Defend your answer.

   B. _____

10. On an AP hip image with accurate positioning taken to demonstrate the hip joint, the (A) _____ and (B) _____ are centered within the collimated field. This is accomplished by centering a (C) _____ central ray 1½ inches (4 cm) (D) _____ to the midpoint of a line connecting the anterior superior iliac spine (ASIS) and superior (E) _____.

11. What anatomical structures are included on an AP hip image with accurate positioning? _____

_____

12. How may the positioning procedure require adjusting if the patient has a prosthesis? _____

_____

13. State whether gonadal shielding should be used for an AP hip image for the following:

   A. Male: _____

   B. Female: _____

For the following descriptions of AP hip images with poor positioning, state how the patient would have been mispositioned for such an image to be obtained.

14. The ischial spine is demonstrated without pelvic brim superimposition, the sacrum and coccyx are not aligned with the symphysis pubis but are rotated away from the affected hip, and the obturator foramen is narrowed.

_____

15. The ischial spine is not aligned with the pelvic brim but is demonstrated closer to the acetabulum, the sacrum and coccyx are not aligned with the symphysis pubis but are rotated toward the affected hip, and the obturator foramen is clearly demonstrated.

_____

16. The femoral neck is completely foreshortened, and the lesser trochanter is demonstrated in profile.

For the following AP hip images with poor positioning, state what anatomical structures are misaligned and how the patient should be repositioned for an optimal image to be obtained.

Figure 6–2

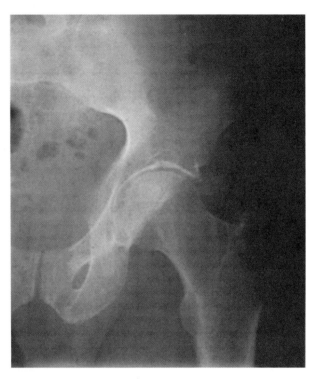

17. (Figure 6-2): _____

_____

_____

_____

_____

_____

Figure 6–3

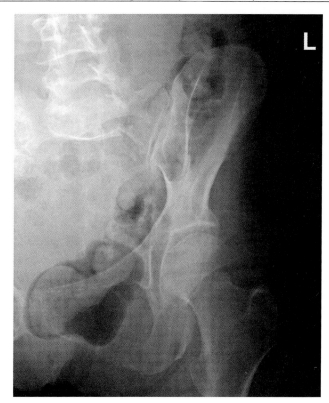

18. (Figure 6-3): _____

_____

_____

_____

_____

_____

_____

Figure 6–4

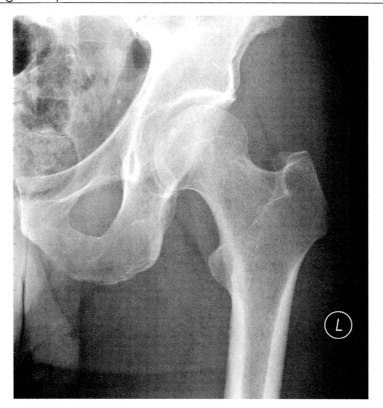

19. (Figure 6-4): _____

_____

_____

_____

_____

_____

_____

Figure 6–5

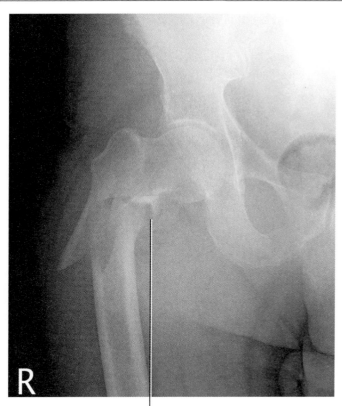

Lesser trochanter

20. (Figure 6-5, fracture): _____

_____

_____

_____

_____

Hip: Mediolateral (Frog-Leg) Projection (Modified Cleaves Method)

1. Identify the labeled anatomy in Figure 6-6.

Figure 6–6

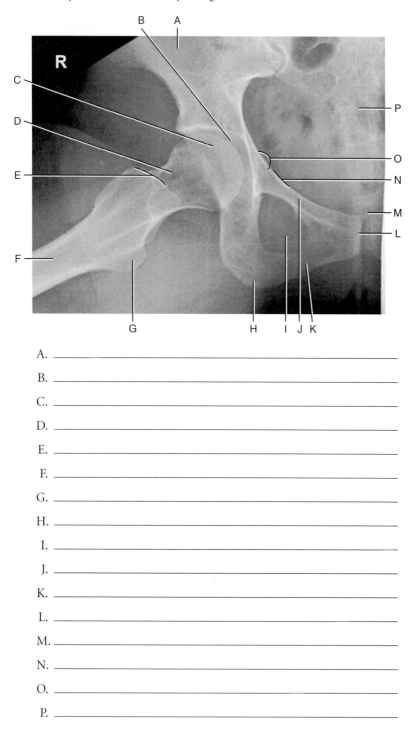

A. _____

B. _____

C. _____

D. _____

E. _____

F. _____

G. _____

H. _____

I. _____

J. _____

K. _____

L. _____

M. _____

N. _____

O. _____

P. _____

2. How can rotation of the pelvis be avoided when positioning a patient for a frog-leg hip image? _____

3. Describe the relationship of the iliac spine to the pelvic brim and the relationship of the sacrum and coccyx to the symphysis pubis on a nonrotated frog-leg hip image.

   A. Sacrum to symphysis pubis: _____

   B. Iliac spine to pelvic brim: _____

4. For the Lauenstein and Hickey lateral hip methods, the patient's pelvis is rotated (A) _____ (toward/away from) the affected hip until the femur is placed (B) _____.

5. On a frog-leg hip image with accurate positioning, the
   (A) _____ trochanter is demonstrated in profile
   (B) _____ (medially/laterally) and the proximal femur is superimposed over the (C) _____ trochanter.

6. The degree of patient knee and hip flexion determines whether or not the greater and lesser trochanter will be in _____.

7. At what degree with the imaging table is the femur placed to accurately position the greater and lesser trochanters on a frog-leg hip image? _____

8. The degree of femoral abduction for a frog-leg hip image will determine what two proximal femur anatomical relationships?

   A. _____

   B. _____

9. Describe the position of the greater trochanter and the degree of femoral neck foreshortening demonstrated on a frog-leg hip image if the femur is abducted as stated for each of the following:

   A. Femur is abducted until it is placed next to the imaging table:

   _____

   B. Femur is abducted to a 45-degree angle with the imaging table:

   _____

   C. Femur is abducted 20 to 30 degrees from vertical:

   _____

10. On a frog-leg hip image with accurate positioning taken to demonstrate the femoral neck, the (A) _____ is centered within the collimated field. This centering is accomplished by centering a (B) _____ central ray (C) _____ inches distal to the midpoint of a line connecting the (D) _____ and superior symphysis pubis.

11. What anatomical structures are included on a frog-leg hip image with accurate positioning? _____

   _____

For the following descriptions of frog-leg hip images with poor positioning, state how the patient would have been mispositioned for such an image to be obtained.

12. The ischial spine is demonstrated without pelvic brim superimposition, the sacrum and coccyx are not aligned with the symphysis pubis but are rotated away from the affected hip, and the obturator foramen is narrowed.

_____

13. The greater trochanter is positioned medially, and the lesser trochanter is obscured.

_____

14. The greater trochanter is positioned laterally.

_____

15. The femoral neck is demonstrated on end, and the greater trochanter is demonstrated on the same transverse level as the femoral head.

_____

For the following frog-leg hip images with poor positioning, state what anatomical structures are misaligned and how the patient should be repositioned for an optimal image to be obtained.

Figure 6–7

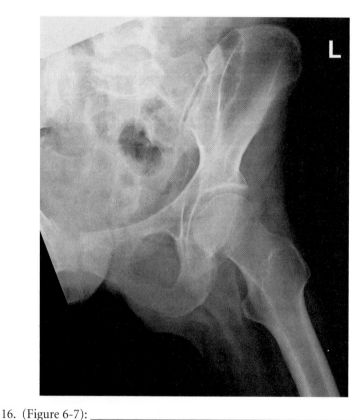

16. (Figure 6-7): _____

_____

_____

_____

Figure 6–8

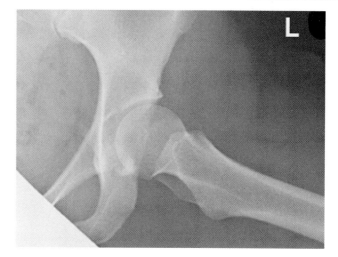

17. (Figure 6-8): _____

_____

_____

_____

Figure 6–9

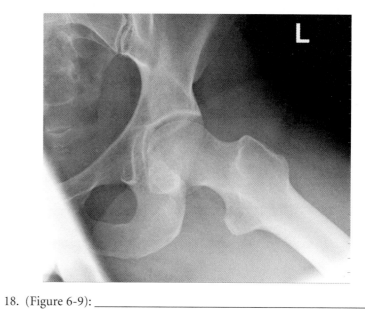

18. (Figure 6-9): _____

_____

_____

_____

Hip: Axiolateral (Inferosuperior) Projection (Danelius-Miller Method)

1. Identify the labeled anatomy in Figure 6-10.

Figure 6–10

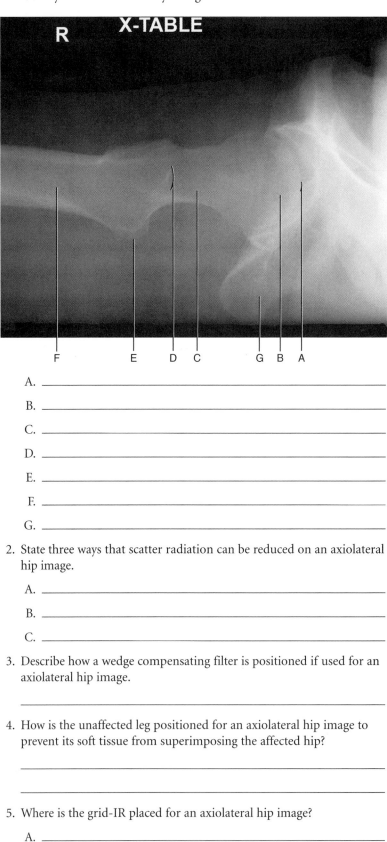

A. _____

B. _____

C. _____

D. _____

E. _____

F. _____

G. _____

2. State three ways that scatter radiation can be reduced on an axiolateral hip image.

   A. _____

   B. _____

   C. _____

3. Describe how a wedge compensating filter is positioned if used for an axiolateral hip image.

   _____

4. How is the unaffected leg positioned for an axiolateral hip image to prevent its soft tissue from superimposing the affected hip?

   _____

   _____

5. Where is the grid-IR placed for an axiolateral hip image?

   A. _____

How is it aligned with the femoral neck?

B. _____

How is the position of the grid-IR changed if the patient has a large amount of lateral soft-tissue thickness?

C. _____

How should the central ray be positioned with respect to the IR and femoral neck?

D. _____

6. Describe how to localize the femoral neck when positioning for an axiolateral hip image.

_____

_____

7. Describe the appearance of the femoral neck and greater trochanter if the central ray is not accurately aligned with the femoral neck for an axiolateral hip image.

A. Femoral neck: _____

B. Greater trochanter: _____

8. On an axiolateral hip image with accurate positioning, the (A) _____ trochanter is demonstrated in profile (B) _____ and the (C) _____ trochanter is superimposed by the femoral shaft.

9. Forced internal rotation of a dislocated hip or fractured proximal femur may cause _____

_____

10. How is the patient's leg positioned to accurately position the lesser trochanter on an axiolateral hip image? _____

_____

11. On an axiolateral hip image with accurate positioning, the _____ is centered within the collimated field.

12. What anatomical structures are included on an axiolateral hip image with accurate positioning?

_____

For the following descriptions of axiolateral hip images with poor positioning, state how the patient or central ray would have been mispositioned for such an image to be obtained.

13. The soft tissue from the unaffected thigh is superimposed over the acetabulum and femoral head of the affected hip.

_____

14. The greater trochanter is demonstrated at a transverse level that is proximal to the lesser trochanter, and the femoral neck is partially foreshortened.

_____

15. The greater trochanter is demonstrated posteriorly, and the lesser trochanter is superimposed over the femoral shaft.

_____

For the following axiolateral hip images with poor positioning, state what anatomical structures are misaligned and how the patient or central ray should be repositioned for an optimal image to be obtained.

Figure 6–11

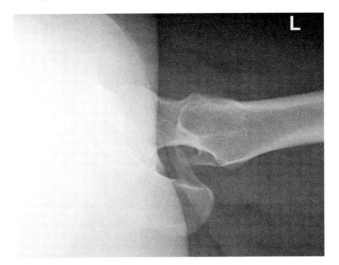

16. (Figure 6-11): _____

_____

_____

_____

_____

Figure 6–12

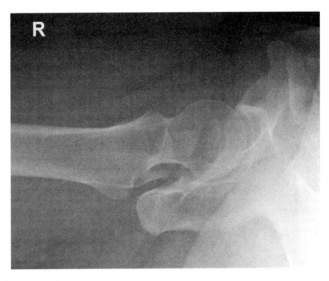

17. (Figure 6-12): _____

_____

_____

_____

Figure 6–13

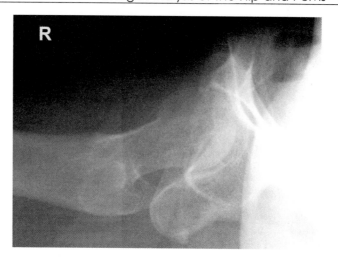

18. Figure (6-13): _____

    _____

    _____

    _____

Figure 6–14

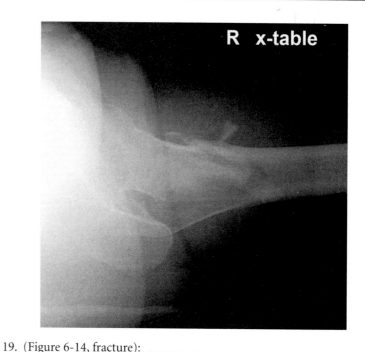

19. (Figure 6-14, fracture): _____

    _____

    _____

    _____

Pelvis: AP Projection

1. Identify the labeled anatomy in Figure 6-15.

Figure 6–15

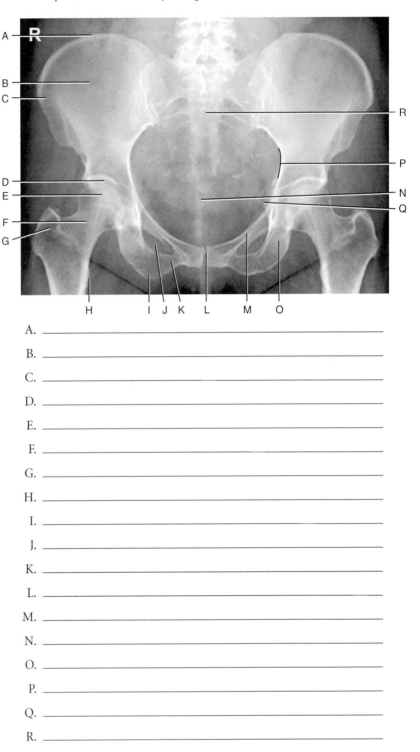

A. _____

B. _____

C. _____

D. _____

E. _____

F. _____

G. _____

H. _____

I. _____

J. _____

K. _____

L. _____

M. _____

N. _____

O. _____

P. _____

Q. _____

R. _____

2. State whether the following pelvis images are from a female or male patient:

Figure 6–16

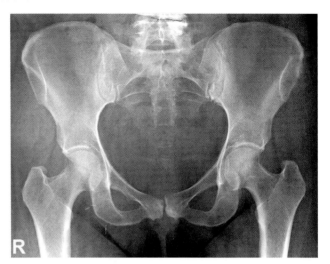

A. (Figure 6-16): _____

Figure 6–17

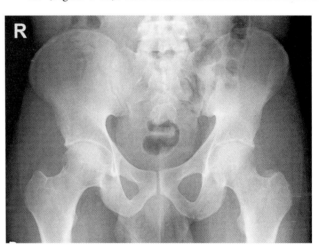

B. (Figure 6-17): _____

3. Complete Table 6-3.

TABLE 6-3 **Male and Female Pelvic Differences**		
	Male	**Female**
Overall shape		
Ala		
Pubic arch angle		
Inlet shape		
Obturator foramen		

4. On an AP pelvic image with accurate positioning, the ischial spines are aligned with the (A) _____ and the sacrum and coccyx are aligned with the (B) _____.

5. How can patient positioning be evaluated to ensure that pelvic rotation is not present on an AP pelvic image? _____

6. Describe the relationship of the sacrum and coccyx to the symphysis pubis and that of the iliac spine to the pelvic brim on an AP pelvic image in which the patient's left side was rotated away from the IR.

_____

_____

7. When the patient's legs are adequately rotated for an AP pelvic image, the femoral necks are demonstrated without (A) _____, the (B) _____ trochanters are demonstrated in profile laterally, and the (C) _____ trochanters are superimposed by the femoral necks.

8. Following are descriptions of the femoral neck appearance on different AP pelvic images. For each description, state the position of the patient's feet and humeral epicondyles that would result in the described image.

   A. Femoral necks without foreshortening: _____

   _____

   B. Femoral necks on end: _____

   _____

   C. Femoral necks partially foreshortened: _____

   _____

9. How are the patient's feet and femoral epicondyles positioned for an AP pelvic image with accurate positioning to be obtained?

_____

_____

10. On an AP pelvic image with accurate positioning, the (A) _____ is centered within the collimated field. This centering is accomplished by centering a (B) _____ central ray to the midsagittal plane at a level halfway between the (C) _____ and an imaginary line connecting the (D) _____.

11. What anatomical structures are included on an AP pelvic image with accurate positioning? _____

_____

For the following descriptions of AP pelvic images with poor positioning, state how the patient would have been mispositioned for such an image to be obtained.

12. The right obturator foramen is narrowed, the right ischial spine is demonstrated without pelvic brim superimposition, and the sacrum and coccyx are rotated toward the left hip.

_____

13. The femoral necks are foreshortened, and the lesser trochanters are demonstrated in profile.

_____

For the following AP pelvic images with poor positioning, state what anatomical structures are misaligned and how the patient should be repositioned for an optimal image to be obtained.

Figure 6–18

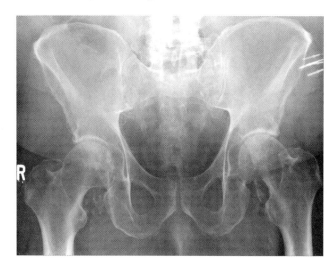

14. (Figure 6-18): _____

_____

_____

_____

_____

Figure 6–19

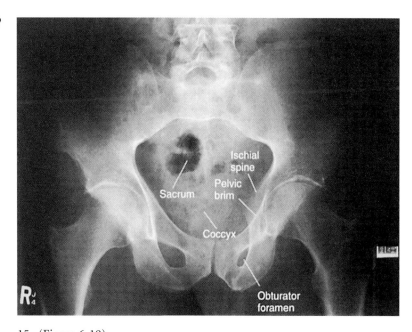

15. (Figure 6-19): _____

_____

_____

_____

Pelvis: AP Oblique (Frog-Leg) Projection (Modified Cleaves Method)

1. Identify the labeled anatomy in Figure 6-20.

Figure 6–20

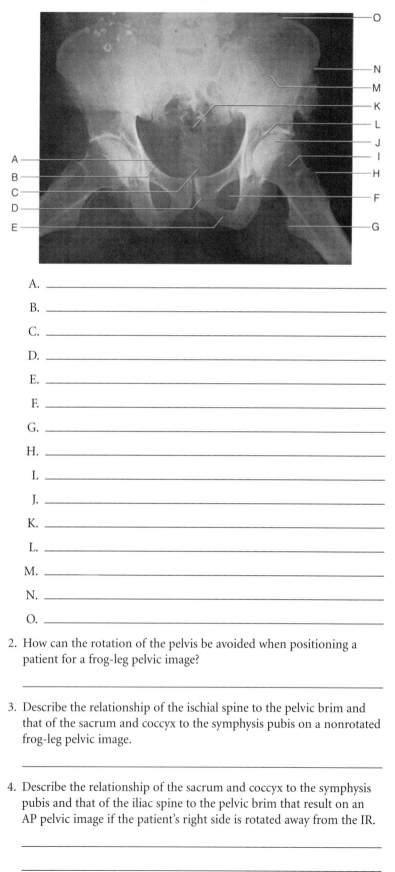

A. _____

B. _____

C. _____

D. _____

E. _____

F. _____

G. _____

H. _____

I. _____

J. _____

K. _____

L. _____

M. _____

N. _____

O. _____

2. How can the rotation of the pelvis be avoided when positioning a patient for a frog-leg pelvic image?

_____

3. Describe the relationship of the ischial spine to the pelvic brim and that of the sacrum and coccyx to the symphysis pubis on a nonrotated frog-leg pelvic image.

_____

4. Describe the relationship of the sacrum and coccyx to the symphysis pubis and that of the iliac spine to the pelvic brim that result on an AP pelvic image if the patient's right side is rotated away from the IR.

_____

_____

5. On a frog-leg pelvic image with accurate positioning, the
   (A) _____ trochanters are demonstrated in profile
   (B) _____ (medially/laterally) and the proximal femurs are
   superimposed over the (C) _____ trochanters.

6. The degree of patient knee and hip flexion determines the position of
   the greater and lesser trochanters to the _____.

7. At what degree with the imaging table are the femurs placed to accurately
   position the greater and lesser trochanters on a frog-leg pelvic image?

   _____

8. The patient's knees and hips were flexed 20 degrees with the imaging
   table for a frog-leg pelvic image. How can this misposition be
   identified on the resulting image?

   _____

9. The degree of femoral abduction for a frog-leg pelvic image
   determines what two anatomical relationships?

   A. _____

   B. _____

10. Describe the position of the greater trochanters and the degree of
    femoral neck foreshortening that are demonstrated on a frog-leg
    pelvic image if the femurs are abducted as follows:

    A. Femurs are abducted until placed against the imaging table:

       _____

    B. Femurs are abducted to a 45-degree angle with the imaging table:

       _____

    C. Femurs are abducted only 20 to 30 degrees from vertical:

       _____

11. On a frog-leg pelvic image with accurate positioning, the
    (A) _____ is centered within the collimated
    field. This centering is accomplished by centering a
    (B) _____ central ray to the (C) _____
    plane at a level halfway between the (D) _____ and
    an imaginary line connecting the (E) _____.

12. What anatomical structures are included on a frog-leg pelvic image
    with accurate positioning? _____

    _____

**For the following descriptions of frog-leg pelvic images with poor posi-
tioning, state how the patient would have been mispositioned for such an
image to be obtained.**

13. The left obturator foramen is narrowed, the left ischial spine is
    demonstrated without pelvic brim superimposition, and the sacrum
    and coccyx are rotated toward the right hip.

    _____

14. The femoral necks are demonstrated on end, and the greater
    trochanters are demonstrated on the same transverse level as the
    femoral heads.

    _____

For the following frog-leg pelvic images with poor positioning, state what anatomical structures are misaligned and how the patient should be repositioned for an optimal image to be obtained.

Figure 6–21

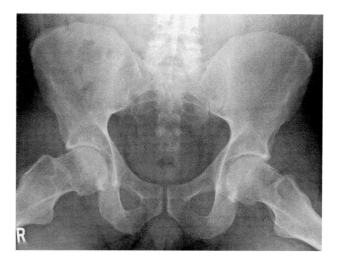

15. (Figure 6-21): _____

_____

_____

_____

Figure 6–22

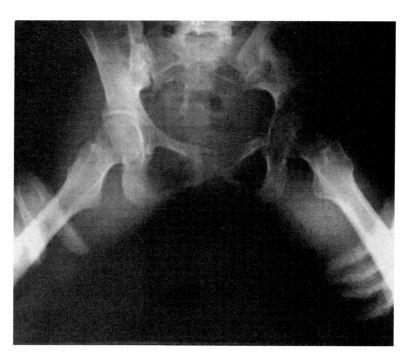

16. (Figure 6-22): _____

_____

_____

_____

Sacroiliac Joints: AP Axial Projection

1. Identify the labeled anatomy in Figure 6-23.

Figure 6–23

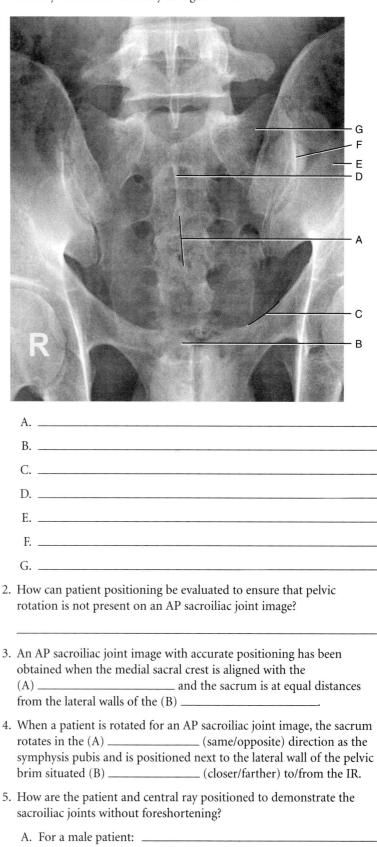

A. _____

B. _____

C. _____

D. _____

E. _____

F. _____

G. _____

2. How can patient positioning be evaluated to ensure that pelvic rotation is not present on an AP sacroiliac joint image?

_____

3. An AP sacroiliac joint image with accurate positioning has been obtained when the medial sacral crest is aligned with the (A) _____ and the sacrum is at equal distances from the lateral walls of the (B) _____.

4. When a patient is rotated for an AP sacroiliac joint image, the sacrum rotates in the (A) _____ (same/opposite) direction as the symphysis pubis and is positioned next to the lateral wall of the pelvic brim situated (B) _____ (closer/farther) to/from the IR.

5. How are the patient and central ray positioned to demonstrate the sacroiliac joints without foreshortening?

A. For a male patient: _____

B. For a female patient: _____

C. For a patient with greater than average lumbosacral curvature:

_____

_____

D. For a patient with less than average lumbosacral curvature:

_____

_____

6. Why is the median sacral crest aligned with the long axis of the collimated field for an AP sacroiliac joint image?

A. _____

B. _____

7. On an AP sacroiliac joint image with accurate positioning, the (A) _____ is centered within the collimated field. This centering is obtained by positioning the central ray to the patient's (B) _____ plane at a level halfway between an imaginary line connecting the (C) _____ and (D) _____.

8. What anatomical structures are included on an AP sacroiliac joint image with accurate positioning? _____

_____

For the following descriptions of sacroiliac joint images with poor positioning, state how the patient or central ray would have been mispositioned for such an image to be obtained.

9. The sacrum is situated closer to the right pelvic brim than to the left.

_____

10. The sacroiliac joints are foreshortened, and the inferior sacrum is demonstrated without symphysis pubis superimposition.

_____

For the following sacroiliac joint images with poor positioning, state what anatomical structures are misaligned and how the patient should be repositioned for an optimal image to be obtained.

Figure 6–24

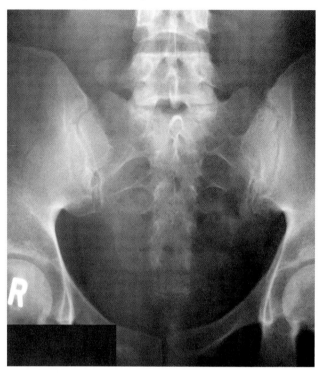

11. (Figure 6-24): _____

_____

_____

_____

_____

Figure 6–25

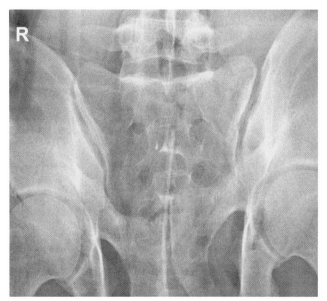

12. (Figure 6-25): _____

_____

_____

_____

_____

_____

Sacroiliac Joints: AP Oblique Projection (LPO and RPO Positions)

1. Identify the labeled anatomy in Figure 6-26.

Figure 6–26

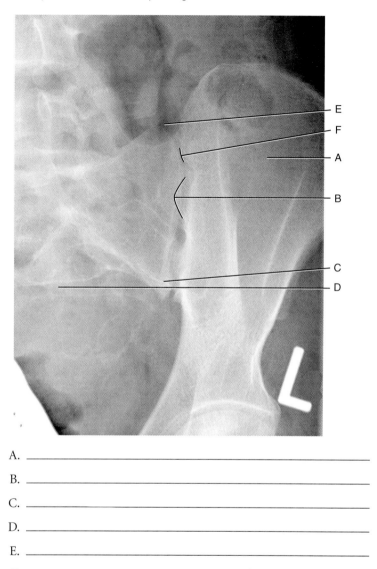

A. _____

B. _____

C. _____

D. _____

E. _____

F. _____

2. What two bony structures articulate to form the sacroiliac joints?

A. _____

B. _____

3. An open sacroiliac joint is obtained when the (A) _____ and (B) _____ are demonstrated without superimposition.

4. For an open sacroiliac joint to be obtained on an oblique sacroiliac joint image, the patient is rotated until the (A) _____ plane is at a (B) _____-degree angle with the imaging table and IR.

5. Which sacroiliac joint is open when the patient is placed in an LPO position?

   A. _____

   Which sacroiliac joint is open if the patient is placed in an RAO position?

   B. _____

6. The affected sacroiliac joint is centered within the collimated field on an oblique sacroiliac joint image with accurate positioning. This centering is obtained by placing the central ray 1 to 1½ inches (A) _____ (medial/lateral) to the elevated (B) _____.

7. What anatomical structures are included on an oblique sacroiliac joint image with accurate positioning?

   _____

   _____

For the following descriptions of sacroiliac joint images with poor positioning, state how the patient would have been mispositioned for such an image to be obtained.

8. The sacroiliac joint is closed, the superior and inferior sacral ala are demonstrated without iliac superimposition, and the lateral sacral ala is superimposed over the iliac tuberosity.

   _____

9. The sacroiliac joint is closed, and the ilium is superimposed over the inferior sacral ala and lateral sacrum.

   _____

For the following sacroiliac joint images with poor positioning, state what anatomical structures are misaligned and how the patient should be repositioned for an optimal image to be obtained.

Figure 6–27

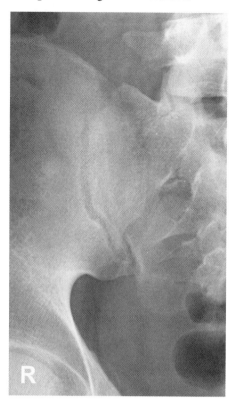

10. (Figure 6-27): _____

_____

_____

_____

_____

Figure 6–28

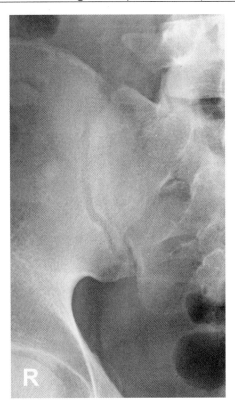

11. (Figure 6-28): _____

_____

_____

_____

CHAPTER 6
STUDY QUESTION ANSWERS

1. A. With the anterior surface upward and the posterior downward. The marker should be correct.
   B. As if the patient is standing in an upright position. The marker should be correct.
   C. As if the patient is standing in an upright position. The marker should be correct. Side positioned away from the IR is marked.
2. Patient's hand
3. A. Patient motion is controlled.
   B. Respiration is halted.
   C. Short object–image receptor distance (OID) is maintained

4. Smallest
5. A. The obturator internus fat plane lies within the pelvic inlet next to the pelvic brim.
   B. The iliopsoas fat plane lies medial to the lesser trochanter.
   C. The pericapsular fat plane is found superior to the femoral neck.
   D. The gluteal fat plane lies superior to the pericapsular fat plane.
   E. They will aid in the detection of intraarticular and periarticular disease.

6. Table 6-1

Position or Projection	kVp	Grid	AEC Chamber(s)	SID
AP projection, hip	70-85	Grid	Center	40-48 inches (100-120 cm)
Mediolateral (frog-leg) projection, hip	70-85	Grid	Center	40-48 inches (100-120 cm)
Axiolateral (inferosuperior) projection, hip	75-85	Grid		40-48 inches (100-120 cm)
AP projection, pelvis	65-85	Grid	Both outside	40-48 inches (100-120 cm)
AP oblique (frog-leg) projection, pelvis	65-85	Grid	Both outside	40-48 inches (100-120 cm)
AP axial projection, sacroiliac joints	80-85	Grid	Center	40-48 inches (100-120 cm)
AP oblique projection, sacroiliac joints	75-85	Grid	Center	40-48 inches (100-120 cm)

AEC, Automatic exposure control; *AP,* anteroposterior; *kVp,* kilovolt peak; *SID,* source–image receptor distance.

7. Table 6-2

Position or Projection	IR Size	Placement or Direction
AP projection, hip	10 × 12 inches (24 × 30 cm)	Lengthwise
Mediolateral (frog-leg) projection, hip	10 × 12 inches (24 × 30 cm)	Lengthwise
Axiolateral (inferosuperior) projection, hip	10 × 12 inches (24 × 30 cm)	Lengthwise
AP projection, pelvis	14 × 17 inches (35 × 43 cm)	Crosswise
AP oblique (frog-leg) projection, pelvis	14 × 17 inches (35 × 43 cm)	Crosswise
AP axial projection, sacroiliac joints	10 × 12 inches (24 × 30 cm)	Lengthwise
AP oblique projection, sacroiliac joints	10 × 12 inches (24 × 30 cm)	Lengthwise

AP, Anteroposterior; *IR,* image receptor.

Hip: AP Projection

1. A. ASIS
   B. Iliac ala
   C. Acetabulum
   D. Femoral head
   E. Femoral neck
   F. Greater trochanter
   G. Lesser trochanter
   H. Ischial tuberosity
   I. Inferior ramus of pubis
   J. Symphysis pubis
   K. Obturator foramen
   L. Superior ramus of pubis
   M. Pelvis brim
   N. Coccyx
   O. Ischial spine
   P. Sacrum
2. A. Pelvic brim
   B. Symphysis pubis
3. Make sure that the ASISs are at equal distances from the imaging table.
4. A. The sacrum would not be aligned with the symphysis pubis but would be rotated toward the affected hip.
   B. The iliac spine would be closer to the acetabulum than the pelvic brim.
5. It will be narrower.
6. A. Foreshortening
   B. Greater

C. Laterally

D. Lesser

7. A. The femoral neck will be demonstrated on end, and the lesser trochanter will be demonstrated in profile medially.

B. The lesser trochanter is in partial profile medially, and the femoral neck is only partially foreshortened.

C. The femoral neck is demonstrated without foreshortening, the greater trochanter is demonstrated in profile laterally, and the lesser trochanter is obscured.

8. The foot should be tilted internally 15 to 20 degrees from vertical, and an imaginary line connecting the epicondyles should be positioned parallel with the imaging table.

9. A. No

B. Forced internal rotation of a fractured or dislocated hip may result in injury to the blood supply and nerves that surround the injured area.

10. A. Femoral head

B. Acetabulum

C. Perpendicular

D. Distal

E. Symphysis pubis

11. The acetabulum, greater and lesser trochanters, femoral head and neck, and one half of the sacrum, coccyx, and symphysis pubis

12. A larger IR and lower central ray centering may be required.

13. A. Yes, no anatomical structures will be covered.

B. Yes, but use a shield that is small enough and is shaped for the female pelvis, to avoid covering any pelvic structures.

14. The patient was rotated toward the affected hip.

15. The patient was rotated away from the affected hip.

16. The patient's leg was in external rotation, with the foot and femoral epicondyles positioned at a 45-degree angle with the imaging table.

17. The ischial spine is demonstrated without pelvic brim superimposition, the sacrum and coccyx are not aligned with the symphysis pubis but are rotated away from the affected hip, and the obturator foramen is narrowed. Rotate the patient toward from the affected hip. The lesser trochanter is demonstrated in profile. Internally rotate the leg until the femoral epicondyles are aligned parallel with the imaging table.

18. The ischial spine is not aligned with the pelvic brim but is demonstrated closer to the acetabulum, the sacrum and coccyx are not aligned with the symphysis pubis but are rotated toward the affected hip, and the iliac ala is narrowed. Rotate the patient toward the affected hip. The lesser trochanter is demonstrated in profile. Internally rotate the leg until femoral epicondyles are aligned parallel with the imaging table.

19. The femoral neck is partially foreshortened, and the lesser trochanter is demonstrated in profile. The patient's leg was externally rotated, bringing the foot vertical and the femoral epicondyles positioned at approximately a 15- to 20-degree angle with the imaging table. Internally rotate the patient's leg until the foot is angled 15 to 20 degrees from vertical and the femoral epicondyles are positioned parallel with the imaging table.

20. The lesser trochanter is in profile, and there is a proximal femur fracture. The leg should not be internally rotated when a femoral or hip fracture is suspected. Adequate positioning is demonstrated.

Hip: Mediolateral (Frog-Leg) Projection (Modified Cleaves Method)

1. A. Iliac ala

B. Acetabulum

C. Femoral head

D. Femoral neck

E. Greater trochanter

F. Femoral shaft

G. Lesser trochanter

H. Ischial tuberosity

I. Obturator foramen

J. Superior ramus

K. Inferior ramus

L. Symphysis pubis

M. Coccyx

N. Pelvic brim

O. Ischial spine

P. Sacrum

2. Position the ASISs at equal distances from the imaging table.

3. A. The sacrum and coccyx would be aligned with the symphysis pubis.

B. The iliac spine would be superimposed by the pelvic brim.

4. A. Toward

B. Against the imaging table

5. A. Lesser

B. Medially

C. Greater

6. Profile

7. 60 to 70 degrees

8. A. The amount of femoral neck foreshortening

B. The transverse level at which the greater trochanter will be demonstrated between the femoral head and lesser trochanter

9. A. Demonstrates the femoral neck on end and the greater trochanter at the same transverse level as the femoral head

B. Demonstrates the femoral neck with only partial foreshortening and positions the greater trochanter at a transverse level halfway between the femoral neck and lesser trochanter

C. Demonstrates the femoral neck without foreshortening and the greater trochanter at the same transverse level as the lesser trochanter

10. A. Femoral neck
    B. Perpendicular
    C. 2½ (6.25 cm)
    D. ASIS
11. The acetabulum, greater and lesser trochanters, femoral head and neck, and one half of the sacrum, coccyx, and symphysis pubis
12. The patient was rotated toward the affected hip.
13. The patient's knee was flexed more than needed, placing the femur at an angle greater than 60 to 70 degrees with the imaging table.
14. The patient's knee was not flexed enough to align the femur at a 60- to 70-degree angle with the imaging table, or the affected leg's foot and ankle were resting on top of the unaffected leg, elevating it off the imaging table.
15. The patient's femur was abducted until it was positioned next to the imaging table.
16. The ischial spine is not aligned with the pelvic brim but is demonstrated closer to the acetabulum; the sacrum and coccyx are not aligned with the symphysis pubis but are rotated toward the affected hip; the iliac ala is narrowed and the obturator foramen widened. Rotate the patient toward the affected hip.
17. The femoral neck is foreshortened, and the greater trochanter is demonstrated at the same transverse level as the femoral head. Adduct the patient's femur until it is aligned at a 45-degree angle with the imaging table.
18. The greater trochanter is positioned laterally. The patient's knee was not flexed enough to align the femur at a 60- to 70-degree angle with the imaging table (20 to 30 degrees from vertical). Increase the knee flexion until the femur is aligned at a 60- to 70-degree angle with the imaging table.

Hip: Axiolateral (Inferosuperior) Projection (Danelius-Miller Method)

1. A. Acetabulum
   B. Femoral head
   C. Femoral neck
   D. Greater trochanter
   E. Lesser trochanter
   F. Femoral shaft
   G. Ischial tuberosity
2. A. Use tight collimation.
   B. Place a flat lead contact strip over the top of the unused half of the IR.
   C. Use a grid.
3. Align the thin end of the filter with the femoral neck and the thicker end with the proximal femur.

4. Place the unaffected leg in maximum flexion and abduction.
5. A. Against the patient's affected side at the level of the iliac crest
   B. Parallel
   C. It should be positioned superior to the iliac crest.
   D. Perpendicular to both
6. Find the center of an imaginary line drawn between the symphysis pubis and the ASIS. Bisect that line and draw a perpendicular line distally. This imaginary line parallels the long axis of the femoral neck.
7. A. Femoral neck will be foreshortened
   B. The greater trochanter will be demonstrated proximal to the lesser trochanter.
8. A. Lesser
   B. Medially
   C. Greater
9. Injury to the blood supply and nerves that surround the injured area
10. Internally rotate the leg until an imaginary line connecting the femoral epicondyles is positioned parallel with the imaging table.
11. Femoral neck
12. The acetabulum, femoral head and neck, greater and lesser trochanters, and ischial tuberosity
13. The unaffected leg was not adequately flexed and abducted.
14. The angle of the central ray to the femur was too great.
15. The patient's leg was in external rotation.
16. Soft tissue from the unaffected thigh is superimposed over the acetabulum and femoral head of the affected hip. Flex and abduct the unaffected leg, drawing it away from the affected acetabulum and femoral head. If the patient is unable to further adjust the unaffected leg, the kVp and mAs can be increased to demonstrate this area. A wedge-type compensating filter may also be added to prevent overexposure of the femoral neck and shaft.
17. The greater trochanter is demonstrated at a transverse level proximal to the lesser trochanter, and the femoral neck is partially foreshortened. Localize the femoral neck. Position the IR parallel with the femoral neck and the central ray perpendicular to the IR and femoral neck.
18. The greater trochanter is demonstrated posteriorly, the lesser trochanter is superimposed over the femoral shaft, the greater trochanter is demonstrated at a transverse level that is proximal to the lesser trochanter, and the femoral neck is foreshortened. Internally rotate the patient's leg and decrease the angle of the central ray to the femur.
19. A fracture of the femoral neck is present. The greater trochanter is demonstrated posteriorly, and

the lesser trochanter is superimposed over the femoral shaft. Do not attempt to adjust the patient's leg position if a fracture of the proximal femur is suspected. No corrective movement is needed.

Pelvis: AP Projection

1. A. Iliac crest
   B. Iliac ala
   C. ASIS
   D. Acetabulum
   E. Femoral head
   F. Femoral neck

   G. Greater trochanter
   H. Lesser trochanter
   I. Ischial tuberosity
   J. Obturator foramen
   K. Inferior ramus of ischium
   L. Symphysis pubis
   M. Superior ramus of pubis
   N. Coccyx
   O. Superior ramus of ischium
   P. Pelvic brim
   Q. Ischial spine
   R. Sacrum
2. A. Female
   B. Male

3. Table 6-3

	Male	Female
Overall shape	Bulkier, deeper, and narrower	Smaller, shallower, and wider
Ala	Narrower, nonflared	Wider, flared
Pubic arch angle	Acute angle	Obtuse angle
Inlet shape	Smaller, heart shaped	Larger, rounded shape
Obturator foramen	Larger	Smaller

4. A. Pelvic brim
   B. Symphysis pubis
5. Make sure that the ASISs are positioned at equal distances from the IR.
6. The sacrum and coccyx would not be aligned with the symphysis pubis but would be rotated toward the left hip; the right iliac spine would be demonstrated within the inlet pelvis without pelvic brim superimposition; and the left iliac spine would be demonstrated next to the left acetabulum.
7. A. Foreshortening
   B. Greater
   C. Lesser
8. A. The patient's legs were internally rotated with the feet at 15 to 20 degrees from vertical and the femoral epicondyles placed parallel with the imaging table.
   B. The patient's legs were externally rotated with the feet at a 45-degree angle from vertical and the femoral epicondyles positioned at a 25- to 30-degree angle with the imaging table.
   C. The patient's legs were externally rotated with the feet vertical and the femoral epicondyles at a 15 to 20 degree angle with the imaging table.
9. The feet are tilted internally 15 to 20 degrees from vertical, and the line connecting the femoral epicondyles is aligned parallel with the imaging table.
10. A. Inferior sacrum
    B. Perpendicular
    C. Symphysis pubis
    D. ASISs

11. The ilia, pubis, ischia, acetabula, femoral necks and heads, and greater and lesser trochanters
12. The pelvis was rotated onto the right side (RPO).
13. The patient's legs were externally rotated, with the feet and an imaginary line connecting the femoral epicondyles positioned at a 45-degree angle with the table.
14. The femoral necks are completely foreshortened, and the lesser trochanters are demonstrated in profile. The patient's legs were externally rotated, with the patient's feet at a 45-degree angle and the femoral epicondyles positioned at a 25- to 30-degree angle with the imaging table. Internally rotate the patient's legs until the feet are angled 15 to 20 degrees from vertical and the femoral epicondyles are positioned parallel with the imaging table.
15. The left obturator foramen is narrower than the right foramen, the left ischial spine is demonstrated without pelvic brim superimposition, and the sacrum and coccyx are rotated toward the right hip. Rotate the patient toward the right hip until the ASISs are positioned at equal distances from the imaging table.

Pelvis: AP Oblique (Frog-leg) Projection (Modified Cleaves Method)

1. A. Ischial spine
   B. Pelvic brim
   C. Coccyx
   D. Symphysis pubis

E. Ischial tuberosity
F. Obturator foramen
G. Lesser trochanter
H. Greater trochanter
I. Femoral neck
J. Femoral head
K. Sacrum
L. Acetabulum
M. Iliac ala
N. ASIS
O. Iliac crest

2. Place the anterior iliac spines at equal distances from the IR.

3. The ischial spines will be aligned and superimposed by the pelvic brim, and the sacrum and coccyx will be aligned with the symphysis pubis.

4. The sacrum and coccyx would not be aligned with the symphysis pubis but would be rotated toward the right hip, the left iliac spine would be demonstrated within the inlet pelvis without pelvic brim superimposition, and the right iliac spine would be demonstrated next to the right acetabulum.

5. A. Lesser
   B. Medially
   C. Greater

6. Proximal femurs

7. 60 to 70 degrees

8. The greater trochanters will be demonstrated lateral to the proximal femur.

9. A. The amount of femoral neck foreshortening
   B. The transverse level at which the greater trochanters will be demonstrated between the femoral heads and lesser trochanters

10. A. The femoral necks would be demonstrated on end, and the greater trochanters would be demonstrated at the same transverse level as the femoral heads.
    B. The femoral necks would be partially foreshortened, and the greater trochanters would be positioned at a transverse level halfway between the femoral necks and lesser trochanters.
    C. The femoral necks would be demonstrated without foreshortening, and the greater trochanters would be positioned at the same transverse level as the lesser trochanters.

11. A. Inferior sacrum
    B. Perpendicular
    C. Midsagittal
    D. Symphysis pubis
    E. ASISs

12. The ilea, pubis, ischia, acetabula, femoral necks and heads, and greater and lesser trochanters

13. The left side of the patient's pelvis was rotated closer to the IR than the right (LPO).

14. The patient's femurs were abducted beyond 45 degrees.

15. The femoral necks are demonstrated "on end." The greater trochanters are demonstrated on the same transverse level as the femoral heads. Consult with reviewers in your facility to determine whether this is an acceptable image. Because the femoral necks cannot be evaluated because of foreshortening, it may be necessary to have the patient position the femurs at a 45-degree angle with the imaging table.

16. The sacrum is rotated toward the right hip, the patient's hands are demonstrated within the collimated field, the right femur is abducted more than the left and the inferior sacrum is not in the center of the image. Rotate the patient toward the right hip, move the patient's hands away from the collimated field, and abduct both femurs equally and accurately center the central ray.

Sacroiliac Joints: AP Axial Projection

1. A. Median sacral crest
   B. Symphysis pubis
   C. Pelvic brim
   D. Second sacral segment
   E. Ilium
   F. Sacroiliac joint
   G. Sacral ala

2. Position the ASISs at equal distances from the imaging table.

3. A. Symphysis pubis
   B. Pelvic brim

4. A. Opposite
   B. Farther

5. A. 30 degrees cephalic
   B. 35 degrees cephalic
   C. Increase the angle over the routine amount used until the central ray and sacroiliac joints are aligned.
   D. Decrease the angle over the routine amount used until the central ray and sacroiliac joints are aligned.

6. A. To obtain tight collimation
   B. To ensure that the central ray is accurately aligned with the sacroiliac joints

7. A. Second sacral segment
   B. Midsagittal
   C. ASISs
   D. Symphysis pubis

8. The sacroiliac joints and first through fourth sacral segments

9. The right side of the patient's pelvis was situated farther away from the IR than the left side (LPO).

10. The central ray was inadequately angled.
11. The sacroiliac joints are foreshortened, and the inferior sacrum is demonstrated without symphysis pubis superimposition. Increase the degree of cephalic central ray angulation.
12. The sacroiliac joints and sacrum are elongated, and the symphysis pubis is superimposed over the inferior aspects of the sacrum and sacroiliac joints. Angle the central ray 30 to 35 degrees cephalad.

Sacroiliac Joints: AP Oblique Projection (LPO and RPO Positions)

1. A. Ileum
   B. Iliac tuberosity
   C. Inferior sacral ala
   D. Sacrum
   E. Superior sacral ala
   F. Sacroiliac joint
2. A. Ileum
   B. Sacrum
3. A. Ileum
   B. Sacrum
4. A. Midcoronal
   B. 25 to 30
5. A. Right
   B. Right
6. A. Medial
   B. ASIS
7. The sacroiliac joint, sacral ala, and ileum
8. The patient was underrotated.
9. The patient was overrotated.
10. The sacroiliac joint is closed. The superior and inferior sacral alae are demonstrated without iliac superimposition, and the lateral sacral ala is superimposed over the iliac tuberosity. Increase the pelvic obliquity.
11. The sacroiliac joint is closed, the ileum is superimposed over the inferior sacral ala and the lateral sacrum. Decrease the degree of pelvic obliquity.

Image Analysis of the Cervical and Thoracic Vertebrae

LEARNING OBJECTIVES

After completion of this chapter you should be able to:

_____ 1. Identify the required anatomy on cervical and thoracic vertebral images.

_____ 2. Describe how to properly position the patient, image receptor (IR), and central ray for cervical and thoracic vertebral images.

_____ 3. State how to properly mark and hang each cervical and thoracic vertebral image.

_____ 4. List the typical artifacts that are found on cervical and thoracic vertebral images.

_____ 5. List the image requirements for cervical and thoracic vertebral images with accurate positioning.

_____ 6. State how to properly reposition the patient when cervical and thoracic vertebral images with poor positioning are produced.

_____ 7. Discuss how to determine the amount of patient or central ray adjustment that is required to improve cervical and thoracic vertebral images with poor positioning.

_____ 8. State the kilovoltage routinely used for cervical and thoracic vertebral images, and describe what anatomical structures are demonstrated when the correct technique factors are used.

_____ 9. Describe how the upper and lower cervical vertebrae can move simultaneously and independently.

_____ 10. Explain how a patient with a suspected subluxation or fracture of the cervical vertebral column is positioned for cervical images.

_____ 11. Discuss the curvature of the cervical vertebrae, and explain how the intervertebral disk spaces slant.

_____ 12. Describe why a 5-degree cephalic central ray angulation is often required for an anteroposterior (AP) open-mouth image of the atlas and axis.

_____ 13. State how the relationship between the dens and atlas's lateral masses changes when the patient's head is rotated.

_____ 14. Describe how the prevertebral fat stripe is used as a diagnostic tool.

_____ 15. Explain how the patient is positioned to demonstrate AP cervical mobility.

_____ 16. Discuss the procedures that are taken if C7 is not demonstrated on a lateral cervical image.

_____ 17. Describe the positioning and image differences that exist between anterior and posterior oblique cervical images.

_____ 18. State why a grid is not used and why a 72-inch (183 cm) source–image receptor distance (SID) is used when the cervical vertebrae are imaged in the oblique and lateral positions.

_____ 19. Discuss when it is necessary to achieve a lateral cervicothoracic position of the cervical vertebrae.

_____ 20. Describe the curvature of the thoracic vertebrae.

_____ 21. List two methods that are used to obtain uniform image density on an AP thoracic vertebral image.

_____ 22. Discuss how scoliosis is differentiated from rotation on AP and lateral thoracic images.

_____ 23. Explain the breathing methods that are used to demonstrate the thoracic vertebrae on a lateral thoracic image.

_____ 24. Describe two methods that are used to offset the sagging of the lower thoracic column that results when the patient is in a lateral position.

STUDY QUESTIONS

1. Describe how the following shoulder images should be hung on a view box or displayed on a CRT monitor.

    A. AP cervical vertebrae: _____

    _____

    B. Right anterior oblique (RAO) cervical vertebrae: _____

    _____

    C. Lateral cervicothoracic: _____

    _____

    D. Lateral thoracic vertebrae: _____

    _____

2. Complete Table 7-1.

TABLE 7-1 **Hip and Pelvic Technical Data**				
Position or Projection	**kVp**	**Grid**	**AEC Chamber**	**SID**
AP axial projection, cervical vertebrae				
AP projection, "open-mouth" C1 and C2				
Lateral position, cervical vertebrae				
AP axial oblique projection, cervical vertebrae				
Lateral "Twining" position, cervicothoracic vertebrae				
AP projection, thoracic vertebrae				
Lateral position, thoracic vertebrae				

AEC, Automatic exposure control; *AP,* anteroposterior; *kVp,* kilovolt peak; *SID,* source–image receptor distance.

3. Complete Table 7-2.

TABLE 7-2 IR Size, Placement, and Direction		
Position or Projection	IR Size	Placement and Direction
AP axial projection, cervical vertebrae		
AP projection, "open-mouth" C1 and C2		
Lateral position, cervical vertebrae	Trauma:	
AP axial oblique projection, cervical vertebrae		
Lateral "Twining" position, cervicothoracic vertebrae		
AP projection, thoracic vertebrae		
Lateral position, thoracic vertebrae		

AP, Anteroposterior; *IR,* image receptor.

Cervical Vertebrae: AP Axial Projection

4. Identify the labeled anatomy in Figure 7-1.

Figure 7–1

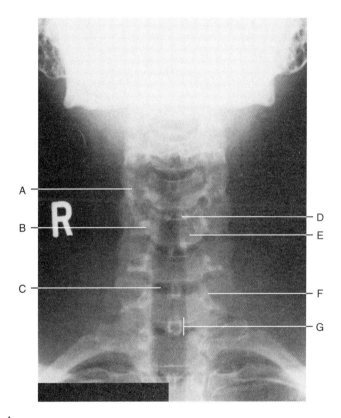

A. _____

B. _____

C. _____

D. _____

E. _____

F. _____

G. _____

5. Define the following terms.

  A. Intervertebral disk space: _____

    _____

  B. Lordotic curvature: _____

    _____

  C. Acanthiomeatal line: _____

    _____

  D. Upper occlusal plane: _____

    _____

6. If the transversely collimated field is coned to a 6-inch (15 cm) field size, where is the marker placed to ensure that it will be within the collimated field? _____

7. How is the patient positioned for an AP cervical image to prevent rotation of the upper and lower cervical vertebrae?

  A. Upper: _____

    _____

  B. Lower: _____

8. On a nonrotated AP cervical image, the (A) _____ are aligned with the midline of the cervical bodies, the (B) _____ and mastoid tips are at equal distances from the cervical vertebrae, and the distances from the (C) _____ to the medial ends of the clavicles are equal.

9. When the patient and cervical vertebrae are rotated away from the AP projection, the vertebral bodies will move toward the side positioned (A) _____ (closer to/farther from) the IR, and the spinous processes will move toward the side positioned (B) _____ (closer to/farther from) the IR.

10. Will rotation on an AP cervical image with poor positioning always be demonstrated throughout the entire cervical column?

  A. _____ (Yes/No)

Defend your answer.

  B. _____

    _____

11. A patient wearing a collar and on a backboard is taken to the x-ray department for a cervical vertebrae series. Should the collar be removed before the x-rays are taken?

  A. _____ (Yes/No)

The patient's head is rotated. Should it be adjusted?

  B. _____ (Yes/No)

Defend your answers to parts A and B.

  C. _____

    _____

12. When the central ray is properly aligned for an AP cervical image, the (A) _____ spaces will be open and each vertebra's spinous process will be demonstrated at the level of its (B) _____.

13. What is the curvature of the cervical vertebral column?

    _____

14. How do the intervertebral disk spaces slant on the cervical vertebrae?

    A. _____

    Is the degree of slant higher when the patient is upright or supine?

    B. _____

    What central ray angulation is used for an AP cervical image in a supine patient?

    C. _____

    In an upright patient?

    D. _____

    What causes this difference?

    E. _____

    _____

15. If the central ray angulation is not adequately angled for an AP cervical image, the intervertebral disk spaces are (A) _____ and each vertebra's spinous process is demonstrated within (B) _____.

16. Where is each vertebra's spinous process demonstrated if the central ray angulation is too cephalad?

    _____

17. Does too much or too little cephalad angulation cause elongation of the uncinate processes on an AP cervical image? _____

18. The third cervical vertebra is demonstrated in its entirety on an AP cervical image with accurate positioning. How was the patient positioned to accomplish this demonstration? _____

    _____

19. On an AP cervical image with accurate positioning, the (A) _____ is centered within the collimated field. This centering is obtained by placing the central ray at the patient's (B) _____ plane at a level halfway between the (C) _____ and (D) _____.

20. What anatomical structures are demonstrated on an AP cervical image with accurate positioning? _____

    _____

For the following descriptions of AP cervical images with poor positioning, state how the patient or central ray would have been mispositioned for such an image to be obtained.

21. The spinous processes are not aligned with the midline of the cervical bodies, and the pedicles and articular pillars are not symmetrically demonstrated lateral to the vertebral bodies. The right mandibular angle is visible, the left mandibular angle is superimposed over the cervical vertebrae, and the medial end of the right clavicle is demonstrated without vertebral column superimposition.

   _____

22. The anteroinferior aspects of the cervical bodies are obscuring the intervertebral disk spaces, and each vertebra's spinous process is demonstrated within the vertebral body.

   _____

23. The posteroinferior aspects of the cervical bodies are obscuring the intervertebral disk spaces, the uncinate processes are elongated, and each vertebra's spinous process is demonstrated within the inferior adjoining vertebral body.

   _____

24. A portion of the third cervical vertebra is superimposed over the posterior occipital bone.

   _____

   _____

25. The mandible is superimposed over a portion of the third cervical vertebra.

   _____

26. The upper cervical vertebra is tilted toward the left side.

   _____

   _____

For the following AP cervical images with poor positioning, state what anatomical structures are misaligned and how the patient should be repositioned for an optimal image to be obtained.

Figure 7–2

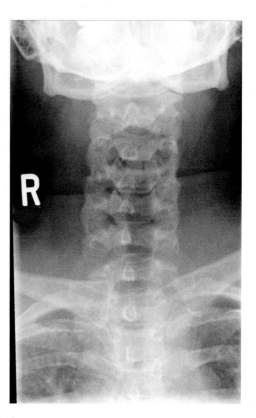

27. (Figure 7-2): _____

_____

_____

_____

Figure 7–3

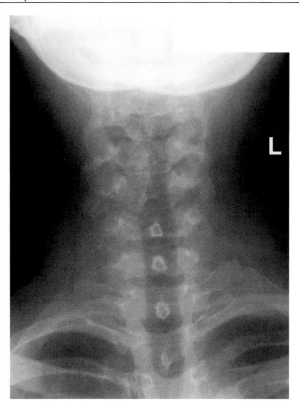

28. (Figure 7-3): _____

_____

_____

_____

Figure 7–4

29. (Figure 7-4): _____

_____

_____

_____

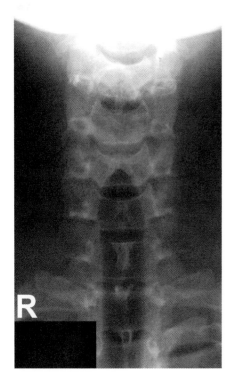

Figure 7–5

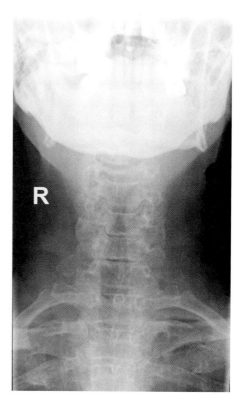

30. (Figure 7-5): _____

_____

_____

_____

Figure 7–6

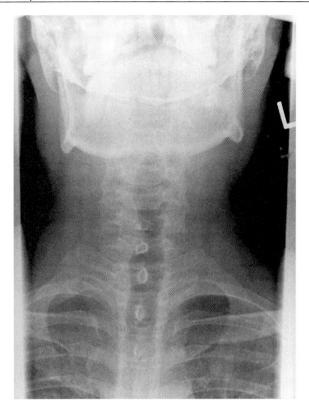

31. (Figure 7-6): _____

_____

_____

_____

Cervical Atlas and Axis: AP Projection (Open mouth)

1. Identify the labeled anatomy in Figure 7-7.

Figure 7–7

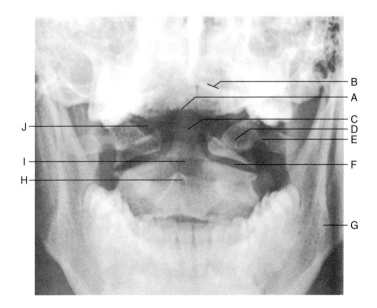

A. _____

B. _____

C. _____

D. _____

E. _____

F. _____

G. _____

H. _____

I. _____

J. _____

2. Define the following terms.

   A. Cervical atlas: _____

   B. Cervical axis: _____

   C. IOML: _____

3. An AP projection of the atlas and axis is obtained when the dens is demonstrated at equal distances from the (A) _____ and the (B) _____ of the axis is aligned with the midline of the axis's body.

4. How is the patient positioned to obtain an AP projection of the atlas and axis without rotation?

   _____

   _____

5. On head rotation the atlas pivots around the dens. This results in the lateral mass located on the side toward which the face is turned being displaced (A) _____ (anteriorly/posteriorly) and the side away from which the face is turned being displaced (B) _____ (anteriorly/posteriorly).

6. How is the patient positioned for an AP projection of the atlas and axis to demonstrate the upper incisor and posterior occiput superior to the dens and atlantoaxial joint?

   A. _____

   _____

   How is a patient without upper teeth positioned?

   B. _____

   _____

7. Why is it necessary to use a 5-degree cephalic central ray angulation on an AP atlas and axis image? _____

   _____

8. Describe how to determine the central ray angulation to use for an AP atlas and axis image on a trauma patient in a collar.

   _____

   _____

9. How can one determine from an AP atlas or axis image that the patient's neck was in flexion for the image?

   A. _____

   _____

   That it was in extension for the image?

   B. _____

   _____

10. On an AP atlas and axis image with accurate positioning, the (A) _____ is centered within the collimated field. This is accomplished by centering the central ray through the open mouth to the (B) _____.

11. What anatomical structures are included on an AP atlas and axis image with accurate positioning?

   _____

   _____

For the following descriptions of AP atlas and axis cervical images with poor positioning, state how the patient or central ray would have been mispositioned for such an image to be obtained.

12. The distances from the atlas's lateral masses to the dens and from the mandibular rami to the dens are narrower on the right side of the patient than on the left side, and the axis's spinous process is shifted from the midline.

   _____

   _____

13. The upper incisors are demonstrated approximately 1 inch (2.5 cm) inferior to the posterior occiput's inferior edge, obscuring the dens and atlantoaxial joint, and the posterior occiput's inferior edge is demonstrated directly superior to the dens. The acanthiomeatal line was aligned perpendicular to the imaging table.

   _____

   _____

14. The upper incisors are superimposed over the dens, and the posterior occiput's inferior edge is demonstrated superior to the dens and upper incisors. A 5-degree cephalic angulation was used to obtain this image.

   A. Patient: _____

   _____

   B. Central ray: _____

15. The dens is superimposed over the posterior occiput, and the upper incisors are demonstrated approximately 2 inches (5 cm) superior to the posterior occiput's inferior edge.

   A. Patient: _____

   _____

   B. Central ray: _____

For the following AP atlas and axis cervical images with poor positioning, state what anatomical structures are misaligned and how the patient should be repositioned for an optimal image to be obtained.

Figure 7–8

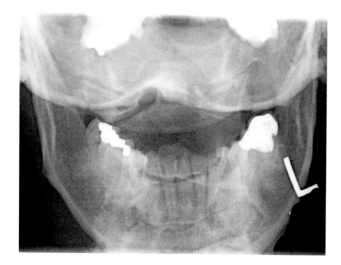

16. (Figure 7-8): _____

_____

_____

_____

Figure 7–9

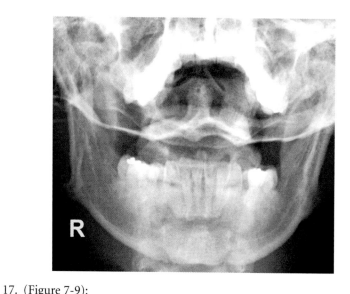

17. (Figure 7-9): _____

_____

_____

_____

Figure 7–10

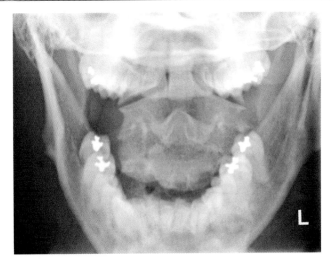

18. (Figure 7-10): _____

_____

_____

_____

Figure 7–11

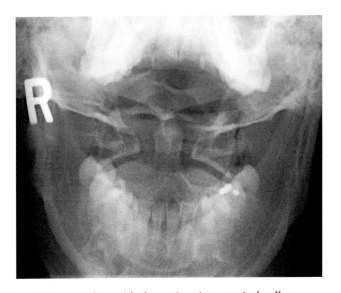

19. Figure 7-11 was taken with the patient in a cervical collar:

_____

_____

_____

_____

Cervical Vertebrae: Lateral Position

1. Identify the labeled anatomy in Figure 7-12.

Figure 7–12

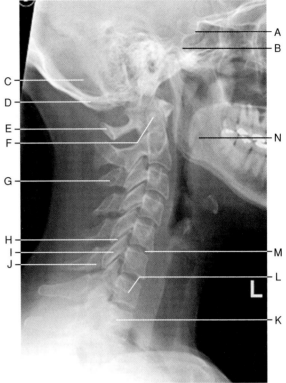

A. _____

B. _____

C. _____

D. _____

E. _____

F. _____

G. _____

H. _____

I. _____

J. _____

K. _____

L. _____

M. _____

N. _____

2. Define the following terms.

A. Infraorbitomeatal line: _____

_____

B. Interpupillary line: _____

_____

C. EAM: _____

D. Air-gap technique: _____

_____

3. What soft-tissue structure found on a lateral cervical image can be used to detect and localize cervical fractures or masses?

_____

4. Why is a long SID used for the lateral cervical vertebrae? _____

_____

5. A nonrotated lateral cervical image demonstrates superimposed right and left (A) _____ and (B) _____.

6. What body plane is positioned perpendicular to the IR for a lateral cervical image? _____

7. What anatomical structures are aligned with the IR to prevent rotation when positioning the patient for a lateral cervical image?

_____

8. How can rotation be identified on a lateral cervical image with poor positioning? _____

_____

9. How must the patient's head be positioned for a lateral cervical image to demonstrate the posterior arch of C1 and the spinous process of C2 in profile without posterior occiput superimposition, and the bodies of C1 and C2 without mandibular rami superimposition?

_____

_____

10. How must the patient's head be positioned for a lateral cervical image to demonstrate superimposed inferior cranial and mandibular cortices and to obtain open superior intervertebral disk spaces?

_____

_____

11. What are two advantages of aligning the long axis of the cervical vertebral column with the long axis of the collimated field?

A. _____

B. _____

12. Why are lateral flexion and extension images of the cervical vertebrae obtained?

_____

13. How is patient positioning adjusted from a neutral lateral position of the cervical vertebrae to achieve a flexed lateral position?

_____

_____

14. How is patient positioning adjusted from a neutral lateral position of the cervical vertebrae to achieve an extended lateral position?

_____

_____

15. On a lateral cervical image with accurate positioning, the (A) _____ is centered within the collimated field. This is accomplished by centering the central ray to the (B) _____ plane at a level halfway between the (C) _____ and (D) _____.

16. What anatomical structures are included on a lateral cervical image with accurate positioning?

_____

_____

17. Why should the clivus be included on all lateral cervical images?

_____

_____

18. It is often difficult to demonstrate C7 on a routine lateral cervical image because of shoulder thickness. How should the patient be positioned to improve C7 demonstration?

A. _____

B. _____

C. _____

19. What special view can be taken to demonstrate C7 when the procedure referred to in question 18 fails? _____

For the following descriptions of lateral cervical images with poor positioning, state how the patient would have been mispositioned for such an image to be obtained.

20. The articular pillars and zygapophyseal joints of one side of the patient are situated anterior to the opposite side's pillars and zygapophyseal joints.

_____

21. Neither the posterior nor the anterior cortices of the cranium nor the mandible are superimposed.

_____

22. The inferior cortices of the cranium and mandible are demonstrated without superimposition, and the vertebral foramen of C1 is demonstrated.

_____

For the following lateral cervical images with poor positioning, state what anatomical structures are misaligned and how the patient should be repositioned for an optimal image to be obtained.

Figure 7–13

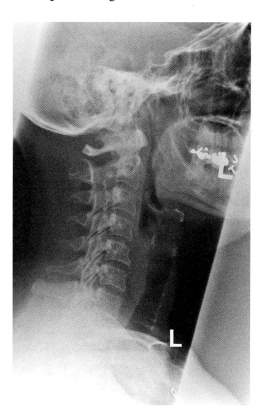

23. (Figure 7-13): _____

_____

_____

_____

Figure 7–14

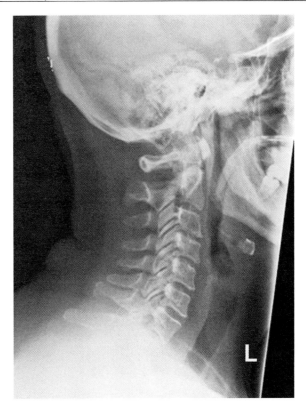

24. (Figure 7-14): _____

_____

_____

_____

Figure 7–15

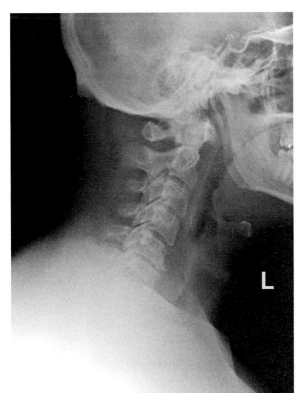

25. (Figure 7-15): _____

_____

_____

_____

Cervical Vertebrae: PA/AP Axial Oblique Projection (Anterior and Posterior Oblique Positions)

1. Identify the labeled anatomy in Figure 7-16.

Figure 7–16

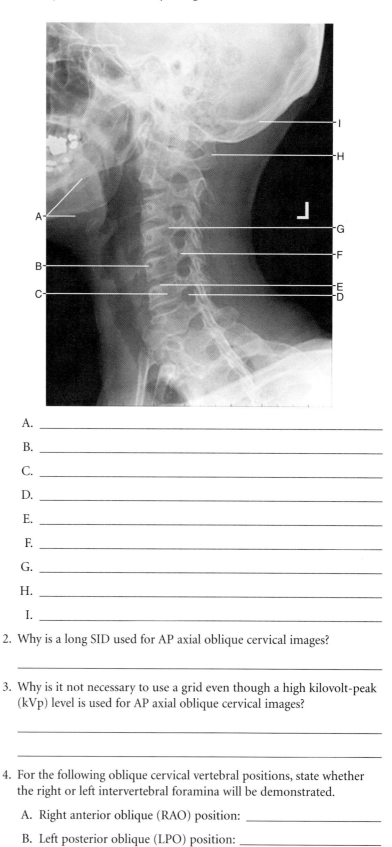

A. _____

B. _____

C. _____

D. _____

E. _____

F. _____

G. _____

H. _____

I. _____

2. Why is a long SID used for AP axial oblique cervical images?

   _____

3. Why is it not necessary to use a grid even though a high kilovolt-peak (kVp) level is used for AP axial oblique cervical images?

   _____

   _____

4. For the following oblique cervical vertebral positions, state whether the right or left intervertebral foramina will be demonstrated.

   A. Right anterior oblique (RAO) position: _____

   B. Left posterior oblique (LPO) position: _____

    C. Left anterior oblique (LAO) position: _____

    D. Right posterior oblique (RPO) position: _____

5. What degree of body rotation is used for oblique cervical images?

    A. _____

What body plane is used to set up the degree of obliquity?

    B. _____.

6. Why is it necessary to use right and left side oblique positions when imaging the cervical vertebrae?

_____

_____

7. Describe how to position the IR beneath a trauma patient to demonstrate the right intervertebral foramina for an oblique cervical image.

    A. _____

_____

How is the central ray angled and positioned?

    B. _____

_____

8. What degree and direction of central ray angulation are used for anterior oblique cervical images?

    A. _____

For posterior oblique cervical images?

    B. _____

Why is it necessary to use an angled central ray for oblique cervical images?

    C. _____

_____

9. How should the patient be positioned to demonstrate the alignment of the right and left posterior cranium and mandible cortices and to demonstrate the upper cervical vertebrae without occipital or mandibular superimposition? _____

_____

10. How should the central ray be adjusted from the routinely used angle for an anterior oblique cervical vertebrae image in a patient who has severe kyphosis to better demonstrate the lower cervical vertebrae?

_____

11. Which cranial and mandibular cortices will be demonstrated inferiorly on a right anterior oblique cervical image?

    A. _____

On a left posterior oblique cervical image?

    B. _____

What aspect of the positioning setup causes these cortices to be projected one superior to the other?

C. _____

_____

12. On an oblique cervical image with accurate positioning, the (A) _____ is centered within the collimated field. This is accomplished by centering the central ray to the (B) _____ plane at a level halfway between the (C) _____ and (D) _____.

13. What anatomical structures are included on an oblique cervical image with accurate positioning? _____

_____

For the following descriptions of oblique cervical images with poor positioning, state how the patient or central ray would have been mispositioned for such an image to be obtained.

14. An LAO cervical image, obtained with the patient's head in an oblique position, demonstrates obscured pedicles and intervertebral foramina, and the vertebral column is superimposed over a portion of the left sternoclavicular joint and medial clavicular end.

_____

15. An RAO cervical image, obtained with the patient's head in a lateral position, demonstrates the intervertebral foramina, the right pedicles (although they are not in true profile), the left pedicles in the midline of the vertebral bodies, and the right zygapophyseal joints.

_____

16. In this LAO cervical image, the intervertebral disk spaces are closed, the vertebral bodies are distorted, the posterior tubercles are demonstrated within the vertebral foramina, the C1 vertebral foramen is not demonstrated, and the inferior mandibular rami and the cranial cortices are demonstrated with superimposition.

_____

17. The upper cervical vertebrae are obscured by the patient's cranium and mandible.

_____

18. The atlas and its posterior arch are obscured. The inferior cranial cortices demonstrate more than ¼ inch (0.6 cm) of distance between them, and the inferior cortices of the mandibular rami demonstrate more than ½ inch (1.25 cm) of distance between them.

_____

For the following oblique cervical images with poor positioning, state what anatomical structures are misaligned and how the patient should be repositioned for such an image to be obtained.

Figure 7–17

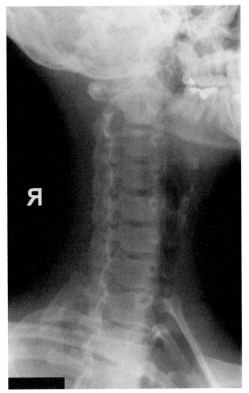

19. (Figure 7-17): _____

_____

_____

Figure 7–18

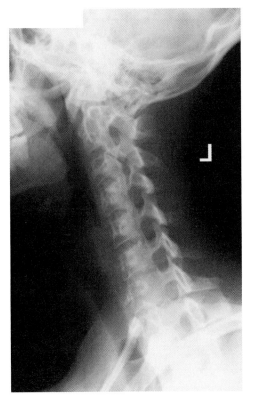

20. (Figure 7-18): _____

_____

_____

Figure 7–19

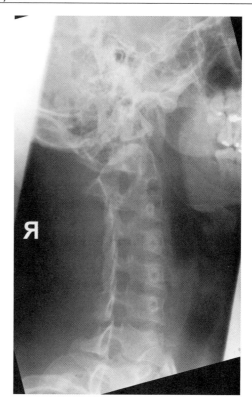

21. (Figure 7-19): _____

_____

_____

Figure 7–20

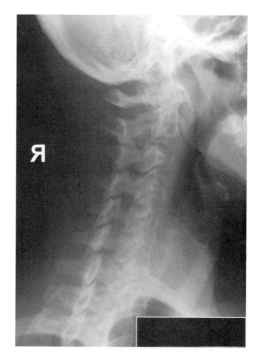

22. (Figure 7-20): _____

_____

_____

Cervicothoracic Vertebrae: Lateral Position (Twining Method)

1. Identify the labeled anatomy in Figure 7-21.

Figure 7–21

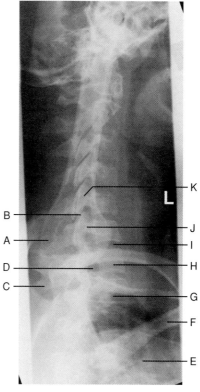

A. _____

B. _____

C. _____

D. _____

E. _____

F. _____

G. _____

H. _____

I. _____

J. _____

K. _____

2. List two situations in which a lateral cervicothoracic position would be indicated.

A. _____

B. _____

_____

3. List three ways to reduce the amount of scatter radiation that reaches the IR when using the lateral cervicothoracic position.

A. _____

B. _____

C. _____

4. What respiration is used for the lateral cervicothoracic position?

    _____

5. A lateral image of the cervicothoracic vertebrae is demonstrated when the right and left (A) _____ joints, (B) _____, and posterior ribs are superimposed.

6. To obtain a lateral cervicothoracic position, how is the arm adjacent to the imaging table positioned?

    A. _____

    How is the arm situated farther from the imaging table positioned?

    B. _____

7. How is the patient positioned to prevent rotation on a lateral cervicothoracic image?

    A. Cervical rotation: _____

    _____

    B. Thoracic rotation: _____

    _____

8. How can rotation be identified on a lateral cervicothoracic image?

    _____

    _____

9. How is the patient positioned for a lateral cervicothoracic image to demonstrate open intervertebral disk spaces and undistorted vertebral bodies?

    _____

    _____

10. On a lateral cervicothoracic image with accurate positioning, the (A) _____ is centered within the collimated field. This is accomplished by centering a perpendicular central ray to the (B) _____ plane at a level 1 inch (2.5 cm) superior to the (C) _____ or at the level of the (D) _____.

11. When should a 5-degree caudal central ray angulation be used with the lateral cervicothoracic position? _____

    _____

12. What anatomical structures are included on a lateral cervicothoracic image with accurate positioning? _____

    _____

For the following descriptions of lateral cervicothoracic images with poor positioning, state how the patient would have been mispositioned for such an image to be obtained.

13. The right and left articular pillars, zygapophyseal joints, and posterior ribs are demonstrated without superimposition. The humerus that was raised and situated closer to the IR is demonstrated posterior to the vertebral column.

    _____

14. The right and left articular pillars, zygapophyseal joints, and posterior ribs are demonstrated without superimposition. The humerus demonstrating the lesser amount of magnification is situated anterior to the vertebral column.

_____

15. The intervertebral disk spaces are closed, and the vertebral bodies are distorted.

_____

For the following lateral cervicothoracic images with poor positioning, state what anatomical structures are misaligned and how the patient should be repositioned for an optimal image to be obtained.

Figure 7–22

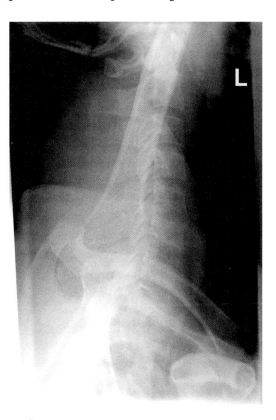

16. (Figure 7-22): _____

_____

_____

Figure 7–23

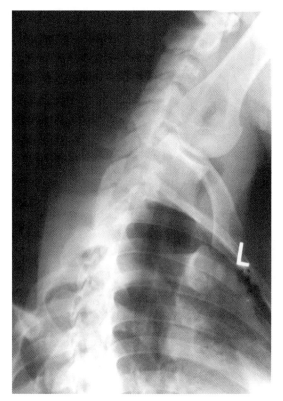

17. (Figure 7-23): _____

_____

_____

Thoracic Vertebrae: AP Projection

1. Identify the labeled anatomy in Figure 7-24.

Figure 7–24

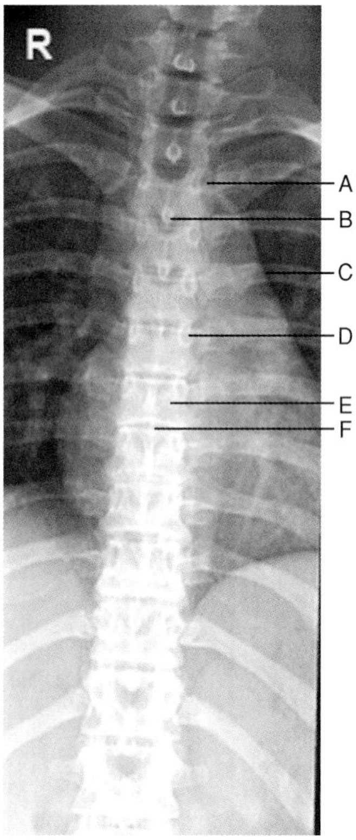

A. _____

B. _____

C. _____

D. _____

E. _____

F. _____

2. How tightly can one safely collimate on an AP projection of the thoracic vertebrae?

   _____

3. List two methods of achieving uniform image density of the thoracic vertebrae on an AP projection.

   A. _____

   B. _____

4. Describe how to accurately position the compensating filter for an AP thoracic image.

   _____

   _____

5. How can the patient be positioned with respect to the x-ray tube for an AP thoracic image to take advantage of the anode-heel effect?

   _____

   _____

6. What patient respiration is used for an AP thoracic image to demonstrate the vertebrae and posterior ribs? _____

7. An AP projection of the thoracic vertebrae is obtained when the (A) _____ are aligned with the midline of the vertebral bodies, the distances from the vertebral column to the sternal ends of the clavicles are (B) _____, and the distances from the pedicles to the spinous processes are (C) _____.

8. How is the patient positioned to ensure that rotation will not be demonstrated on an AP thoracic image? _____

   _____

9. When rotation is present on an AP thoracic image, the side demonstrating the greater distance between the spinous processes and pedicles will be _____ (closer to/farther from) the IR.

10. What patient condition can simulate rotation on an AP thoracic image?

    A. _____

    Describe how this condition can be distinguished from rotation.

    B. _____

    _____

11. What type of curvature does the thoracic vertebral column demonstrate?

    A. _____

    How can the patient be positioned to reduce this curvature and better align the x-ray beams with the intervertebral disk spaces?

    B. _____

    _____

12. On an AP thoracic image with accurate positioning, the

(A) _____ is centered within the collimated field. This is accomplished by centering the central ray to the (B) _____ plane at a level halfway between the (C) _____ and xiphoid.

13. What anatomical structures are included on an AP thoracic image with accurate positioning? _____

_____

For the following descriptions of AP thoracic images with poor positioning, state how the patient would have been mispositioned for such an image to be obtained.

14. The lower thoracic intervertebral disk spaces are obscured, and the vertebral bodies are distorted.

_____

15. The distance from the left pedicles to the spinous processes is greater than the distance from the right pedicles to the spinous processes.

_____

16. The upper thoracic vertebrae are overexposed, and the lower thoracic vertebrae demonstrate adequate density.

_____

For the following AP thoracic images with poor positioning, state what anatomical structures are misaligned and how the patient should be repositioned for an optimal image to be obtained.

Figure 7–25

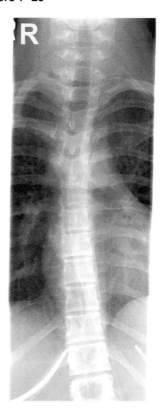

17. (Figure 7-25): _____

_____

_____

Figure 7–26

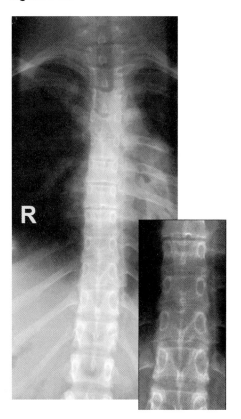

18. (Figure 7-26): _____

_____

_____

Thoracic Vertebrae: Lateral Position

1. Identify the labeled anatomy in Figure 7-27.

Figure 7–27

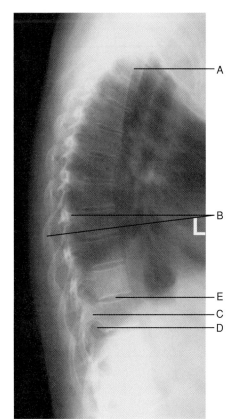

A. _____

B. _____

C. _____

D. _____

E. _____

2. Define the following terms.

   A. Breathing technique: _____

   _____

   B. Kyphotic curvature: _____

   _____

3. What advantage does using a breathing technique over a nonbreathing technique have when imaging the thoracic vertebrae in the lateral position? _____

   _____

4. If patient motion cannot be avoided on a lateral thoracic image when using a breathing technique, what respiration should be used?

   _____

5. A lateral thoracic image will demonstrate the intervertebral (A) _____ , superimposed posterior vertebral bodies, and no more than ½ inch (1.25 cm) of space between the (B) _____ .

6. List two reasons why the patient's arms should be positioned at a 90-degree angle with the body for a lateral thoracic image.

   A. _____

   _____

   B. _____

   _____

7. How is the patient positioned to prevent rotation on a lateral thoracic image?

   _____

   _____

8. How can rotation be identified on a lateral thoracic image?

   _____

   _____

9. How can scoliosis be distinguished from rotation on a lateral thoracic image? _____

   _____

10. When the thoracic vertebrae are in a lateral position, the posterior ribs are positioned on top of each other. Why does the resulting image demonstrate the posterior ribs approximately ½ inch (1.25 cm) apart?

    _____

    _____

11. How is the patient positioned to obtain open intervertebral disk spaces on a lateral thoracic image ?

    _____

12. Describe the patient body form that demonstrates the greatest thoracic vertebral sagging when the patient is placed in a lateral position.

    A. _____

    _____

    State where the radiolucent sponge is positioned to offset this sagging.

    B. _____

    _____

    State how the central ray can be adjusted to offset this sagging.

    C. _____

13. On a lateral thoracic vertebral image with accurate positioning, the (A) _____ is centered within the collimated field. This is accomplished by centering the central ray to the (B) _____ when the patient's arm is positioned at a 90-degree angle with the body.

14. What anatomical structures are included on a lateral thoracic image with accurate positioning?

    _____

15. List two methods of confirming which thoracic vertebra is the twelfth on a lateral thoracic image.

    A. _____

    B. _____

    _____

16. List two methods of confirming which thoracic vertebra is the first on a lateral thoracic image.

    A. _____

    B. _____

17. If the first, second, or third thoracic vertebra is not included on a routine lateral thoracic image, what supplementary position is used to demonstrate these vertebrae?

    _____

For the following descriptions of lateral thoracic images, with poor positioning state how the patient would have been mispositioned for such an image to be obtained.

18. The posterior surfaces of the vertebral bodies are demonstrated without superimposition, and more than ½ inch (1.25 cm) of space is demonstrated between the posterior ribs.

    _____

19. The posterior surfaces of the vertebral bodies are demonstrated without superimposition, and the posterior ribs are superimposed.

    _____

20. The eighth through twelfth thoracic intervertebral disk spaces are obscured, and the vertebral bodies are distorted.

    _____

For the following lateral thoracic images, with poor positioning state what anatomical structures are misaligned and how the patient should be repositioned for an optimal image to be obtained.

Figure 7–28

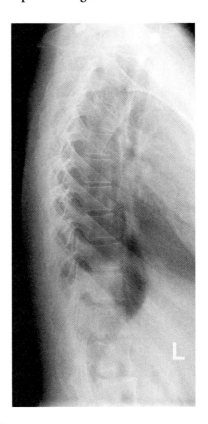

21. (Figure 7-28): _____

_____

_____

Figure 7–29

L

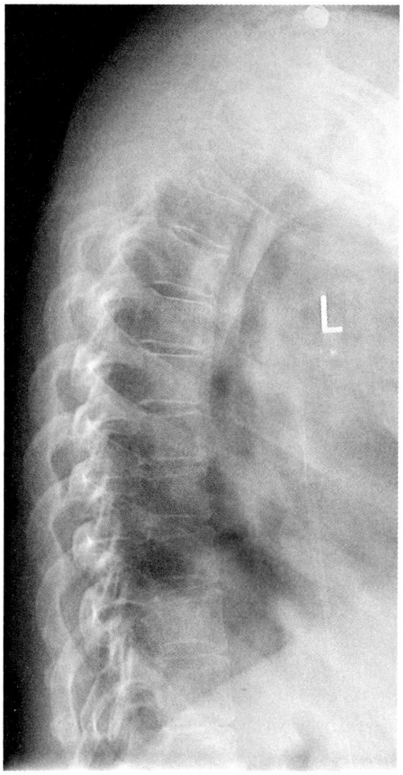

22. (Figure 7-29): ______________________________

____

____

____

____

Figure 7–30

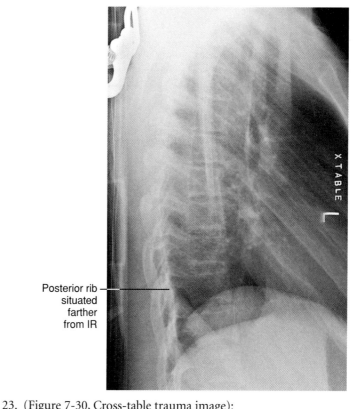

X TABLE
L
Posterior rib situated farther from IR

23. (Figure 7-30, Cross-table trauma image): ______________________________

____

____

CHAPTER 7
STUDY QUESTION ANSWERS

1. A. As if the patient is standing in an upright position. The marker is correct.

  B. As if the patient is standing in an upright position. The marker is reversed.
  C. As if the patient is standing in an upright position. The marker is correct.
  D. As if the patient is standing in an upright position. The marker is correct.

2. Table 7-1

Position or Projection	kVp	Grid	AEC Chamber	SID
AP axial projection, cervical vertebrae	70-80	Grid	Center	40-48 inches (100-120 cm)
AP projection, "open-mouth" C1 and C2	70-80	Grid		40-48 inches (100-120 cm)
Lateral position, cervical vertebrae	70-80	Optional air gap	Center	72 inches (150-180 cm)
AP axial oblique projection, cervical vertebrae	70-80	Optional air gap	Center	72 inches (150-180 cm)
Lateral "Twining" position, cervicothoracic vertebrae	65-85	Grid		40-48 inches (100-120 cm)
AP projection, thoracic vertebrae	75-85	Grid	Center	40-48 inches (100-120 cm)
Lateral position, thoracic vertebrae	80-90	Grid	Center	40-48 inches (100-120 cm)

AEC, Automatic exposure control; AP, anteroposterior; kVp, kilovolt peak; SID, source–image receptor distance.

3. Table 7-2

Position or Projection	IR Size	Placement and Direction
AP axial projection, cervical vertebrae	8 × 10 inches (18 × 24 cm)	Lengthwise
AP projection, "open-mouth" C1 and C2	8 × 10 inches (18 × 24 cm)	Lengthwise
Lateral position, cervical vertebrae	8 × 10 inches (18 × 24 cm) Trauma: 10 × 12 inches (24 × 30 cm)	Lengthwise
AP axial oblique projection, cervical vertebrae	8 × 10 inches (18 × 24 cm)	Lengthwise
Lateral "Twining" position, cervicothoracic vertebrae	10 × 12 inches (24 × 30 cm)	Lengthwise
AP projection, thoracic vertebrae	14 × 17 inches (35 × 43 cm)	Lengthwise
Lateral position, thoracic vertebrae	14 × 17 inches (35 × 43 cm)	Lengthwise

AP, Anteroposterior; IR, image receptor.

Cervical Vertebrae: AP Axial Projection

4. A. Articular pillar
  B. Pedicle
  C. Sixth to seventh intervertebral disk space
  D. Fourth spinous process
  E. Fifth vertebral body
  F. Seventh uncinate process
  G. Air-filled trachea
5. A. Space that is formed between two vertebral bodies
  B. Backward (posterior) curvature of the spine
  C. Imaginary line connecting the point at which the upper lip and nose meet the external ear opening
  D. Chewing surface of the maxillary teeth
6. No more than 3 inches (7.5 cm) from the IR center
7. A. Position the mastoid tips and mandibular angles at equal distances from the imaging table.
  B. Position the shoulders at equal distances from the imaging table.
8. A. Spinous processes

  B. Mandibular angles
  C. Vertebral column
9. A. Closer to
  B. Farther from
10. A. No
  B. The upper and lower cervical vertebrae can move independently of each other.
11. A. No
  B. No
  C. Spinal cord injury may be caused by moving the patient when a fracture is suspected.
12. A. Intervertebral disk
  B. Inferior intervertebral disk space
13. Lordotic
14. A. Upwardly, anteriorly to posteriorly
  B. Higher when upright
  C. 15 degrees cephalad
  D. 20 degrees cephalad
  E. The gravitational pull on the vertebrae that results when the patient is supine
15. A. Closed
  B. Its vertebral body

16. Within the inferior adjoining vertebral body
17. Too much
18. The patient's chin was tucked or elevated until an imaginary line connecting the upper occlusal plane and the posterior occiput's inferior edge was aligned perpendicular to the imaging table or until the acanthiomeatal line was aligned perpendicular to the imaging table.
19. A. Fourth cervical vertebra
    B. Midsagittal
    C. External auditory meatus (EAM)
    D. Jugular notch
20. The third through seventh cervical vertebrae, first thoracic vertebra, and surrounding soft tissue
21. The patient's head was turned, and the torso was rotated toward the right side.
22. The central ray was not angled cephalically enough.
23. The central ray was angled too cephalically.
24. The chin was not adequately tucked, positioning the upper occlusal plane superior to the posterior occiput's inferior edge.
25. The chin was overtucked, positioning the upper occlusal plane inferior to the base of the occiput.
26. The patient's head and upper cervical vertebrae's midsagittal plane was not aligned with the lower cervical vertebrae.
27. The spinous processes are not aligned with the midline of the cervical bodies but are closer to the right side, and the medial end of the right clavicle is superimposed over the vertebral column. Rotate the patient toward the right side until the shoulders are at equal distances from the imaging table or upright grid holder.
28. The anteroinferior aspects of the cervical bodies are obscuring the intervertebral disk spaces, and each vertebra's spinous process is demonstrated within its vertebral body. Increase the amount of cephalic central ray angulation.
29. The posteroinferior aspects of the cervical bodies are obscuring the intervertebral disk spaces, the uncinate processes are elongated, and each vertebra's spinous process is demonstrated within the inferior adjoining vertebral body. Decrease the amount of cephalic central ray angulation.
30. A portion of the third cervical vertebra is superimposed over the posterior occipital bone, preventing clear visualization of the third cervical vertebra. Tuck the chin half the distance demonstrated between the base of the skull and the mandibular mentum or until an imaginary line connecting the upper occlusal plane and the base of the skull is aligned perpendicular to the imaging table or upright grid holder.
31. The mandible is superimposed over a portion of the third cervical vertebra, the anteroinferior aspects of the cervical bodies are obscuring the intervertebral disk spaces, and each vertebra's spinous process is demonstrated within its

vertebra body. Raise the chin half the distance demonstrated between the base of the skull and the mandibular mentum or until an imaginary line connecting the upper occlusal plane and the inferior base of the posterior occiput is aligned perpendicular to the imaging table or upright grid holder, and increase the degree of cephalic central ray angulation.

Cervical Atlas and Axis: AP Projection (Open mouth)

1. A. Upper incisors
   B. Posterior occipital bone
   C. Dens
   D. C1 lateral mass
   E. Transverse process
   F. Atlantoaxial joint
   G. Mandibular ramus
   H. C2 spinous process
   I. C2 body
   J. Occipitoatlantal joint
2. A. First cervical vertebra
   B. Second cervical vertebra
   C. Imaginary line connecting the inferior orbital rim and the external ear opening
3. A. Atlas's lateral masses
   B. Spinous process
4. Position the patient's shoulders, mandibular angles, and mastoid tips at equal distances from the imaging table.
5. A. Posteriorly
   B. Anteriorly
6. A. Tuck the patient's chin until an imaginary line connecting the upper occlusal plane and the posterior occiput's inferior edge is aligned perpendicular to the imaging table or until the acanthiomeatal line is perpendicular to the imaging table.
   B. Imagine where the occlusal plane would be if the patient had teeth, and position the patient in the same manner.
7. To offset the magnification of the upper incisors that is caused by the long object–image receptor distance (OID)
8. Angle the central ray until it is aligned parallel with the infraorbitomeatal line (IOML).
9. A. The atlantoaxial joint will be closed, and the axis's spinous process will demonstrate an increased superior location to the dens.
   B. The atlantoaxial joint will be closed, and the axis's spinous process will demonstrate an increased inferior location to the dens.
10. A. Dens
    B. Midsagittal plane
11. The atlantoaxial and occipitoatlantal joints, atlas's lateral masses and transverse processes, and axis's dens and body

12. The patient's face was rotated toward the left side.
13. The central ray was not angled 5 degrees cephalad.
14. A. The patient's chin was tucked more than needed to position the acanthiomeatal line perpendicular to the imaging table.
    B. The central ray was angled too caudally.
15. A. The patient's chin was not tucked enough to position the acanthiomeatal line perpendicular to the imaging table.
    B. The central ray was angled too cephalically.
16. The distances from the atlas's lateral masses to the dens and from the mandibular rami to the dens are narrower on the left side than on the right side, and the dens is superimposed over the posterior occiput. Rotate the face toward the left side until the mandibular angles and mastoid tips are positioned at equal distances from the imaging table or upright grid holder, and tuck the chin toward the chest until an imaginary line connecting the upper occlusal plane with the base of the skull is aligned perpendicular to the IR.
17. The dens is superimposed over the posterior occiput. The upper incisors are demonstrated directly superior to the dens. Tuck the chin toward the chest until an imaginary line connecting the upper occlusal plane with the base of the skull is aligned perpendicular to the IR. A 5-degree cephalad angulation should be used.
18. The upper incisors are demonstrated inferior to the base of the skull, superimposing the dens and atlantoaxial articulation. The base of the skull is demonstrated directly superior to the dens. If the upper occlusal plane and the base of the skull were aligned perpendicular to the imaging table, and a perpendicular central ray was used for this image, do not adjust patient positioning; simply direct the central ray 5 degrees cephalad. If a 5-degree cephalad angulation was used for this image, do not adjust patient positioning; simply increase the cephalad angulation by 5 degrees.
19. The upper incisors are demonstrated superior to the dens and the base of the skull, and the dens is superimposed over the posterior occiput. Adjust the central ray angulation caudally until it is aligned parallel with the IOML.

Cervical Vertebrae: Lateral Position

1. A. Sella turcica
   B. Clivus
   C. Posterior occipital bone
   D. Inferior cranial cortices
   E. Posterior arch
   F. Dens
   G. Third spinous process
   H. Fifth through sixth zygapophyseal joints
   I. Articular pillars
   J. Sixth lamina
   K. First thoracic vertebra
   L. Seventh cervical vertebra
   M. Intervertebral disk space
   N. Mandibular rami
2. A. An imaginary line connecting the inferior orbital bone with the external ear opening
   B. An imaginary line connecting the eye pupils when they are looking forward
   C. External auditory meatus
   D. When the OID is long, scatter radiation that would expose the IR at a short OID is scattered away from the IR. Because less scatter reaches the IR, a grid is not needed.
3. Prevertebral fat stripe
4. Using a long SID will decrease the cervical magnification that results from the long OID that is created between the cervical vertebrae and IR.
5. A. Articular pillars
   B. Zygapophyseal joints
6. Midcoronal
7. Align the shoulders, mastoid tips, and mandibular rami.
8. The articular right or left pillars and zygapophyseal joints will be demonstrated one anterior to the other.
9. Position the head's midsagittal plane parallel with the IR and the IOML parallel with the floor.
10. Position the midsagittal plane parallel with the IR and the interpupillary line perpendicular to the IR.
11. A. Places the cervical vertebrae in a neutral position
    B. Allows for tight transverse collimation
12. To demonstrate AP vertebral mobility
13. Instruct the patient to tuck the chin against the chest as tightly as possible.
14. Instruct the patient to extend the chin up and backward as far as possible.
15. A. Fourth cervical vertebra
    B. Midcoronal
    C. EAM
    D. Jugular notch
16. The sella turcica, clivus, first through seventh cervical vertebrae, superior half of the first thoracic vertebra, and surrounding soft tissue
17. The clivus with the dens can be used to evaluate cervical injury.
18. A. Take the image with the patient in an upright position.
    B. Have the patient hold weights on each arm to depress the shoulders.
    C. Take the exposure on suspended expiration.
19. Lateral cervicothoracic (Twining method)
20. The patient was rotated.
21. The patient's head was rotated.
22. The patient's head and upper cervical vertebrae were tilted toward the IR.

23. The articular pillars and zygapophyseal joints on one side of the patient are situated anterior to those on the other side. Rotate the patient until the midcoronal plane is aligned perpendicular to the IR.

24. Neither the inferior nor the posterior cortices of the cranium nor the mandible is superimposed, the posterior arch of C1 is demonstrated in profile, and the right and left articular pillars and zygapophyseal joints demonstrate a superoinferior separation. Rotate the head until the midsagittal plane is aligned parallel with the IR, and then tilt the head toward the IR until the interpupillary line is perpendicular to the IR.

25. The vertebral body of C7 is not demonstrated in its entirety, and the superior body of T1 is not demonstrated. Have the patient hold 5- to 10-lb weights on each arm to depress the shoulders. If the patient cannot hold weights or if the weights do not sufficiently drop the shoulders, a special image known as the cervicothoracic lateral (Twining method) should be taken to demonstrate this area.

Cervical Vertebrae: PA/AP Axial Oblique Projection (Anterior and Posterior Oblique Positions)

1. A. Inferior mandibular cortices
   B. Pedicle
   C. Sixth vertebral body
   D. Intervertebral foramen
   E. Intervertebral disk space
   F. Pedicle
   G. Fourth uncinate process
   H. Posterior arch
   I. Inferior cranial cortices

2. To offset the magnification that would result because of the long OID used for the examination

3. When a long OID is used, causing scatter radiation to be diverged away from the IR and decreasing the amount of scatter radiation that reaches the IR

4. A. Right
   B. Right
   C. Left
   D. Left

5. A. 45 degrees
   B. Midcoronal

6. To demonstrate the intervertebral foramina located on the right and left sides of the cervical vertebrae

7. A. Align the left mastoid tip with the longitudinal axis of the IR and the right gonion with the transverse axis of the IR.
   B. Direct it 45 degrees medially and 15 degrees cephalically. Center it to the right side of the patient's neck halfway between the AP

surfaces of the neck at the level of the thyroid cartilage.

8. A. 15 to 20 degrees caudally
   B. 15 to 20 degrees cephalically
   C. To open the intervertebral disk spaces and demonstrate undistorted vertebral bodies

9. Position the skull's midsagittal plane parallel with the IR and the acanthiomeatal line parallel with the floor.

10. Increase the degree of central ray angulation.

11. A. Left
    B. Left
    C. The angulation of the central ray projects the mandible situated farther from the IR inferiorly on anterior oblique images and superiorly on posterior oblique images.

12. A. Fourth cervical vertebra
    B. Midsagittal plane
    C. EAM
    D. Jugular notch

13. The first through seventh cervical vertebrae, first thoracic vertebra, and surrounding soft tissue

14. The patient was rotated less than 45 degrees.

15. The patient was rotated more than 45 degrees.

16. The central ray was not angled enough caudally.

17. The patient's head was not turned to a lateral position.

18. The head and upper cervical vertebrae were tilted away from the IR.

19. This patient was in an RAO position, with the head in an oblique position. The right pedicles and intervertebral foramina are obscured. Increase patient obliquity until the midcoronal plane is placed at a 45-degree angle with the IR.

20. This patient was in an LAO position, with the head in a lateral position. The intervertebral foramina are demonstrated, the left pedicles are visible (although they are not in true profile), the right pedicles are demonstrated in the midline of the vertebral bodies, and the left zygapophyseal joints are demonstrated. Decrease patient rotation until the midcoronal plane is placed at a 45-degree angle with the IR.

21. This patient was in an RAO position, with the head in a lateral position. The atlas and its posterior arch are obscured. The inferior cranial cortices demonstrate more than ¼ inch (0.6 cm) between them, and the inferior cortices of the mandibular rami demonstrate more than ½ inch (1.25 cm) between them. The first thoracic vertebra is not included in its entirety. Tilt the patient's head toward the IR until the interpupillary line is aligned perpendicular to the IR, and move the central ray and IR inferiorly.

22. This patient was in an RAO position, with the head in a lateral position. The intervertebral disk spaces are closed, the cervical bodies are distorted,

the posterior tubercles are demonstrated within the intervertebral foramina, the C1 vertebral foramen is not demonstrated, and the inferior mandibular rami and the cranial cortices are demonstrated with superimposition. The central ray was directed perpendicular to the IR. Angle the central ray 15 to 20 degrees caudally for anterior oblique images.

Cervicothoracic Vertebrae: Lateral Position (Twining Method)

1. A. Humeral head
   B. Zygapophyseal joints
   C. C7 spinous process
   D. Intervertebral foramen
   E. Humeral head
   F. Clavicle
   G. T1 vertebra
   H. C7 vertebral body
   I. Intervertebral disk space
   J. Pedicles
   K. Articular pillars
2. A. When the routine lateral cervical image demonstrates the seventh vertebra
   B. When the routine lateral thoracic image does not demonstrate the first through third thoracic vertebrae
3. A. Use tight collimation.
   B. Use a high ratio grid.
   C. Align a lead contact shield or apron along the posterior edge of the collimated field.
4. Expiration
5. A. Zygapophyseal
   B. Articular pillars
6. A. The arm is elevated above the patient's head as high as possible.
   B. The arm is against the patient's side and should be depressed.
7. A. Position the patient's head in a lateral position.
   B. Position the patient to superimpose the shoulders and inferior posterior ribs.
8. The right and left articular pillars, posterior ribs, and zygapophyseal joints will be demonstrated without superimposition.
9. The cervical and vertebral column should be positioned parallel with the IR.
10. A. First thoracic vertebra
    B. Midcoronal
    C. Jugular notch
    D. Vertebral prominens
11. When the patient is unable to depress the shoulder positioned farther from the IR
12. The fifth through seventh cervical vertebrae and first through third thoracic vertebrae

13. The shoulder that was depressed and positioned farther from the IR was rotated anteriorly.
14. The shoulder that was depressed and positioned farther from the IR was rotated posteriorly.
15. The patient's vertebral column was not positioned parallel with the IR.
16. The intervertebral disk spaces are closed, and the vertebral bodies are distorted. The patient's cervical vertebral column was not positioned parallel with the IR. Position the midsagittal plane of the head and cervical vertebral column parallel with the IR. It may be necessary to prop the head on a sponge to help the patient maintain the position.
17. The right and left articular pillars, zygapophyseal joints, and posterior ribs are demonstrated without superimposition. The patient's thorax was rotated. The humerus that was raised and situated closer to the IR is demonstrated anterior to the vertebral column. Rotate the shoulder positioned farther from the IR anteriorly until your flat palms placed against the shoulders and the posterior ribs, respectively, are aligned perpendicular to the imaging table and upright IR.

Thoracic Vertebrae: AP Projection

1. A. Medial clavicular end
   B. Spinous process
   C. Posterior rib
   D. Pedicle
   E. Vertebral body
   F. Intervertebral disk space
2. To an 8-inch (20-cm) transverse field size
3. A. Use the anode-heel effect.
   B. Use a wedge compensating filter.
4. Position the thin edge of the filter at the inferior sternum where it begins to decline. The thick end will be directed toward the cervical vertebrae.
5. Position the patient's head and upper thoracic vertebrae at the anode end of the tube, and the lower thoracic vertebrae at the cathode end of the tube.
6. Suspended expiration
7. A. Spinous processes
   B. Equal
   C. Equal
8. Position the shoulders and anterior superior iliac spines at equal distances from the imaging table.
9. Closer to
10. A. Scoliosis
    B. A rotated thoracic image will demonstrate rotation of the thoracolumbar vertebrae and either the upper thoracic or lower lumbar vertebrae, whereas scoliosis will demonstrate

rotation of the thoracolumbar vertebrae without corresponding rotation of the upper thoracic or lower lumbar vertebrae.

11. A. Kyphotic
    B. Position the patient's head on a thin pillow and bend his or her knees, placing the feet flat against the imaging table.

12. A. Seventh thoracic vertebra
    B. Midsagittal
    C. Jugular notch

13. The seventh cervical vertebra, first through twelfth thoracic vertebrae, first lumbar vertebra, and 2½ inches (6.25 cm) of the posterior ribs and mediastinum on each side of the vertebral column

14. The patient's legs were extended.

15. The left side of the patient was positioned closer to the IR than was the right side (LPO).

16. The patient's head was positioned at the cathode end of the tube, and a compensating filter was not positioned over the upper thoracic vertebrae.

17. The upper thoracic vertebrae demonstrate more distance from the left pedicle to the spinous process than from the right pedicle to the spinous process, and the left medial clavicle is demonstrated away from the vertebral column. Rotate the patient toward the right side until the shoulders are at equal distances from the imaging table.

18. The eighth through twelfth intervertebral disk spaces are obscured, and the vertebral bodies distorted. Flex the patient's hips and knees, placing the feet and back firmly against the imaging table.

Thoracic Vertebrae: Lateral Position

1. A. First thoracic vertebra
   B. Posterior ribs
   C. Pedicles
   D. Intervertebral foramen
   E. Intervertebral disk space

2. A. A method of blurring out unwanted structures to better visualize needed structures by using a long exposure time and allowing the patient to costal breathe during the exposure
   B. Forward curve

3. It will blur the ribs and lung markings.

4. Suspended expiration

5. A. Foramina
   B. Posterior ribs

6. A. To prevent the humeri or their soft tissue from obscuring the thoracic vertebrae
   B. So the inferior scapular angle can be used to locate the seventh thoracic vertebra

7. Align the shoulders, posterior ribs, and posterior pelvic wings on top of each other.

8. By evaluating the superimposition of the right and left posterior surfaces of the vertebral bodies and the degree of posterior rib superimposition

9. The posterior ribs demonstrate differing degrees of rotation.

10. X-ray divergence will cause the posterior ribs that are situated farther from the IR to demonstrate more magnification than those situated closer to the IR.

11. The vertebral column should be positioned parallel with the IR.

12. A. A patient who has wide hips and a narrow waist
    B. Between the patient's lateral body surface and the imaging table, just superior to the iliac crest
    C. Angle the central ray 5 to 10 degrees cephalically.

13. A. Seventh thoracic vertebra
    B. Inferior scapular angle

14. The seventh cervical vertebra, first through twelfth thoracic vertebrae, and first lumbar vertebra

15. A. The vertebra that has the last rib attached to it is the twelfth.
    B. Follow the posterior vertebral bodies of the lower thoracic and upper lumbar vertebrae, locating the subtle change from kyphotic to lordotic that takes place between T12 and L1.

16. A. Counting up from the twelfth thoracic vertebra
    B. Locate the first vertebral prominens.

17. Cervicothoracic lateral (Twining method) position

18. The elevated side of the thorax was rotated posteriorly.

19. The elevated side of the thorax was rotated anteriorly.

20. The thoracic vertebral column was not aligned parallel with the imaging table.

21. The posterior surfaces of the vertebral bodies are demonstrated without superimposition, and the posterior ribs are superimposed. Rotate the elevated thorax posteriorly until a flat palm placed against the shoulder, posterior ribs, and posterior pelvic wings is aligned perpendicular to the imaging table.

22. The posterior surfaces of the vertebral bodies are demonstrated without superimposition, and more than ½ inch (1.25 cm) of space is demonstrated between the posterior ribs. Rotate the elevated thorax anteriorly until a flat palm placed against the shoulders and the posterior ribs is perpendicular to the imaging table. The T8 to T12 intervertebral disk spaces are obscured, and the vertebral bodies are distorted. Position a radiolucent sponge between the lateral body surface and the imaging table just superior to the patient's iliac crest, aligning the thoracic and lumbar vertebral column parallel with the imaging table.

23. The T8 to T12 intervertebral disk spaces are obscured, and the vertebral bodies are distorted. The vertebral column was not positioned parallel with the IR. The inferior posterior ribs situated farther from the IR are projected superior to the posterior ribs situated closer to the IR, indicating that the lower vertebral column was situated farther from the IR than the upper. Shift the lower half of the patient's body toward the IR until the vertebral column is parallel with the imaging table.

Image Analysis of the Lumbar Vertebrae, Sacrum, and Coccyx

LEARNING OBJECTIVES

After completion of this chapter you should be able to:

_____ 1. Identify the required anatomy on lumbar, sacral, and coccygeal images.

_____ 2. Describe how to properly position the patient, image receptor (IR), and central ray for lumbar, sacral, and coccygeal images.

_____ 3. State how to properly mark and hang lumbar, sacral, and coccygeal images.

_____ 4. List the typical artifacts that are found on lumbar, sacral, and coccygeal images.

_____ 5. List the image requirements for lumbar, sacral, and coccygeal images with accurate positioning.

_____ 6. State how to properly reposition the patient when lumbar, sacral, and coccygeal images with poor positioning are produced.

_____ 7. Discuss how to determine the amount of patient or central ray adjustment that is required to improve lumbar, sacral, and coccygeal images with poor positioning.

_____ 8. State the kilovolt-peak (kVp) level routinely used for lumbar, sacral, and coccygeal images, and describe what anatomical structures are demonstrated when the correct technique factors are used.

_____ 9. Describe how the upper and lower lumbar vertebrae can move simultaneously and independently.

_____ 10. Describe how spinal scoliosis is distinguished from rotation on an anteroposterior (AP) lumbar image.

_____ 11. State the curvature of the lumbar vertebrae, sacrum, and coccyx.

_____ 12. Discuss when gonadal radiation protection is used on AP lumbar, sacral, and coccygeal images.

_____ 13. State which zygapophyseal joints are demonstrated when posterior and anterior oblique lumbar images are produced.

_____ 14. List the anatomical structures that make up the parts of the "Scottie dogs" that are demonstrated on an oblique lumbar image with accurate positioning.

_____ 15. Explain what procedures are taken to produce lateral lumbar, L5-S1 spot, sacral, and coccygeal images with the least amount of scatter radiation reaching the IR.

_____ 16. State two methods of positioning the long axis of the lumbar column parallel with the long axis of the imaging table for a lateral lumbar image.

_____ 17. Describe how the patient is positioned to demonstrate AP mobility of the lumbar vertebral column.

_____ 18. Describe how to position a flat contact shield to protect the gonads for lateral lumbar, L5-S1, sacral, and coccygeal images.

_____ 19. State why the patient is instructed to empty the bladder and colon before an AP sacral or coccygeal image is taken.

_____ 20. List the procedures that can be taken to obtain sharply defined recorded details on sacral and coccygeal images.

STUDY QUESTIONS

1. Describe how the following shoulder images should be hung on a view box or displayed on a cathode ray tube (CRT) monitor.

   A. AP lumbar vertebrae: _____

   B. Right posterior oblique (RPO) lumbar vertebrae: _____

   _____

   C. Lateral coccyx: _____

2. List four methods of obtaining sharply defined recorded details on an AP coccygeal image.

   A. _____

   B. _____

   C. _____

   D. _____

3. Complete Table 8-1.

TABLE 8-1 **Lumbar, Sacrum, and Coccyx Technical Data**				
Position or Projection	**kVp**	**Grid**	**AEC Chamber**	**SID**
AP projection, lumbar vertebrae				
AP oblique projection, lumbar vertebrae				
Lateral position, lumbar vertebrae				
Lateral position, L5-S1 lumbosacral junction				
AP axial projection, sacrum				
Lateral position, sacrum				
AP axial projection, coccyx				
Lateral position, coccyx				

AEC, Automatic exposure control; *AP,* anteroposterior; *kVp,* kilovolt peak; *SID,* source–image receptor distance.

4. Complete Table 8-2.

TABLE 8-2 IR Size, Placement, and Direction		
Position or Projection	**IR Size**	**Placement and Direction**
AP projection, lumbar vertebrae		
AP oblique projection, lumbar vertebrae		
Lateral position, cervical vertebrae		
Lateral position, L5-S1 lumbosacral junction		
AP axial projection, sacrum		
Lateral position, sacrum		
AP axial projection, coccyx		
Lateral position, coccyx		

AP, Anteroposterior; *IR,* image receptor.

Lumbar Vertebrae: AP Projection

1. Identify the labeled anatomy in Figure 8-1.

Figure 8–1

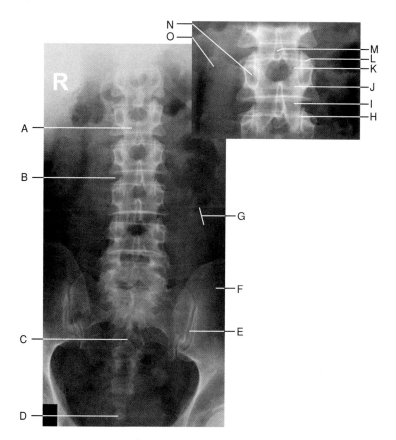

A. _____

B. _____

C. _____

D. _____

E. _____

F. _____

G. _____

H. _____

I. _____

J. _____

K. _____

L. _____

M. _____

N. _____

O. _____

2. What soft-tissue structures are included on an AP lumbar image when proper contrast and density exist?

A. _____

Where are these structures located?

B. _____

3. An AP projection of the lumbar vertebrae is achieved when the (A) _____ are aligned with the midline of the vertebral bodies and the distances from the pedicles to the (B) _____ are equal on both sides. The sacrum and coccyx are aligned with the (C) _____.

4. How is the patient positioned to prevent rotation on an AP lumbar image? _____

_____

5. How is rotation identified on an AP lumbar image?

_____

_____

6. How can a rotated AP lumbar image be distinguished from an AP lumbar image in a patient with subtle scoliosis? _____

_____

_____

7. How is the patient positioned to ensure that open intervertebral disk spaces and undistorted vertebral bodies are obtained?

_____

_____

8. What is the curvature of the lumbar vertebral column?

_____

9. What is the relationship of the iliac spine to the pelvic brim on an AP lumbar image that was taken with the patient's legs extended?

_____

_____

10. What anatomical structures can be used to ensure that the long axis of the lumbar vertebral column is aligned with the collimated field when positioning for an AP lumbar vertebral image?

   A. _____

   _____

   Why is the patient's naval not a reliable structure to use when locating the lumbar vertebral column?

   B. _____

   _____

11. An AP lumbar image demonstrates the vertebral column deviating laterally at the level of the second through fourth lumbar vertebrae; the sacrum is centered within the pelvic inlet, and the distances from the pedicles to the spinous processes of the eleventh thoracic vertebra and the fifth lumbar vertebra are nearly equal. What has caused the appearance of this image?_____

12. On an AP lumbar image with accurate positioning taken on an 11- × 14-inch (28- × 35-cm) lengthwise IR, the (A) _____ is centered within the collimated field. This is accomplished by centering the central ray to the (B) _____ plane at a level 1½ inches (4 cm) (C) _____ to the (D) _____.

13. What anatomical structures are included on an AP lumbar image with accurate positioning taken on an 11- × 14-inch (28- × 35-cm) lengthwise IR?

   _____

14. On an AP lumbar image with accurate positioning taken on a 14- × 17-inch (35- × 43-cm) lengthwise IR, the (A) _____ is centered within the collimated field. This is accomplished by centering the central ray to the (B) _____ plane at the level of the (C) _____.

15. What anatomical structures are included on an AP lumbar image with accurate positioning taken on a 14- × 17-inch (35- × 43-cm) lengthwise IR? _____

   _____

16. How tightly can the transversely collimated field be coned and still include all the required anatomical structures?

   _____

17. When is gonadal shielding not used for an AP lumbar image of a female patient?

   _____

For the following descriptions of AP lumbar images with poor positioning, state how the patient would have been mispositioned for such an image to be obtained.

18. The distance from the right pedicles to the spinous processes is less than the distance from the left pedicles to the spinous processes, and the sacrum and coccyx are rotated toward the right lateral inlet pelvis.

_____

19. The first through third lumbar vertebrae are demonstrated without rotation, the fourth and fifth vertebrae are rotated, and the sacrum and coccyx are rotated toward the patient's left side.

_____

20. The intervertebral disk spaces between the twelfth thoracic vertebra and the third lumbar vertebra are closed, and these lumbar bodies are distorted. The iliac spines are demonstrated without pelvic brim superimposition.

_____

For the following AP lumbar images with poor positioning, state what anatomical structures are misaligned and how the patient should be repositioned for an optimal image to be obtained.

Figure 8–2

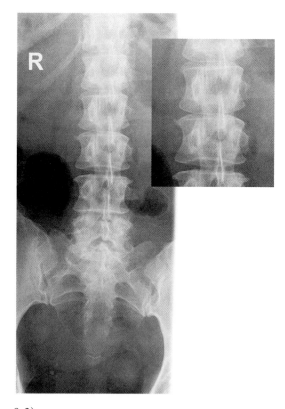

21. (Figure 8-2): _____

_____

_____

Figure 8–3

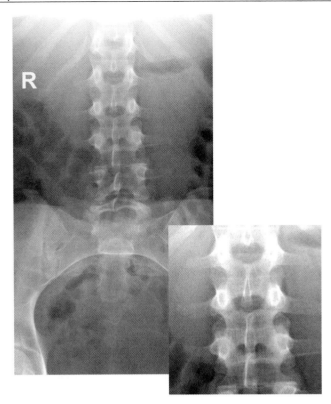

22. (Figure 8-3): _____

_____

_____

_____

_____

_____

Lumbar Vertebrae: AP Oblique Projection (RPO and LPO Positions)

1. Identify the labeled anatomy in Figure 8-4.

Figure 8–4

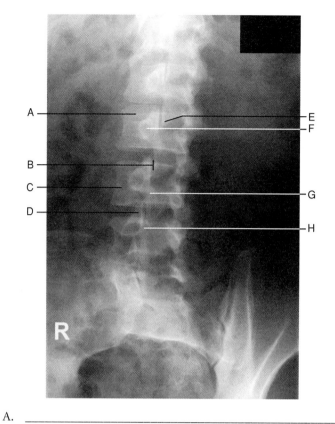

A. _____

B. _____

C. _____

D. _____

E. _____

F. _____

G. _____

H. _____

2. For the following positions, state whether the right or left
   zygapophyseal joints are demonstrated on an oblique lumbar image.

A. RAO: _____

B. LPO: _____

C. RPO: _____

D. LAO: _____

3. An AP oblique lumbar image with accurate positioning will demonstrate the (A) _____ and (B) _____ articular processes in profile, open (C) _____ joints, and the pedicles midway between the midpoint of the vertebral bodies and the (D) _____.

4. What body plane is used to determine patient obliquity for an AP oblique lumbar image?

   A. _____

   How much is the patient's torso rotated for an AP oblique lumbar image?

   B. _____

5. Name the anatomical structures of the lumbar vertebrae that correspond with the parts of the "Scottie dog" listed below.

   A. Ear: _____

   B. Nose: _____

   C. Body: _____

   D. Eye: _____

   E. Front leg: _____

6. On an AP oblique lumbar image with proper imaging, the (A) _____ is centered within the collimated field. This is accomplished by centering the central ray 2 inches (5 cm) (B) _____ to the elevated (C) _____ at a level 1½ inches (4 cm) superior to the (D) _____.

7. What anatomical structures are included on an AP oblique lumbar image with accurate positioning? _____

For the following descriptions of AP oblique lumbar images with poor positioning, state how the patient would have been mispositioned for such an image to be obtained.

8. The vertebrae's superior and inferior articular processes are not demonstrated in profile, their corresponding zygapophyseal joint spaces are closed, and their pedicles are demonstrated adjacent to the vertebrae's lateral vertebral body borders.

---

9. The vertebrae's superior and inferior articular processes are not demonstrated in profile, their corresponding zygapophyseal joint spaces are closed, their laminae are obscured, and their pedicles are shown at the midpoint of the vertebral bodies.

For the following oblique lumbar images with poor positioning, state what anatomical structures are misaligned and how the patient should be repositioned for an optimal image to be obtained.

Figure 8–5

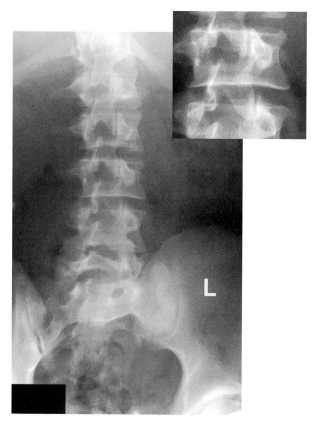

10. (Figure 8-5): _____

_____

_____

Figure 8–6

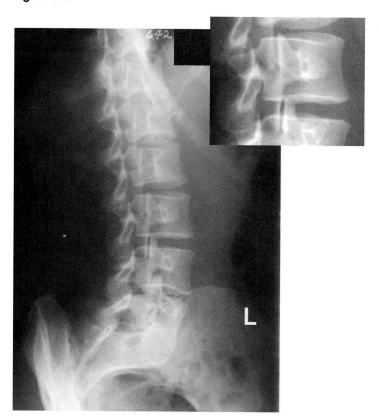

11. (Figure 8-6): _____

_____

_____

Lumbar Vertebrae: Lateral Position

1. Identify the labeled anatomy in Figure 8-7.

Figure 8–7

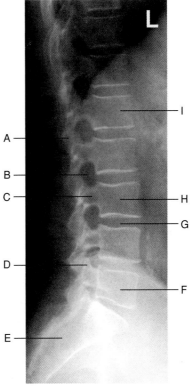

A. _____

B. _____

C. _____

D. _____

E. _____

F. _____

G. _____

H. _____

I. _____

2. List three methods of controlling the amount of scatter radiation that reaches the IR when a lateral lumbar image is produced.

   A. _____

   B. _____

   C. _____

3. Controlling the amount of scatter radiation that reaches the IR will provide a (A) _____ (higher/lower) contrast image and will (B) _____ (increase/decrease) the visibility of recorded details.

4. A lateral lumbar image with accurate positioning demonstrates the (A) _____ and spinous processes in profile, and the right and left pedicles and posterior surfaces of the vertebral bodies are (B) _____.

5. How is the patient positioned to prevent rotation on a lateral lumbar image?

_____

_____

6. For a lateral lumbar image, the patient may be placed on the imaging table in a left or right recumbent position unless the patient has what spinal condition?

   A. _____

   For this condition, how are the central ray and vertebral column positioned?

   B. _____

7. What is accomplished by placing a pillow or sponge between the patient's legs for a lateral lumbar image? _____

_____

8. How can rotation be detected on a rotated lateral lumbar image?

_____

_____

9. Will the upper and lower vertebrae on a lateral lumbar image always demonstrate simultaneous rotation?

   A. _____ (Yes/No)

   Defend your answer.

   B. _____

   _____

10. Why is it difficult to determine which side of the body has been rotated anteriorly or posteriorly when a lateral lumbar image demonstrates rotation?

_____

11. How is the patient positioned to ensure open intervertebral disk spaces and undistorted vertebral bodies on a lateral lumbar image?

_____

12. Describe the body shape that requires a radiolucent sponge to be used to position the lumbar vertebral column parallel with the imaging table.

   A. _____

   Where is the sponge placed for such a patient?

   B. _____

   _____

   If a sponge cannot be used with such a patient, what alternative method can be used?

   C. _____

13. Why are flexion and extension lateral lumbar images requested?

_____

14. Describe how patient positioning is adjusted from a neutral lateral position to place the patient in maximum flexion for a lateral lumbar image.

    A. _____

    Describe how patient positioning is adjusted from a neutral lateral position to place the patient in maximum extension for a lateral lumbar image?

    B. _____

    _____

15. The lordotic curvature on a lumbar image is (A) _____ (increased/decreased) when the patient is positioned in maximum flexion and is (B) _____ (increased/decreased) when the patient is positioned in maximum extension.

16. Describe how one can find the AP location of the lumbar vertebral column.

    _____

    _____

17. On a lateral lumbar image with accurate positioning, the (A) _____ is centered within the collimated field when an 11- × 14-inch (28- × 35-cm) lengthwise IR is used. This is accomplished by centering the central ray to the (B) _____ plane located halfway between the elevated (C) _____ and (D) _____ at a level 1½ inches (4 cm) superior to the (E) _____.

18. What anatomical structures are included on a lateral lumbar image with accurate positioning taken on an 11- × 14-inch (28- × 35-cm) lengthwise IR?

    _____

19. On a lateral lumbar image with accurate positioning, the (A) _____ are centered within the collimated field when a 14- × 17-inch (35- × 43-cm) lengthwise IR is used. This is accomplished by centering the central ray to the (B) _____ plane located halfway between the elevated (C) _____ and (D) _____ at the level of the (E) _____.

20. What anatomical structures are included on a lateral lumbar image with accurate positioning taken on a 14- × 17-inch (35- × 43-cm) lengthwise IR?

    _____

21. Describe two situations in which a tightly collimated lateral view of the L5-S1 lumbar region is indicated after the lateral lumbar image has been reviewed.

    A. _____

    B. _____

22. Explain how the shield is positioned for a lateral lumbar image to protect the patient's gonads.

    _____

    _____

For the following descriptions of lateral lumbar images with poor positioning, state how the patient would have been mispositioned for such an image to be obtained.

23. The posterior surfaces of the first through fourth vertebral bodies and the posterior ribs are demonstrated without superimposition. The most magnified ribs are demonstrated anteriorly.

    _____

24. The L4-5 and L5-S1 intervertebral disk spaces are closed, and the third through fifth vertebral bodies are distorted.

    _____

For the following lateral lumbar images with poor positioning, state what anatomical structures are misaligned and how the patient should be repositioned for an optimal image to be obtained.

Figure 8–8

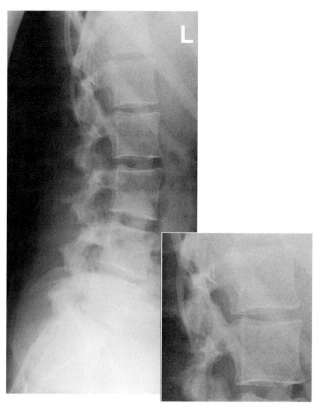

25. (Figure 8-8): _____

    _____

    _____

    _____

    _____

Figure 8–9

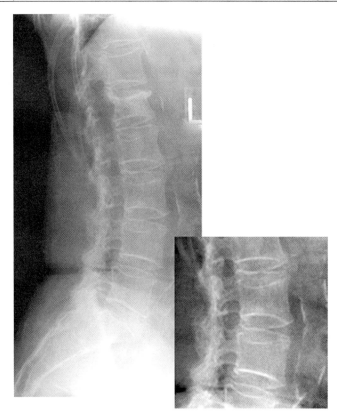

26. (Figure 8-9): _____

    _____

    _____

Figure 8–10

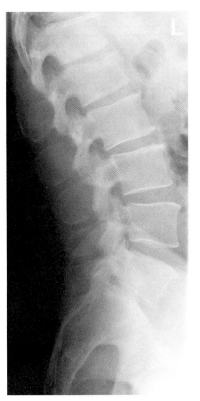

27. (Figure 8-10): _____

    _____

    _____

L5-S1 Lumbosacral Junction: Lateral Position

1. Identify the labeled anatomy in Figure 8-11.

Figure 8–11

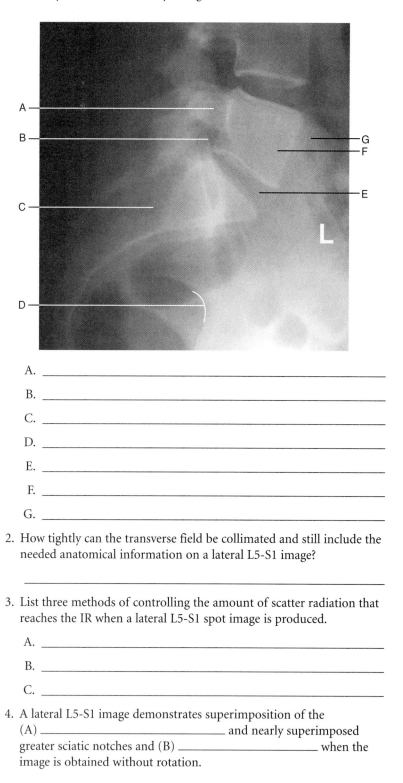

A. _____

B. _____

C. _____

D. _____

E. _____

F. _____

G. _____

2. How tightly can the transverse field be collimated and still include the needed anatomical information on a lateral L5-S1 image?

_____

3. List three methods of controlling the amount of scatter radiation that reaches the IR when a lateral L5-S1 spot image is produced.

A. _____

B. _____

C. _____

4. A lateral L5-S1 image demonstrates superimposition of the (A) _____ and nearly superimposed greater sciatic notches and (B) _____ when the image is obtained without rotation.

5. How is the patient positioned to prevent rotation on a lateral L5-S1 image?

_____

_____

6. What is accomplished by placing a pillow or sponge between the patient's legs for a lateral L5-S1 image?

_____

_____

7. How can rotation be detected on a rotated lateral L5-S1 image?

_____

_____

8. How is the patient positioned to obtain open intervertebral disk spaces and undistorted vertebral bodies on a lateral L5-S1 image?

_____

9. What patient body shape requires that a radiolucent sponge be used to position the lumbar vertebral column parallel with the imaging table?

A. _____

_____

Where is the sponge placed on such a patient?

B. _____

If a sponge cannot be used on such a patient, what alternative method can be used?

C. _____

10. How should the central ray be adjusted to obtain an open L5-S1 joint space in a patient whose vertebral column curves upwardly?

_____

11. On a lateral L5-S1 image with accurate positioning, the (A) _____ is centered within the collimated field. This is accomplished by centering the central ray to a point 2 inches (5 cm) (B) _____ to the elevated (C) _____ and 1½ inches (4 cm) (D) _____ to the (E) _____.

12. What anatomical structures are included on a lateral L5-S1 image with accurate positioning?

_____

13. Describe how the gonads of male and female patients can be protected when a lateral L5-S1 image is taken.

_____

_____

For the following descriptions of lateral L5-S1 lumbar images with poor positioning, state how the patient would have been mispositioned for such an image to be obtained.

14. The L5-S1 intervertebral foramen is obscured, and the greater sciatic notches and femoral heads are not superimposed.

_____

15. The L5-S1 intervertebral disk space is closed, and the pelvic alae are not superimposed.

_____

For the following lateral L5-S1 lumbar images with poor positioning, state what anatomical structures are misaligned and how the patient should be repositioned for an optimal image to be obtained.

Figure 8–12

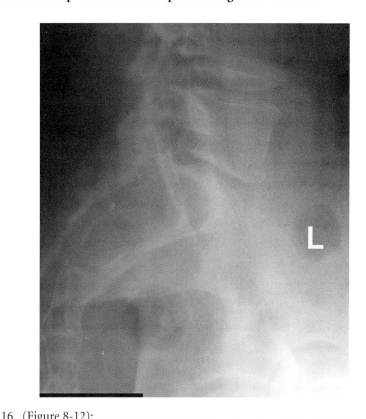

16. (Figure 8-12): _____

_____

_____

Figure 8–13

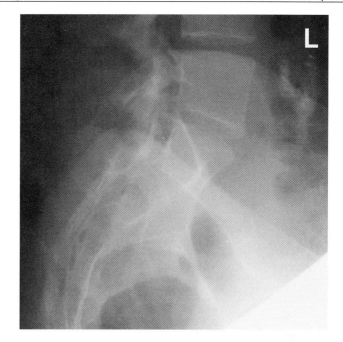

17. (Figure 8-13): _____

_____

_____

Sacrum: AP Axial Projection

1. Identify the labeled anatomy in Figure 8-14.

Figure 8–14

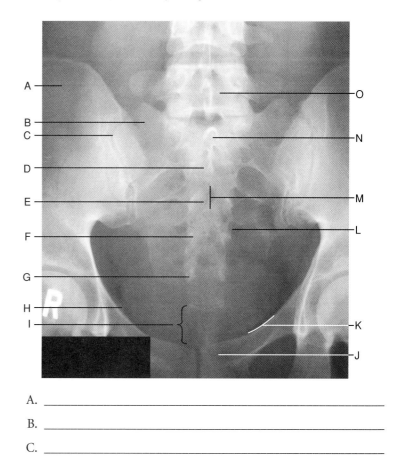

A. _____

B. _____

C. _____

D. _____

E. _____

F. _____

G. _____

H. _____

I. _____

J. _____

K. _____

L. _____

M. _____

N. _____

O. _____

2. Why is the patient instructed to empty the bladder and colon before an AP sacral image is taken? _____

_____

3. How can patient positioning be evaluated to ensure that pelvic rotation will not be present on an AP sacral image?

_____

4. An AP sacral image with accurate positioning is obtained when the medial sacral crest is aligned with the (A) _____ and the ischial spines are equally demonstrated and aligned with the (B) _____.

5. When a patient is rotated for an AP sacral image, the sacrum rotates in the (A) _____ (opposite/same) direction as the symphysis pubis and is positioned next to the lateral pelvic brim situated (B) _____ (closer/farther) to/from the IR.

6. What is the curvature of the sacrum? _____

7. How must the patient and central ray be positioned to demonstrate the sacrum without foreshortening?

_____

_____

8. Why is the median sacral crest aligned with the long axis of the collimated field for an AP sacral image? _____

_____

9. On an AP sacral image with accurate positioning, the (A) _____ is centered within the collimated field. This centering is accomplished by positioning the central ray to the (B) _____ plane at a level halfway between (C) _____ and the (D) _____.

10. What anatomical structures are included on an AP sacral image with accurate positioning? _____

_____

11. Is gonadal protection shielding used on all AP sacral images?

   A. _____ (Yes/No)

   Defend your answer.

   B. _____

   _____

For the following descriptions of AP sacral images with poor positioning, state how the patient or central ray would have been mispositioned for such an image to be obtained.

12. The left ischial spine is demonstrated without pelvic brim superimposition, and the median sacral crest and coccyx are rotated toward the right hip.

   _____

13. The first, second, and third sacral segments are foreshortened.

   _____

14. The sacrum is elongated, and the symphysis pubis is superimposed over the fifth sacral segment.

   _____

For the following AP sacral images with poor positioning, state what anatomical structures are misaligned and how the patient should be repositioned for an optimal image to be obtained.

Figure 8–15

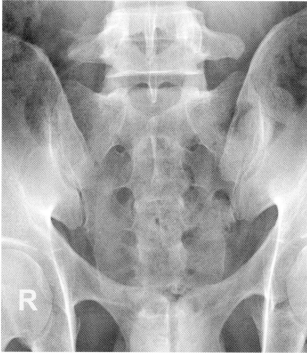

15. (Figure 8-15): _____

   _____

   _____

Figure 8–16

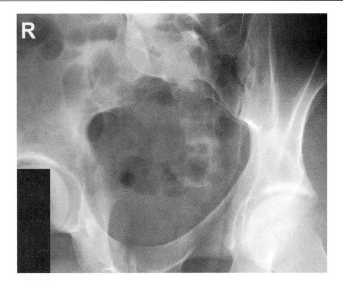

16. (Figure 8-16): _____

_____

_____

_____

Figure 8–17

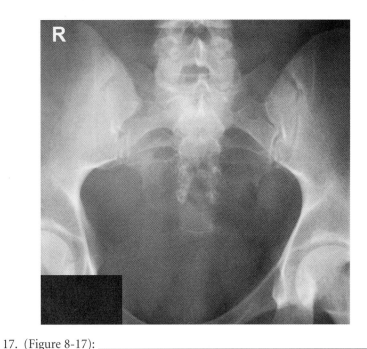

17. (Figure 8-17): _____

_____

_____

_____

Sacrum: Lateral Position

1. Identify the labeled anatomy in Figure 8-18.

Figure 8–18

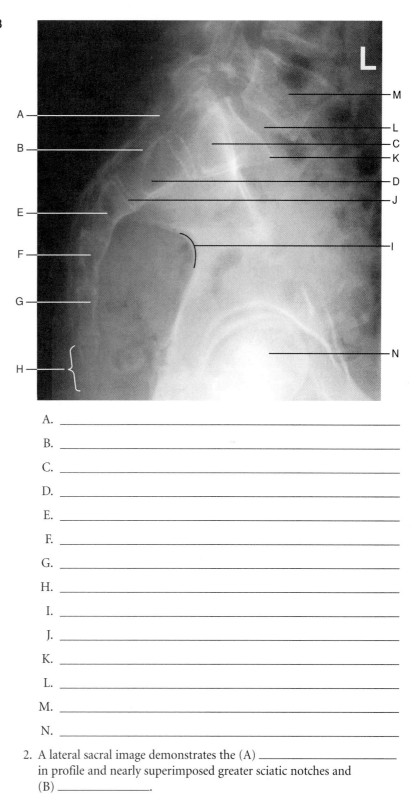

A. _____

B. _____

C. _____

D. _____

E. _____

F. _____

G. _____

H. _____

I. _____

J. _____

K. _____

L. _____

M. _____

N. _____

2. A lateral sacral image demonstrates the (A) _____ in profile and nearly superimposed greater sciatic notches and (B) _____.

3. How is the patient positioned to prevent rotation on a lateral sacral image?

_____

_____

4. What is accomplished by placing a pillow or sponge between the patient's legs for a lateral sacral image?

_____

_____

5. How can rotation be detected on a rotated lateral sacral image?

_____

_____

6. When a lateral sacral image demonstrates rotation and the femoral heads are demonstrated on the image, the hip that is projected inferiorly is situated _____ (closer to/farther away from) the IR.

7. How is the patient positioned to obtain an open L5-S1 disk space and an undistorted fifth lumbar body on a lateral sacral image?

_____

_____

8. What patient body shape requires that a radiolucent sponge be used to position the lumbar vertebral column parallel with the imaging table for a lateral sacral image?

A. _____

Where is the sponge placed on such a patient?

B. _____

_____

If a sponge cannot be used on such a patient, what alternative method can be used?

C. _____

_____

9. How should the central ray be adjusted to obtain an open L5-S1 intervertebral joint space in a patient whose vertebral column curves upwardly?

_____

10. On a lateral sacral image with accurate positioning, the (A) _____ is centered within the collimated field. This is accomplished by centering the central ray to the (B) _____ plane located 3 to 4 inches (7.5 to 10 cm) posterior to the elevated (C) _____.

11. What anatomical structures are included on a lateral sacral image with accurate positioning? _____

_____

12. Describe how the gonads of male and female patients can be protected when a lateral sacral image is taken.

_____

_____

For the following descriptions of lateral sacral images with poor positioning, state how the patient would have been mispositioned for such an image to be obtained.

13. The greater sciatic notches are demonstrated without superimposition, the median sacral crest is not in profile, and the inferiorly located femoral head is rotated posteriorly.

_____

14. The L5-S1 intervertebral disk space is closed, the fifth lumbar vertebra and sacrum are foreshortened, and the greater sciatic notches are demonstrated without superimposition.

_____

For the following lateral sacral images with poor positioning, state what anatomical structures are misaligned and how the patient should be repositioned for an optimal image to be obtained.

Figure 8–19

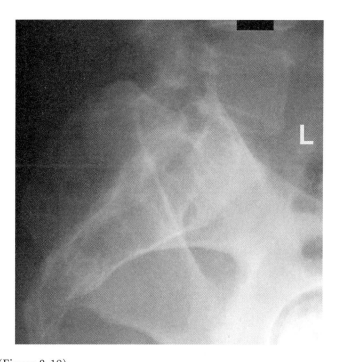

15. (Figure 8-19): _____

_____

_____

Figure 8–20

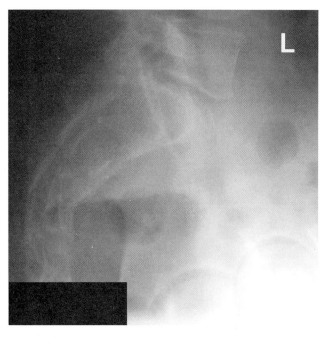

16. (Figure 8-20): _____

_____

_____

Coccyx: AP Axial Projection

1. Identify the labeled anatomy in Figure 8-21.

Figure 8–21

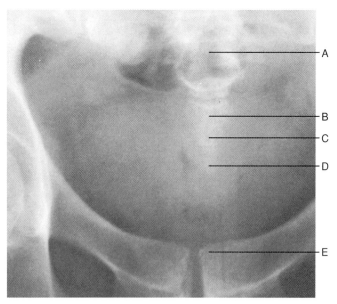

A. _____

B. _____

C. _____

D. _____

E. _____

2. How much can the transverse field be safely collimated and still include the required anatomical structures for an AP coccygeal image?

   _____

3. Where is the marker placed on an AP coccygeal image that is collimated to a 6-inch (15 cm) field size?

   _____

4. Why is the patient instructed to empty the bladder and colon before an AP sacral image is taken? _____

   _____

5. How can patient positioning be evaluated to ensure that pelvic rotation is not present on an AP coccygeal image?

   _____

   _____

6. An AP coccygeal image with accurate positioning is obtained when the coccyx is aligned with the (A) _____ and is at equal distances from the lateral walls of the (B) _____.

7. When a patient is rotated for an AP coccygeal image, the coccyx rotates in the (A) _____ (opposite/same) direction as the symphysis pubis and is positioned next to the lateral pelvic wall situated (B) _____ (closer/farther) to/from the IR.

8. How must the patient and central ray be positioned for an AP coccygeal image to demonstrate the coccyx without foreshortening?

   _____

9. What is the curvature of the coccyx? _____

10. On an AP coccygeal image with accurate positioning, the (A) _____ is centered within the collimated field. This is accomplished by positioning the central ray to the (B) _____ plane at a level 2 inches (5 cm) superior to the (C) _____.

11. What anatomical structures are included on an AP coccygeal image with accurate positioning?

   _____

12. Should the gonads of male and female patients be shielded for an AP coccygeal image?

   A. _____ (Yes/No)

   Defend your answer.

   B. _____

   _____

For the following descriptions of AP coccygeal images with poor positioning, state how the patient or central ray would have been mispositioned for such an image to be obtained.

13. The urinary bladder is dense and creating a shadow over the coccyx.

   _____

14. The coccyx is not aligned with the symphysis pubis but is situated closer to the left lateral pelvic wall.

_____

15. The symphysis pubis is superimposed over the coccyx, and the second and third coccygeal vertebrae are foreshortened.

_____

For the following AP coccygeal images with poor positioning, state what anatomical structures are misaligned and how the patient should be repositioned for an optimal image to be obtained.

Figure 8–22

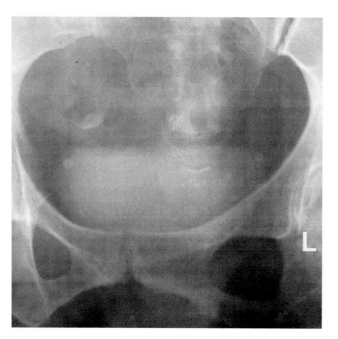

16. (Figure 8-22): _____

_____

_____

Figure 8–23

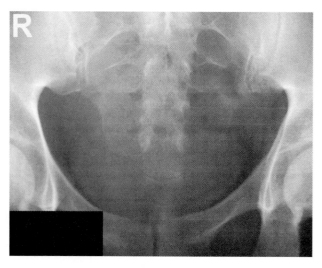

17. (Figure 8-23): _____

_____

_____

COCCYX: LATERAL POSITION

1. Identify the labeled anatomy in Figure 8-24.

Figure 8–24

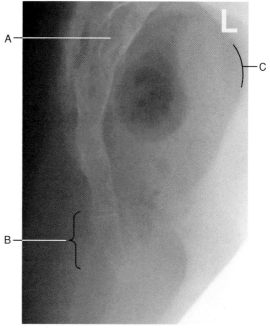

A. _____

B. _____

C. _____

2. List three methods of reducing the amount of scatter radiation that reaches the IR when a lateral coccygeal image is produced.

A. _____

B. _____

C. _____

3. A lateral coccygeal image demonstrates the _____ in profile and nearly superimposed greater sciatic notches.

4. How is the patient positioned to prevent rotation on a lateral coccygeal image?

_____

5. What is accomplished by placing a pillow or sponge between the patient's legs for a lateral coccygeal image?

_____

_____

6. How can rotation be detected on a rotated lateral coccygeal image?

_____

7. How is the patient positioned to prevent foreshortening of the coccyx on a lateral coccygeal image? _____

_____

8. On a lateral coccygeal image with accurate positioning, the (A) _____ is centered within the collimated field. This is accomplished by centering a perpendicular central ray approximately 3½ inches (9 cm) (B) _____ and 2 inches (5 cm) (C) _____ to the (D) _____.

9. How tightly can one safely collimate on a lateral coccygeal image without fear of clipping any portion of the coccyx?

_____

10. What anatomical structures are included on a lateral coccygeal image with accurate positioning?

_____

For the following description of a lateral coccygeal image with poor positioning, state how the patient would have been mispositioned for such an image to be obtained.

11. The greater sciatic notches are demonstrated without superimposition, and the ischium is nearly superimposed over the third coccygeal segment.

_____

For the following lateral coccygeal image with poor positioning, state what anatomical structures are misaligned and how the patient should be repositioned for an optimal image to be obtained.

Figure 8–25

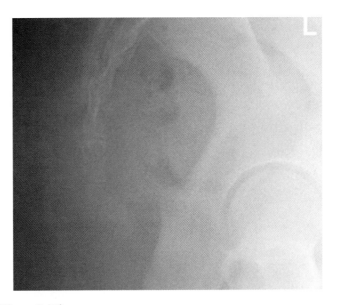

12. (Figure 8-25): _____

_____

_____

CHAPTER 8

STUDY QUESTION ANSWERS

1. A. As if the patient is standing in an upright position. The marker is correct.
   B. As if the patient is standing in an upright position. The marker is correct.
   C. As if the patient is standing in an upright position. The marker is correct.

2. A. Patient motion is controlled.
   B. Respiration is halted.
   C. A short OID is maintained.
   D. The smallest possible IR is used for digital images.

3. Table 8-1

Position or Projection	kVp	Grid	AEC Chamber	SID
AP projection, lumbar vertebrae	75-80	Grid	Center	40-48 inches (100-120 cm)
AP oblique projection, lumbar vertebrae	75-85	Grid	Center	40-48 inches (100-120 cm)
Lateral position, lumbar vertebrae	85-95	Grid	Center	40-48 inches (100-120 cm)
Lateral position, L5-S1 lumbosacral junction	95-100	Grid	Center	40-48 inches (100-120 cm)
AP axial projection, sacrum	75-80	Grid	Center	40-48 inches (100-120 cm)
Lateral position, sacrum	85-95	Grid	Center	40-48 inches (100-120 cm)
AP axial projection, coccyx	75-80	Grid	Center	40-48 inches (100-120 cm)
Lateral position, coccyx	80-85	Grid		40-48 inches (100-120 cm)

AEC, Automatic exposure control; *AP*, anteroposterior; *kVp*, kilovolt peak; *SID*, source–image receptor distance.

4. Table 8-2

Position or Projection	IR Size	Placement and Direction
AP projection, lumbar vertebrae	14 × 17 inches (35 × 43 cm) or 11 × 14 inches (28 × 35 cm)	Lengthwise
AP oblique projection, lumbar vertebrae	11 × 14 inches (28 × 35 cm)	Lengthwise
Lateral position, cervical vertebrae	14 × 17 inches (35 × 43 cm) or 11 × 14 inches (28 × 35 cm)	Lengthwise
Lateral position, L5-S1 lumbosacral junction	8 × 10 inches (18 × 24 cm)	Lengthwise
AP axial projection, sacrum	10 × 12 inches (24 × 30 cm)	Lengthwise
Lateral position, sacrum	10 × 12 inches (24 × 30 cm)	Lengthwise
AP axial projection, coccyx	8 × 10 inches (18 × 24 cm)	Lengthwise
Lateral position, coccyx	8 × 10 inches (18 × 24 cm)	Lengthwise

AP, Anteroposterior; *IR*, image receptor.

Lumbar Vertebrae: AP Projection

1. A. First lumbar vertebra
   B. Intervertebral disk space
   C. Sacrum
   D. Coccyx
   E. Sacroiliac (SI) joint
   F. Ilium
   G. Lateral edge of psoas major muscle
   H. Zygapophyseal joint
   I. Lamina
   J. Pars interarticularis
   K. Inferior articular process
   L. Superior articular process
   M. Spinous process
   N. Pedicle
   O. Transverse process

2. A. Psoas major muscles
   B. Lateral to the lumbar vertebrae, originating at the first lumbar vertebra on each side and extending to the corresponding side's lesser trochanter

3. A. Spinous processes
   B. Spinous processes
   C. Symphysis pubis

4. Position the shoulders and anterior superior iliac spines (ASISs) at equal distances from the imaging table.
5. By comparing the distance between each pedicle to the spinous process on the same vertebra and comparing the distance between each SI joint to the spinous processes
6. Rotated lumbar vertebrae will demonstrate corresponding upper or lower lumbar rotation as well as middle lumbar rotation, whereas a scoliotic patient may demonstrate a rotated appearance in the middle of the vertebral column without corresponding upper or lower vertebrae rotation.
7. Flex the patient's knees and hips until the lower back rests firmly against the imaging table.
8. Lordotic
9. Iliac spines will be demonstrated without pelvic brim superimposition.
10. A. Use the xiphoid and a point halfway between the ASISs.
    B. It is often shifted to one side and not located directly above the lumbar vertebrae.
11. The patient has scoliosis.
12. A. L3-4 intervertebral disk space
    B. Midsagittal
    C. Superior
    D. Iliac crest
13. The twelfth thoracic vertebra, first through fifth lumbar vertebrae, sacroiliac joints, and psoas major major muscles
14. A. L4-5 intervertebral disk space
    B. Midsagittal
    C. Iliac crest
15. The twelfth thoracic vertebra, first through fifth lumbar vertebrae, sacroiliac joints, sacrum, coccyx, and psoas major muscles
16. 8 inches (20 cm)
17. When the sacrum and coccyx are not of interest
18. The patient was rotated onto the left side (LPO).
19. The upper torso was accurately positioned, and the pelvis was rotated toward the right side.
20. The patient's legs were extended.
21. The distances from the left pedicles to the spinous processes of L1-4 are less than the distances from the right pedicles to the spinous processes, and the intervertebral disk spaces between T12 and L3 are closed. Rotate the patient toward the left side, and flex the hips and knee until the lower back rests firmly against the imaging table.
22. The intervertebral disk spaces between T12 and L3 are closed. Flex the patient's hips and knees until the lower back rests firmly against the imaging table.

Lumbar Vertebrae: AP Oblique Projection (RPO and LPO Positions)

1. A. Second lumbar vertebra
   B. Zygapophyseal joint
   C. Transverse process
   D. Superior articular process
   E. Inferior articular process
   F. Pedicle
   G. Lamina
   H. Pars interarticularis
2. A. Left
   B. Left
   C. Right
   D. Right
3. A. Superior
   B. Inferior
   C. Zygapophyseal
   D. Vertebral body's lateral border
4. A. Midcoronal
   B. 45 degrees
5. A. Superior articular process
   B. Transverse process
   C. Lamina
   D. Pedicle
   E. Inferior articular process
6. A. Third lumbar vertebra
   B. Medial
   C. ASIS
   D. Iliac crest
7. The twelfth thoracic vertebra, first through fifth lumbar vertebrae, first and second sacral segments, and SI joints
8. The patient's lumbar vertebrae were rotated less than 45 degrees.
9. The patient's upper lumbar vertebrae were rotated more than 45 degrees.
10. The first and second lumbar vertebrae are accurately positioned, but the third through fifth lumbar vertebrae's superior and inferior articular processes are not demonstrated in profile, their corresponding zygapophyseal joint spaces are closed, and their pedicles are demonstrated adjacent to the vertebrae's lateral vertebral body border. While maintaining the degree of thoracic and upper lumbar vertebral obliquity, increase the lower lumbar vertebral and pelvic rotation.
11. The lumbar vertebrae's superior and inferior articular processes are not demonstrated in profile, their corresponding zygapophyseal joint spaces are closed, their laminae are obscured, and their pedicles are aligned with the midline of the vertebral bodies. Decrease the degree of lumbar vertebrae rotation to 45 degrees.

Lumbar Vertebrae: Lateral Position

1. A. Pars interarticularis
   B. Intervertebral foramen
   C. Pedicle

   D. Zygapophyseal joint
   E. Sacrum
   F. Fifth lumbar vertebra
   G. Intervertebral disk space
   H. Third lumbar vertebra
   I. First lumbar vertebra
2. A. Use tight collimation.
   B. Use a high ratio grid.
   C. Place a flat contact shield on the imaging table along the posterior edge of the collimated field.
3. A. Higher
   B. Increase
4. A. Intervertebral foramina
   B. Superimposed
5. Align the shoulders, posterior ribs, and posterior pelvic wings perpendicular to the imaging table.
6. A. Scoliosis
   B. The patient should be positioned on the table so the central ray is directed into the spinal curve.
7. It prevents the side of the patient positioned farther from the IR from rotating anteriorly.
8. By evaluating the superimposition of the right and left posterior surfaces of the vertebral bodies
9. A. No
   B. The upper and lower lumbar vertebrae can rotate independently or simultaneously.
10. Because the right and left sides are mirror images of each other
11. Align the lumbar column parallel with the imaging table.
12. A. Wide hips and a narrow waist
    B. Between the patient's lateral body surface and the imaging table just superior to the iliac crest
    C. Angle the central ray 3 to 5 degrees caudally.
13. To demonstrate AP vertebral mobility
14. A. Flex the shoulders, upper thorax, and knees anteriorly, rolling into a tight ball.
    B. Arch the back by extending the shoulders, upper thorax, and legs as far posteriorly as possible.
15. A. Decreased
    B. Increased
16. It is located halfway between the ASIS and posterior wing of the patient's side situated farther from the IR.
17. A. Third lumbar vertebra
    B. Coronal
    C. ASIS
    D. Posterior wing
    E. Iliac crest
18. The twelfth thoracic vertebra, first through fifth lumbar vertebrae, and L5-S1 intervertebral disk space
19. A. Fourth lumbar vertebra and iliac crest
    B. Coronal
    C. ASIS
    D. Posterior wing
    E. Iliac crest

20. The eleventh and twelfth thoracic vertebrae, first through fifth lumbar vertebrae, and sacrum
21. A. The L5-S1 area on a lateral lumbar image is too light.
    B. The L5-S1 intervertebral disk spaces are closed on a lateral lumbar image.
22. Position the edge of a flat contact shield against an imaginary line drawn between the coccyx and a point 1 inch (2.5 cm) posterior to the elevated ASIS.
23. The side of the patient situated farther from the IR was rotated anteriorly.
24. The lumbar vertebral column was not aligned parallel with the imaging table.
25. The posterior surfaces of the first through fourth vertebral bodies and the posterior ribs are demonstrated one anterior to the other. The posterior ribs demonstrating the greater magnification were positioned posteriorly. Rotate the side positioned farther from the IR anteriorly until the posterior ribs are superimposed, while maintaining posterior pelvic wing superimposition.
26. The L4-L5 and L5-S1 intervertebral disk spaces are closed, and the third through fifth vertebral bodies are distorted. Position a radiolucent sponge between the patient's lateral body surface and the imaging table just superior to the iliac crest. The sponge should be only thick enough to align the lumbar column parallel with the imaging table and IR.
27. The lumbar vertebral column demonstrates excess lordotic curvature. The patient was in an extended position. If a neutral lateral position is desired, flex the shoulders, upper thorax, and legs anteriorly until the posterior thorax and pelvic wings are aligned with the long axis of the imaging table.

L5-S1 Lumbosacral Junction: Lateral Position

1. A. Pedicles
   B. Intervertebral foramen
   C. Sacrum
   D. Greater sciatic notches
   E. L5-S1 disk space
   F. Fifth lumbar vertebra
   G. Pelvic wing
2. 8 inches (10 cm)
3. A. Use tight collimation.
   B. Use a high ratio grid.
   C. Place a flat contact shield on the imaging table along the posterior edge of the collimated field.
4. A. Right and left pedicles
   B. Pelvic wings

5. Align the shoulders, posterior ribs, and posterior pelvic wings perpendicular to the imaging table.

6. It prevents the side positioned farther from the IR from rotating anteriorly.

7. By evaluating the openness of the intervertebral foramen and the superimposition of the greater sciatic notches and the femoral heads when demonstrated.

8. Position the vertebral column parallel with the imaging table.

9. A. Wide hips and a narrow waist
   B. Between the patient's lateral body surface and the imaging table just superior to the iliac crest
   C. The central ray can be angled 3 to 5 degrees caudally.

10. Angle the central ray cephalically until it parallels the interiliac line.

11. A. L5-S1 intervertebral disk space
    B. Posterior
    C. ASIS
    D. Inferior
    E. Iliac crest

12. The fifth lumbar vertebra and the first and second sacral segments

13. Position the edge of a flat contact shield against an imaginary line drawn between the coccyx and a point 1 inch (2.5 cm) posterior to the elevated ASIS.

14. The patient was rotated.

15. The vertebral column was not aligned parallel with the IR.

16. The L5-S1 intervertebral foramen is obscured, and the greater sciatic notches and the femoral heads are demonstrated without superimposition. The femoral head positioned closer to the IR was rotated anteriorly. Rotate the patient's hip that was positioned farther from the IR toward the opposite hip until the posterior ribs and the posterior pelvic wings are superimposed.

17. The L5-S1 intervertebral disk space is closed, and the pelvic alae are not superimposed. Neither the long axis of the lumbar vertebral column nor the sacrum was aligned parallel with the imaging table, nor were the iliac crests positioned at different transverse levels. Position a radiolucent sponge between the patient's lateral body surface and the imaging table just superior to the patient's iliac crest. The sponge should be just thick enough to align the long axis of the vertebral column and sacrum parallel with the imaging table and place the iliac crests at the same transverse levels.

Sacrum: AP Axial Projection

1. A. Ilium
   B. Sacral ala
   C. SI joint
   D. Second sacral segment
   E. Third sacral segment
   F. Fourth sacral segment
   G. Fifth sacral segment
   H. Ischial spine
   I. Coccyx
   J. Symphysis pubis
   K. Pelvic brim
   L. Sacral foramen
   M. Median sacral crest
   N. Sacral body
   O. Fifth lumbar vertebra

2. It prevents urine, gas, and fecal material from obscuring the sacrum.

3. Position the ASISs at equal distances from the IR.

4. A. Symphysis pubis
   B. Pelvic brim

5. A. Opposite
   B. Farther

6. Kyphotic

7. Position the patient supine with the legs extended, and angle the central ray 15 degrees cephalically.

8. It will allow for tight collimation and ensure that the central ray is aligned correctly with the sacrum.

9. A. Third sacral segment
   B. Midsagittal
   C. An imaginary line drawn between the ASISs
   D. Symphysis pubis

10. The fifth lumbar vertebra, first through fifth sacral segments, first coccygeal vertebra, symphysis pubis, and SI joints

11. A. No
    B. Using gonadal shielding on female patients will cover sacral information.

12. The patient's left side was positioned closer to the IR than was the right side.

13. The central ray was not angled enough cephalically.

14. The central ray was angled too cephalically.

15. The sacrum is elongated, and the symphysis pubis is superimposed over the fifth sacral segment. Either the central ray was angled too cephalically or the patient's legs were not fully extended and a 15-degree central ray angle was used. If the patient's legs were extended, decrease the central ray. If the patient's legs were flexed and a 15-degree central ray angle was used, fully extend the patient's legs and use the same angulation.

16. The right ischial spine is demonstrated without pelvic brim superimposition, and the median sacral crest and coccyx are rotated toward the left hip. The patient was rotated onto the right side (RPO). Rotate the patient toward the left hip until the ASISs are positioned at equal distances from the imaging table.

17. The right ischial spine is demonstrated without pelvic brim superimposition, and the first, second, and third sacral segments are foreshortened. Rotate the patient toward the left hip until the ASISs are positioned at equal distances from the imaging table and the patient's legs are fully extended, then angle the central ray 15 degrees cephalad.

Sacrum: Lateral Position

1. A. Median sacral crest
   B. Sacral canal
   C. First sacral segment
   D. Second sacral segment
   E. Third sacral segment
   F. Fourth sacral segment
   G. Fifth sacral segment
   H. Coccyx
   I. Greater sciatic notches
   J. Transverse ridges
   K. Sacral promontory
   L. L5-S1 disk space
   M. Fifth lumbar vertebra
   N. Femoral heads
2. A. Medial sacral crest
   B. Pelvic wings
3. Align the shoulders, posterior ribs, and posterior pelvic wings perpendicular to the imaging table.
4. It prevents the side of the patient positioned farther from the IR from rotating anteriorly.
5. By evaluating the superimposition of the greater sciatic notches and pelvic wings
6. Farther away from
7. Position the long axis of the vertebral column parallel with the imaging table.
8. A. Wide hips and a narrow waist
   B. Between the patient's lateral body surface and the imaging table just superior to the iliac crest
   C. Angle the central ray 5 degrees caudally for male patients and 8 degrees for female patients.
9. Angle the central ray cephalically until it is parallel with the interiliac line.
10. A. Third sacral segment
    B. Coronal
    C. ASIS
11. The fifth lumbar vertebra, first through fifth sacral segments, promontory, and first coccygeal vertebra
12. Position the edge of a flat contact shield against an imaginary line drawn between the coccyx and a point 1 inch (2.5 cm) posterior to the elevated ASIS.
13. The patient was not in a lateral position. The side of the patient that was situated farther from the IR (right) was rotated posteriorly.
14. The long axis of the lumbar vertebral column was not positioned parallel with the imaging table.

15. The L5-S1 intervertebral disk space is closed, the sacrum is foreshortened, and the greater sciatic notches are demonstrated without superoinferior superimposition. The patient's long axis was not aligned parallel with the imaging table. Position the long axis of the lumbar vertebral column and sacrum parallel with the IR. It may be necessary to place a radiolucent sponge between the patient's lateral body surface and the imaging table just superior to the iliac crest. The sponge should be just thick enough to align the lumbar column parallel with the imaging table.
16. The L5-S1 intervertebral foramen is obscured, and the greater sciatic notches and the femoral heads are demonstrated without superimposition. The femoral head positioned closer to the IR was rotated anteriorly. Rotate the patient's hip that was positioned farther from the IR (right) toward the opposite hip until the posterior ribs and the posterior pelvic wings are superimposed.

Coccyx: AP Axial Projection

1. A. Sacrum
   B. First coccygeal segment
   C. Second coccygeal segment
   D. Third coccygeal segment
   E. Symphysis pubis
2. 6 inches (15 cm)
3. No more than 3 inches (7.5 cm) from the center of the IR
4. It will prevent urine, gas, and fecal material from obscuring the coccyx.
5. Position the ASISs at equal distances from the imaging table.
6. A. Symphysis pubis
   B. Inlet pelvis
7. A. Opposite
   B. Farther
8. The patient should be supine with the legs extended, and the central ray should be angled 10 degrees caudally.
9. Kyphotic
10. A. Coccyx
    B. Midsagittal
    C. Symphysis pubis
11. The fifth sacral segment, three coccygeal vertebrae, symphysis pubis, and inlet pelvis
12. A. No
    B. Shielding a female patient will obscure the coccyx.
13. The patient did not empty the bladder.
14. The patient was rotated toward the right side.
15. The central ray was not angled enough caudally.
16. The urinary bladder is dense and creating a shadow over the coccyx. The coccyx is not aligned with the symphysis pubis but is situated closer to

the left lateral wall of the inlet pelvis. Have the patient empty the urinary bladder, and rotate the patient toward the left side until the ASISs are positioned at equal distances from the imaging table and IR.

17. The symphysis pubis is superimposed over the inferior coccyx, and the coccyx is foreshortened. Angle the central ray 10 degrees caudally.

Coccyx: Lateral Position

1. A. Sacrum
    B. Coccyx
    C. Greater sciatic notches
2. A. Use tight collimation.
    B. Use a high ratio grid.
    C. Place a flat contact shield on the imaging table along the posterior edge of the collimated field.
3. Median sacral crest
4. Align the shoulders, posterior ribs, and posterior pelvic wings perpendicular to the imaging table.
5. It prevents the side of the patient positioned farther from the imaging table from rotating anteriorly.
6. By evaluating the superimposition of the greater sciatic notches
7. Position the vertebral column parallel with and the iliac line perpendicular to the imaging table.
8. A. Coccyx
    B. Posteriorly
    C. Inferiorly
    D. ASIS
9. 4 inches (10 cm)
10. The fifth sacral segment, first through third coccygeal vertebrae, and inferior medial sacral crest
11. The patient was rotated.
12. The greater sciatic notches are demonstrated one anterior to the other, and the ischium is nearly superimposed over the third coccygeal segment. When rotation has occurred, it is most common for the elevated side of the patient to have been rotated anteriorly. Rotate the elevated pelvic wing posteriorly until the posterior pelvic wings are aligned perpendicular to the IR. It may be necessary to position a sponge or pillow between the patient's knees to help maintain this positioning.

Image Analysis of the Sternum and Ribs

LEARNING OBJECTIVES After completion of this chapter you should be able to:

_____ 1. Identify the required anatomy on sternal and rib images.

_____ 2. Describe how to properly position the patient, image receptor (IR), and central ray on sternal and rib images.

_____ 3. State how to properly mark and hang sternal and rib images.

_____ 4. List the typical artifacts that are found on sternal and rib images.

_____ 5. List the image requirements for sternal and rib images with accurate positioning.

_____ 6. State how to properly reposition the patient when sternal and rib images with poor positioning are produced.

_____ 7. Discuss how to determine the amount of patient or central ray adjustment that is required to improve sternal and rib images with poor positioning.

_____ 8. State the kilovolt-peak (kVp) level routinely used for sternal and rib images, and describe what anatomical structures are shown when the correct technique factors are used.

_____ 9. Describe how the patient is positioned to achieve homogeneous density on right anterior oblique (RAO) sternal images.

_____ 10. Explain why a 30-inch (76 cm) source–image distance (SID) is used on RAO sternal images.

_____ 11. Define _costal breathing_, and discuss the advantages of using it for RAO sternal images.

_____ 12. Describe how thoracic thickness affects how far the sternum is positioned from the vertebral column when the patient is rotated.

_____ 13. List ways of reducing the amount of scatter radiation that reaches the IR when the sternum is imaged in the lateral position.

_____ 14. Discuss when it is appropriate to take an anteroposterior (AP) projection of the ribs rather than a posteroanterior (PA) projection.

_____ 15. Describe why the kVp used for above-diaphragm ribs is different from that used for below-diaphragm ribs.

_____ 16. Explain why the respiration used for above-diaphragm ribs is different than that used for below-diaphragm ribs.

_____ 17. Discuss why the posterior oblique position is preferred over the anterior oblique position when the axillary ribs are imaged.

STUDY QUESTIONS

Sternum

1. Describe how the following shoulder images should be hung on a view box or displayed on a cathode ray tube (CRT) monitor.

   A. PA oblique (RAO) sternum: _____

   B. Lateral sternum: _____

   C. Left AP oblique: _____

2. Complete Table 9-1.

TABLE 9-1 **Sternum and Rib Technical Data**			
Position or Projection	**kVp**	**Grid**	**SID**
PA oblique projection, sternum			
Lateral position, sternum			
AP/PA projection, upper ribs			
AP/PA projection, lower ribs			
AP/PA oblique, upper ribs			
AP/PA oblique, lower ribs			

AP, Anteroposterior; *kVp,* kilovolt peak; *PA,* posteroanterior; *SID,* source–image receptor distance.

3. Complete Table 9-2.

TABLE 9-2 **IR Size, Placement, and Direction**		
Position or Projection	**IR Size**	**Placement and Direction**
PA oblique projection, sternum		
Lateral position, sternum		
AP/PA projection, ribs		
AP/PA oblique, ribs		

AP, Anteroposterior; *IR,* image receptor; *PA,* posteroanterior.

Sternum: PA Oblique Projection (RAO Position)

4. Identify the labeled anatomy in Figure 9-1.

Figure 9–1

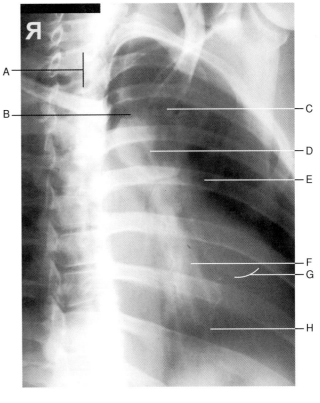

A. _____

B. _____

C. _____

D. _____

E. _____

F. _____

G. _____

H. _____

5. Define the following terms.

A. Homogeneous: _____

B. Costal breathing: _____

6. Why is a PA oblique (RAO) projection chosen over a PA oblique (left anterior oblique [LAO]) projection when imaging the sternum?

_____

7. Keeping the entire sternum within the heart shadow for the PA oblique (RAO) position provides a sternal image with _____ density.

8. List four structures that overlay the sternum in a PA oblique (RAO) sternal image.

A. _____

B. _____

C. _____

D. _____

9. A short SID is used when imaging the sternum in the PA oblique (RAO) position to magnify the (A) _____ and (B) _____. Using a short SID will result in (C) _____ patient entrance skin dosage.

10. Using a long exposure time and (A) _____ breathing for the PA oblique (RAO) sternal image will (B) _____ the lung markings and (C) _____.

11. If the patient breathes deeply during the exposure for a PA oblique (RAO) sternal image, the resulting image demonstrates a _____ sternum.

12. The sternum is rotated from beneath the thoracic vertebrae for a PA oblique (RAO) sternal image by rotating the patient until the (A) _____ plane is aligned (B) _____ degrees with the IR.

13. Any portion of the sternum that is positioned outside the heart shadow on a PA oblique (RAO) sternal image demonstrates _____ (more/less) density than that positioned within the heart shadow.

14. On a PA oblique (RAO) sternal image with accurate positioning, the _____ is centered within the collimated field.

15. Proper centering for a PA oblique (RAO) sternal image is accomplished by centering the central ray (A) _____ inches to the left of the (B) _____ and placing the top of the IR approximately 1½ inches superior to the (C) _____.

16. When the patient is rotated for a PA oblique (RAO) sternal image, the (A) _____ (superior/inferior) portion of the sternum remains situated closer to the thoracic vertebrae than the (B) _____ (superior/inferior) portion.

17. Because the long axis of the sternum does not align with the long axis of the IR in the PA oblique (RAO) projection, transverse collimation should be limited to the (A) _____ and (B) _____.

18. Adequate RAO obliquity is obtained on a PA oblique (RAO) sternal image when the (A) _____ and (B) _____ are no longer superimposed.

For the following description of a PA oblique (RAO) sternal image with poor positioning, state how the patient would have been mispositioned for such an image to be obtained.

19. The right sternoclavicular (SC) joint and right side of the manubrium are superimposed by the thoracic vertebrae.

_____

For the following PA oblique (RAO) sternal images with poor positioning, state what anatomical structures are misaligned and how the patient should be repositioned for an optimal image to be obtained.

Figure 9–2

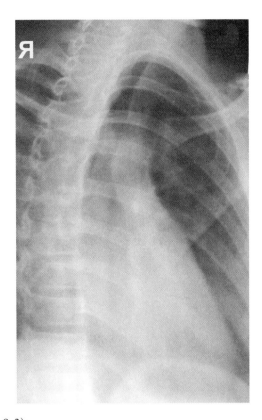

20. (Figure 9-2): _____

_____

_____

Figure 9–3

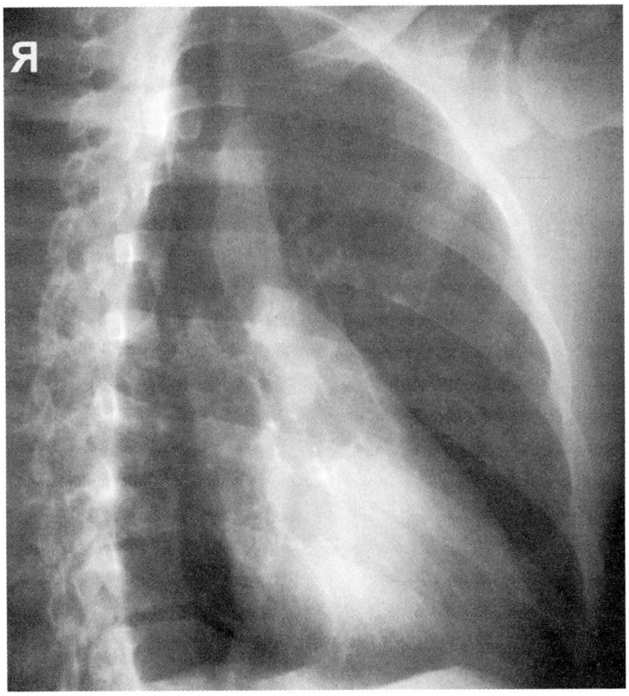

21. (Figure 9-3): _____

_____

_____

_____

Sternum: Lateral Position

1. Identify the labeled anatomy in Figure 9-4.

Figure 9–4

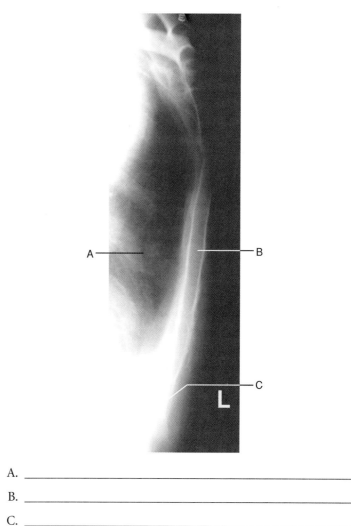

A. _____

B. _____

C. _____

2. Identify the labeled anatomy in Figure 9-5.

Figure 9–5

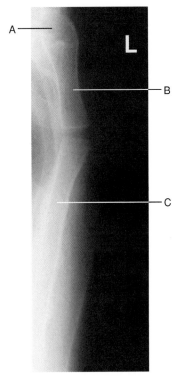

A. _____

B. _____

C. _____

3. Why is it often difficult to demonstrate the superior and inferior sternum simultaneously on a lateral sternal image?

_____

_____

4. List three methods of controlling the amount of scatter radiation that reaches the IR on a lateral sternal image.

A. _____

B. _____

C. _____

5. How is rotation avoided when positioning the patient for a lateral sternal image? _____

_____

6. How is rotation identified on a lateral sternal image? _____

_____

7. Describe how one can determine on a lateral sternal image with poor positioning that the patient's right thorax is rotated anteriorly.

_____

_____

8. Deep suspended respiration draws the sternum away from the

   _____.

9. How is the patient positioned to prevent humeral soft tissue from superimposing the sternum? _____

   _____

10. On a lateral sternal image with accurate positioning, the (A) _____ is centered within the collimated field. This is accomplished by placing the top edge of the IR (B) _____ inches above the (C) _____ and aligning the receptor's long axis and a (D) _____ central ray to the midsternum.

11. Why is a 72-inch (180-cm) SID used for a lateral sternum image?

   _____

   _____

12. What anatomical structures are included on a lateral sternal image with accurate positioning?

   _____

For the following descriptions of lateral sternal images with poor positioning, state how the patient would have been mispositioned for such an image to be obtained.

13. The anterior ribs are demonstrated without superimposition, the sternum is not in profile, and the superior heart shadow extends beyond the sternum and into the anteriorly situated lung.

   _____

14. The anterior ribs are demonstrated without superimposition, the sternum is not in profile, and the superior heart shadow does not extend beyond the sternum.

   _____

For the following lateral sternal image with poor positioning, state what anatomical structures are misaligned and how the patient should be repositioned for an optimal image to be obtained.

Figure 9–6

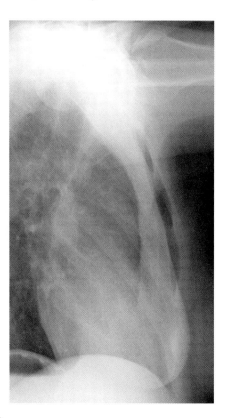

15. (Figure 9-6): _____

_____

_____

_____

_____

Ribs: Anteroposterior or Posteroanterior Projection (above or below Diaphragm)

1. Identify the labeled anatomy in Figure 9-7.

Figure 9–7

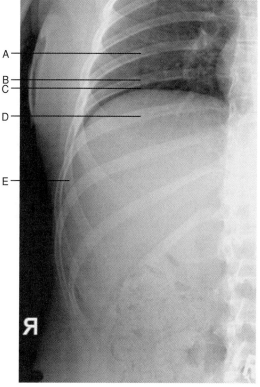

A. _____

B. _____

C. _____

D. _____

E. _____

2. Why do some facilities require the technologist to tape a rib marker (lead "BB") on the patient's skin near the area where the ribs are tender? _____

_____

3. A. What patient respiration is used when imaging ribs located above the diaphragm?

_____

B. What patient respiration is used when imaging ribs located below the diaphragm?

_____

4. Explain why a higher kVp is used when imaging below-diaphragm ribs versus above-diaphragm ribs? _____

_____

5. What soft-tissue structures are evaluated for associated injury on the following rib images?

A. Upper ribs: _____

_____

B. Lower ribs: _____

6. If the patient complains of anterior rib pain, what projection of the ribs should be taken?

A. _____ (AP/PA)

When the patient indicates posterior rib pain, what projection of the ribs should be taken?

B. _____ (AP/PA)

If the opposite is taken for these two situations, what difference would result?

C. _____

7. If the thorax is demonstrated without rotation on an AP or PA rib image, the sternum and (A) _____ are superimposed and the distance from the vertebral column to the sternal ends of the clavicles is (B) _____.

8. How is spinal scoliosis identified on PA and AP rib images?

_____

_____

9. Describe how the patient is positioned to prevent thoracic rotation for the following projections of the ribs.

A. AP: _____

_____

B. PA: _____

_____

10. For each of the following projections, describe how the patient is positioned to obtain an image of the ribs with the scapula placed outside the lung field.

A. AP: _____

_____

B. PA: _____

11. If an AP or PA supine rib image is taken in full suspended inspiration, how many ribs are demonstrated above the diaphragm? _____

12. What ribs are demonstrated below the diaphragm when an AP or PA rib image is taken on expiration? _____

13. On an above-diaphragm AP or PA rib image with accurate positioning, the (A) _____ is at the center of the collimated field. This is accomplished on an AP projection by centering the central

ray halfway between the (B) _____ and affected lateral body surface at a level halfway between the (C) _____ and (D) _____. This centering is accomplished on a PA projection by placing the central ray halfway between the (E) _____ and lateral rib surface at the level of the (F) _____.

14. What anatomical structures are included on an above-diaphragm AP or PA rib image with accurate positioning?

   _____

15. On a below-diaphragm AP or PA rib image with accurate positioning, the (A) _____ is at the center of the collimated field. This centering is accomplished by placing the lower border of the IR at the (B) _____, centering a perpendicular central ray to the IR, and moving the patient side to side until the longitudinal collimator light line is aligned halfway between the (C) _____ and lateral body surface.

   How should this centering be adjusted for a hypersthenic patient?

   D. _____

16. What anatomical structures are included on an AP or PA below-diaphragm rib image with accurate positioning?

   _____

For the following descriptions of AP or PA rib images with poor positioning, state how the patient would have been mispositioned for such an image to be obtained.

17. The sternum and SC joints are demonstrated to the left of the patient's vertebral column on an AP projection taken because of left rib pain.

   _____

18. The left scapula is superimposed over the upper lateral rib field on a PA projection.

   _____

19. The tenth through twelfth posterior ribs are demonstrated below the diaphragm on a below-diaphragm image.

   _____

For the following AP or PA rib images with poor positioning, state what anatomical structures are misaligned and how the patient should be repositioned for an optimal image to be obtained.

Figure 9–8

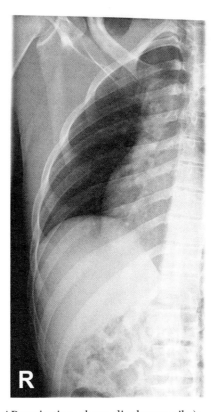

20. (Figure 9-8, AP projection, above-diaphragm ribs): _____

_____

_____

_____

_____

Figure 9–9

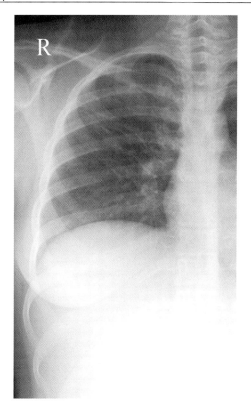

21. (Figure 9-9, AP projection, above-diaphragm ribs): _____

_____

_____

Figure 9–10

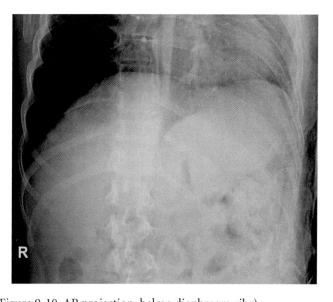

22. (Figure 9-10, AP projection, below-diaphragm ribs): _____

_____

_____

_____

Ribs: Anteroposterior Oblique Projection (Posterior Oblique Position, above or below Diaphragm)

1. Identify the labeled anatomy in Figure 9-11.

Figure 9–11

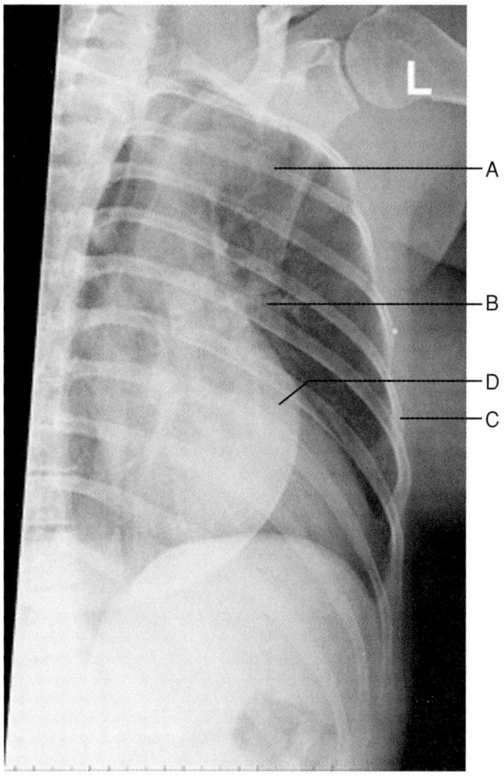

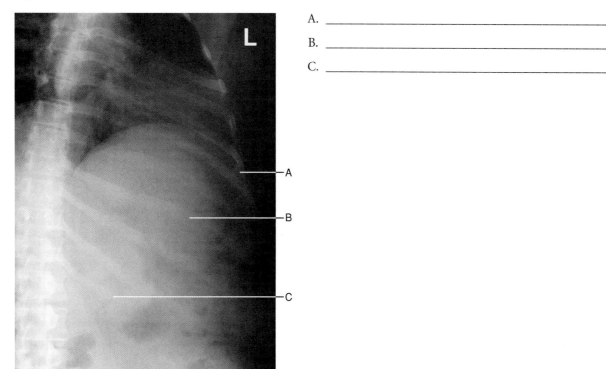

A. _____

B. _____

C. _____

D. _____

2. Identify the labeled anatomy in Figure 9-12.

Figure 9–12

A. _____

B. _____

C. _____

3. Which oblique position demonstrates the sharper axillary rib details?

    A. _____ (Anterior/Posterior)

    Defend your answer.

    B. _____

    _____

4. What degree of patient rotation is used for AP oblique rib images?

    A. _____

    What body plane is used to align this angle?

    B. _____

5. For the following positions, state whether the patient is rotated toward or away from the affected side to demonstrate the axillary ribs in the AP oblique position.

    A. AP (posterior) oblique: _____

    B. PA (anterior) oblique: _____

6. How can one determine from an AP oblique rib image if the patient has been rotated 45 degrees? _____

7. What patient respiration is used when imaging ribs located above the diaphragm? _____

8. What patient respiration is used when imaging ribs located below the diaphragm? _____

_____

9. On an above-diaphragm posterior oblique rib image with accurate positioning, the (A) _____ is centered within the collimated field. This is accomplished by centering a (B) _____ central ray halfway between the midsagittal plane and (C) _____, at a level halfway between the (D) _____ and (E) _____.

10. What anatomical structures are included on an above-diaphragm oblique rib image with accurate positioning? _____

_____

11. On a below-diaphragm posterior oblique rib image with accurate positioning, the (A) _____ is centered within the collimated field. This is accomplished by positioning the lower IR border at the patient's (B) _____ and centering the central ray halfway between the (C) _____ and lateral rib surface.

12. What anatomical structures are included on a below-diaphragm oblique rib image? _____

_____

For the following descriptions of AP oblique rib images with poor positioning, state how the patient would have been mispositioned for such an image to be obtained.

13. The axillary ribs demonstrate increased self-superimposition, and the sternum is rotated toward the patient's left side on an image taken for right side rib pain.

_____

14. The sternal body is demonstrated adjacent to the vertebral column.

15. An above-diaphragm anterior oblique rib image demonstrates the first through seventh posterior ribs above the diaphragm.

For the following AP oblique rib images with poor positioning, state what anatomical structures are misaligned and how the patient should be repositioned for an optimal image to be obtained.

Figure 9–13

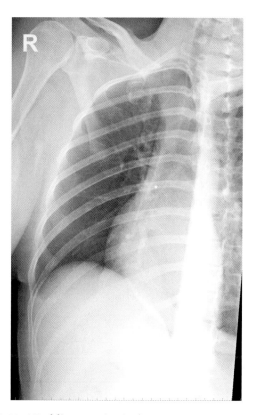

16. (Figure 9-13, AP oblique projection): _____

_____

_____

Figure 9–14

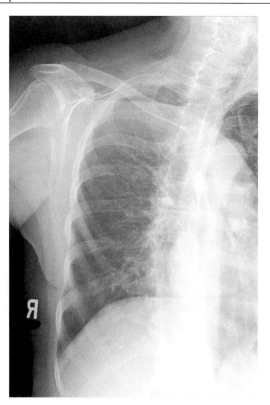

17. (Figure 9-14, PA oblique projection): _____

_____

_____

_____

_____

CHAPTER 9
STUDY QUESTION ANSWERS
Sternum

1. A. As if the patient is in an upright position; the marker is reversed.
   B. As if the patient is in an upright position; the marker is correct.
   C. As if the patient is in an upright position; the marker is correct.

2. Table 9-1

Position or Projection	kVp	Grid	SID
PA oblique projection, sternum	60-70	Grid	30-40 inches (75-100 cm)
Lateral position, sternum	70-75	Grid	72 inches (180 cm)
AP/PA projection, upper ribs	65-70	Grid	40-48 inches (100-120 cm)
AP/PA projection, lower ribs	70-80	Grid	40-48 inches (100-120 cm)
AP/PA oblique, upper ribs	70-75	Grid	40-48 inches (100-120 cm)
AP/PA oblique, lower ribs	70-80	Grid	40-48 inches (100-120 cm)

AP, Anteroposterior; *kVp,* kilovolt peak; *PA,* posteroanterior; *SID,* source–image receptor distance.

3. Table 9-2

Position or Projection	IR Size	Placement and Direction
PA oblique projection, sternum	10 × 12 inches (24 × 30 cm)	Lengthwise
Lateral position, sternum	10 × 12 inches (24 × 30 cm) or 11 × 14 inches (28 × 35 cm)	Lengthwise
AP/PA projection, ribs	14 × 17 inches (35 × 43 cm)	Lengthwise
AP/PA oblique, ribs	14 × 17 inches (35 × 43 cm)	Lengthwise

AP, Anteroposterior; *IR,* image receptor; *PA,* posteroanterior.

Sternum: PA Oblique Projection (RAO Position)

4. A. Thoracic vertebral column
   B. Jugular notch
   C. SC joint
   D. Manubrium
   E. Posterior rib
   F. Sternal body
   G. Inferior scapular angle
   H. Xiphoid process
5. A. Uniform in quality
   B. Shallow breathing
6. Because it superimposes the heart shadow over the sternum
7. Homogeneous
8. A. Posterior ribs
   B. Lung markings
   C. Heart shadow
   D. Left inferior scapula
9. A. Posterior ribs
   B. Left scapula
   C. Increased

10. A. Costal
    B. Blur
    C. Posterior ribs
11. Blurred
12. A. Midcoronal
    B. 15 to 20
13. More
14. Midsternum
15. A. 3 inches (7.5 cm)
    B. Thoracic spinous processes
    C. Jugular notch
16. A. Superior
    B. Inferior
17. A. Thoracic spinous processes
    B. Left inferior angle of the scapula
18. A. Sternum
    B. Thoracic vertebrae
19. The patient was rotated less than 15 to 20 degrees.
20. The sternum and lung markings are blurry and unidentifiable. Instruct the patient to breathe shallowly instead of deeply. If the patient is unable to costal breathe, take the exposure on expiration.

21. The sternum is positioned to the left of the heart shadow. Decrease the degree of patient obliquity.

Sternum: Lateral Position

1. A. Anterior rib
   B. Sternal body
   C. Xiphoid process
2. A. Jugular notch
   B. Manubrium
   C. Sternal body
3. Because the pectoral muscles and female breast tissue are superimposed over the inferior sternum but not the superior sternum
4. A. Use a grid.
   B. Collimate tightly.
   C. Position a flat contact strip anterior to the sternum close to the shadow of the anterior skinline.
5. Align the shoulders, posterior ribs, and posterior pelvic wings perpendicular to the IR.
6. By evaluating the degree of anterior rib and sternal superimposition
7. The superior heart shadow will not continue into the anteriorly situated lung but will end at the sternum.
8. Anterior ribs
9. Extend the patient's arms behind the back, and clasp the hands.
10. A. Midsternum
    B. 1½
    C. Jugular notch
    D. Perpendicular
11. To reduce the magnification that would result from the long OID
12. The jugular notch, sternal body, and xiphoid process
13. The patient's left side is positioned anterior to the right side.
14. The patient's right side is positioned anterior to the left side.
15. The anterior ribs are demonstrated without superimposition, the sternum is not in profile, the superior heart shadow does not extend beyond the sternum and into the anteriorly situated lung, and the humeri soft tissue is superimposed over the manubrium. Position the left thorax slightly anteriorly, extend the patient's arms behind the back, and clasp the hands.

Ribs: Anteroposterior or Posteroanterior Projection (above or below Diaphragm)

1. A. Seventh posterior rib
   B. Eighth posterior rib
   C. Diaphragm
   D. Ninth posterior rib
   E. Eighth anterior rib
2. To aid the reviewer in pinpointing the exact location of the potential injury
3. A. Full suspended inspiration
   B. Full suspended expiration
4. Higher kVp is needed to penetrate the denser abdominal structures and demonstrate the ribs.
5. A. Upper thorax, axillary and neck soft tissues, and vascular lung markings.
   B. Upper abdominal tissue
6. A. Posteroanterior
   B. Anteroposterior
   C. The ribs of interest would demonstrate increased magnification.
7. A. Vertebral column
   B. Equal
8. In a rotated patient the distances from the vertebral column to the lateral edge will be uniform down the length of the lung field, and in a patient with scoliosis the distances from the vertebral column to the lateral lung edge will vary.
9. A. Flex the patient's knees, placing the feet flat against the imaging table and positioning the shoulders at equal distances from the IR.
   B. Place the patient's chin on a sponge so the patient can look straight ahead, and position the patient's shoulders and anterior superior iliac spines (ASISs) at equal distances from the imaging table.
10. A. Place the back of the patient's hands on the hips, and rotate the elbows and shoulders anteriorly.
    B. Internally rotate the patient's arms, forcing the shoulders to rotate anteriorly.
11. Nine
12. Ninth through twelfth
13. A. Seventh posterior rib
    B. Midsagittal plane
    C. Jugular notch
    D. Xiphoid process
    E. Midsagittal plane
    F. Inferior scapular angle

14. The first through ninth ribs and vertebral column
15. A. Tenth posterior rib
    B. Iliac crest
    C. Midsagittal plane
    D. Place the lower IR border 2 inches (5 cm) above the iliac crest.
16. The vertebral column and eighth through twelfth ribs
17. The patient's right side was positioned farther away from the IR than was the left side.
18. The patient's left arm was not adequately internally rotated.
19. The image was taken on inspiration.
20. The sternum is demonstrated to the right of the patient's vertebral column. Flex the patient's knees and rotate the thorax toward the left side until the shoulders are at equal distances from the IR. Seven posterior ribs are demonstrated above the diaphragm. Obtain the image after full suspended inspiration.
21. Eight posterior ribs are demonstrated above the diaphragm. Obtain the image after full suspended inspiration.
22. The distance from the spinous process to the pedicles on the right side is narrower than that on the left side. Rotate the patient toward the right side until the shoulders and ASISs are at equal distances from the IR.

Ribs: Anteroposterior Oblique Projection (Posterior Oblique Position, above or below Diaphragm)

1. A. Third axillary rib
   B. Inferior scapular angle
   C. Fifth anterior rib
   D. Sternum
2. A. Sixth anterior rib
   B. Ninth axillary rib
   C. Twelfth rib
3. A. Posterior
   B. When posterior oblique ribs are taken, the axillary ribs are positioned closer to the IR, resulting in less magnification.
4. A. 45 degrees
   B. Midcoronal
5. A. Toward the affected side
   B. Away from the affected side
6. The inferior sternal body will be located halfway between the lateral body surface and vertebral column.
7. Full suspended inspiration
8. Full suspended expiration
9. A. Seventh axillary rib
   B. Perpendicular
   C. Affected lateral rib surface
   D. Jugular notch
   E. Xiphoid process
10. The first through ninth axillary ribs of the affected side and thoracic vertebral column
11. A. Tenth axillary rib
    B. Iliac crest
    C. Midsagittal plane
12. The vertebral column and ninth through twelfth axillary ribs of the affected side
13. The patient was rotated the wrong direction (toward the left side).
14. The patient was rotated less than 45 degrees.
15. The image was not taken on full inspiration.
16. The sternum is situated next to the vertebral column. Increase the degree of patient obliquity to 45 degrees.
17. The axillary ribs demonstrate increased superimposition. The patient was rotated the wrong direction. The patient should be rotated away from the affected ribs when a PA oblique image is obtained. The ribs demonstrate increased magnification. Obtain the image in an AP projection to decrease rib magnification.

Image Analysis of the Cranium

LEARNING OBJECTIVES

After completion of this chapter you should be able to:

_____ 1. Identify the required anatomy on cranial, facial bone, mandible, mastoid, and sinus images.

_____ 2. Describe how to properly position the patient, image receptor (IR), and central ray on cranial, facial bone, mandible, mastoid, and sinus images.

_____ 3. State how to properly mark and hang cranial, facial bone, mandible, mastoid, and sinus images.

_____ 4. List the typical artifacts that are found on cranial, facial bone, mandible, mastoid, and sinus images.

_____ 5. List the analysis requirements for cranial, facial bone, mandible, mastoid, and sinus images with accurate positioning.

_____ 6. State how to properly reposition the patient when cranial, facial bone, mandible, mastoid, and sinus images with poor positioning are produced.

_____ 7. Discuss how to determine the amount of patient or central ray adjustment that is required to improve cranial, facial bone, mandible, mastoid, and sinus images with poor positioning.

_____ 8. State the kilovoltage routinely used for cranial, facial bone, mandible, mastoid, and sinus images, and describe what anatomical structures are visible when the correct technique factors are used.

_____ 9. State how the central ray is adjusted to obtain accurate cranial positioning when the patient has a suspected cervical injury or is unable to adequately align the head with the IR.

_____ 10. Define and state the common abbreviations used for the cranial positioning lines.

_____ 11. Discuss why the parietoacanthial (Waters) projection is taken with the patient's mouth open.

_____ 12. Explain how the patient and central ray are positioned to demonstrate accurate air-fluid levels in the sinus cavities.

STUDY QUESTIONS

Cranium, Facial Bones, Mandible, Sinuses, and Petromastoid Portion

1. Describe how the following images should be hung on a view box or displayed on a cathode ray tube (CRT) monitor.

    A. Anteroposterior (AP) cranium:

    _____

    B. Parietoacanthial sinuses: _____

    C. Submentovertex (SMV) (Schueller) mandible:

    _____

    D. AP axial (Caldwell) cranium: _____

2. Complete Table 10-1.

TABLE 10-1 Cranium, Facial Bones, Mandible, Sinuses, and Petromastoid Technical Data						
Position or Projection	**Structure**	**kVp**	**Grid**	**AEC Chamber(s)**	**SID**	
AP or PA projection	Cranium					
	Mandible					
PA axial (Caldwell) projection	Cranium					
	Facial bones					
	Sinuses					
AP axial (Towne) projection	Cranium					
	Mandible					
	Petromastoid portion					
Lateral position	Cranium					
	Facial bones					
	Sinuses					
	Nasal bones					
Submentovertex (Schueller) projection	Cranium					
	Mandible					
	Sinuses					
	Zygomatic arches					
Parietoacanthial (Waters) projection	Facial bones					
	Sinuses					
Parietoorbital oblique (Rhese) projection	Optic canal and foramen					
Tangential (superoinferior) projection	Nasal bones					
Axiolateral oblique (modified Law) projection	Petromastoid portion					
Axiolateral oblique (Stenvers) projection	Petromastoid portion					

AEC, Automatic exposure control; *AP*, anteroposterior; *kVp*, kilovolt-peak; *PA*, posteroanterior; *SID*, source–image receptor distance.

3. Complete Table 10-2.

TABLE 10-2 IR Size, Placement, and Direction

Position or Projection	Structure	IR Size	Placement and Direction
AP or PA projection	Cranium		
	Mandible		
PA axial (Caldwell) projection	Cranium		
	Facial bones		
	Sinuses		
AP axial (Towne) projection	Cranium		
	Mandible		
	Petromastoid portion		
Lateral position	Cranium		
	Facial bones		
	Sinuses		
	Nasal bones		
Submentovertex (Schueller) projection	Cranium		
	Mandible		
	Sinuses		
Parietoacanthial (Waters) projection	Facial bones		
	Sinuses		
Parietoorbital oblique (Rhese) projection	Optic canal and foramen		
Tangential (superoinferior) projection	Nasal bones		
Axiolateral oblique (modified Law) projection	Petromastoid portion		
Axiolateral oblique (Stenvers) projection	Petromastoid portion		

AP, Anteroposterior; *IR,* image receptor; *PA,* posteroanterior.

Cranium and Mandible: PA or AP Projection

4. Identify the labeled anatomy in Figure 10-1.

Figure 10–1

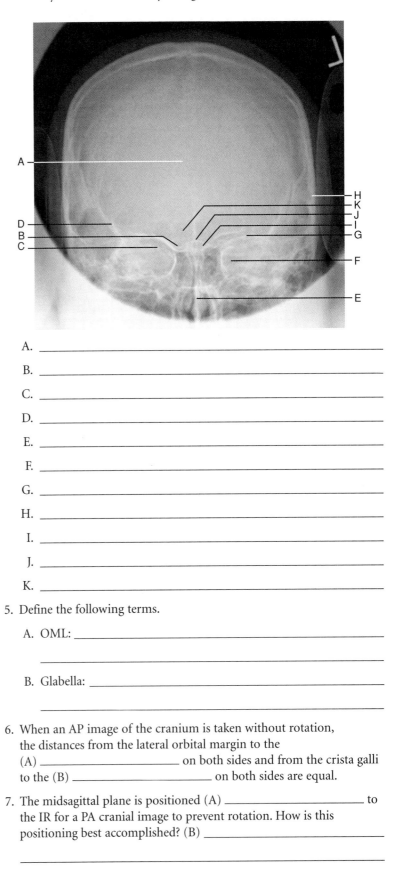

A. _____

B. _____

C. _____

D. _____

E. _____

F. _____

G. _____

H. _____

I. _____

J. _____

K. _____

5. Define the following terms.

A. OML: _____

_____

B. Glabella: _____

_____

6. When an AP image of the cranium is taken without rotation,
the distances from the lateral orbital margin to the
(A) _____ on both sides and from the crista galli
to the (B) _____ on both sides are equal.

7. The midsagittal plane is positioned (A) _____ to
the IR for a PA cranial image to prevent rotation. How is this
positioning best accomplished? (B) _____

_____

8. How is cranial rotation identified on a rotated PA skull image?

_____

9. How is the patient's head position adjusted to prevent rotation on an AP skull image taken in a patient with a suspected cervical injury?

_____

10. PA and AP skull images demonstrate different magnified anatomical structures. Which of these projections demonstrates the greater orbital magnification?

   A. _____

   Which projection demonstrates the greater parietal bone magnification?

   B. _____

11. A PA cranial image with accurate positioning demonstrates the anterior clinoids and dorsum sellae superior to the
   (A) _____, the petrous ridges superimposed over the (B) _____, and the internal auditory canals aligned horizontally through the (C) _____.
   What patient positioning line is used to obtain these anatomical relationships on the PA image? (D) _____ How is this line positioned with respect to the imaging table?
   (E) _____

12. If the patient is unable to accurately position the OML to the IR for a PA cranial image, how is the central ray adjusted to compensate?

_____

13. When the patient's chin is tucked for a PA cranial image, in which direction will the supraorbital margins move with respect to the petrous ridges? _____ (Inferiorly/Superiorly)

14. If the patient is unable to adjust the degree of chin elevation for an AP trauma cranial image, how is the central ray used to compensate?

_____

15. A PA skull image with poor positioning demonstrates approximately 1 inch (2.5 cm) of space between the petrous ridges and supraorbital margins. The ridges are inferior. Where are the dorsum sellae and anterior clinoids demonstrated with respect to the ethmoid sinuses on this image? _____

16. On a trauma AP cranial image with poor positioning, the petrous ridges are demonstrated superior to the supraorbital margins. The distance between them is approximately ½ inch (1.25 cm). Will there be an increase or decrease in the amount of dorsum sella and anterior clinoid superimposition above the ethmoid sinuses on this image?

_____

17. What two anatomical structures are aligned with the long axis of the image if the patient's midsagittal plane is accurately aligned with the collimated field on a PA or AP cranial image?

   A. _____

   B. _____

18. On a PA or AP cranial image with accurate positioning, the
    (A) _____ is centered within the collimated field.
    This centering is obtained when the central ray is centered to the
    (B) _____.

19. What anatomical structures are included on a PA or AP cranial image
    with accurate positioning?

    _____

20. On a PA or AP mandible image with accurate positioning, the
    (A) _____
    is centered within the collimated field. This centering is obtained
    when the central ray is centered to (B) _____.

21. What anatomical structures are included on a PA or AP cranial image
    with accurate positioning?

    _____

**For the following descriptions of PA cranial images with poor position-
ing, state how the patient or central ray would have been mispositioned
for such an image to be obtained.**

22. The distance from the lateral orbital margins to the lateral cranial
    cortex and from the crista galli to the lateral cranial cortex on the left
    side is greater than on the right side.

    _____

23. The petrous ridges are demonstrated inferior to the supraorbital
    margins, and the dorsum sellae and anterior clinoids are superimposed
    over the ethmoid sinuses. How was the patient mispositioned?

    A. _____

    If this were a trauma AP projection, how would the central ray have
    been mispositioned?

    B. _____

24. The petrous ridges are demonstrated superior to the supraorbital
    margins. How was the patient mispositioned?

    A. _____

    If this were a trauma AP projection, how would the central ray have
    been mispositioned?

    B. _____

For the following PA cranial images with poor positioning, state what anatomical structures are misaligned and how the patient should be repositioned for an optimal image to be obtained.

Figure 10–2

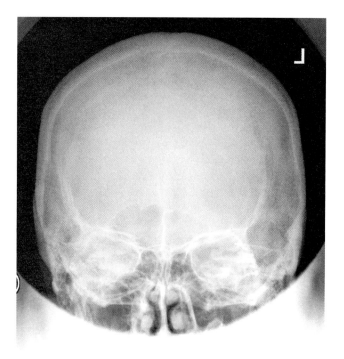

25. (Figure 10-2, PA projection): _____

_____

_____

_____

Figure 10–3

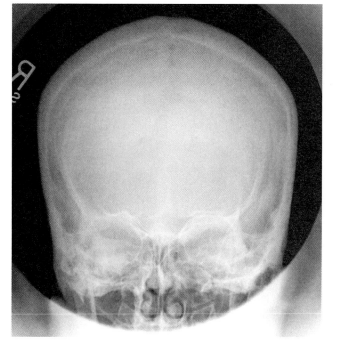

26. (Figure 10-3, PA projection): _____

_____

_____

_____

_____

_____

Figure 10–4

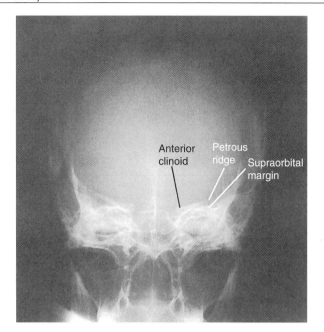

27. (Figure 10-4, PA projection): _____

_____

_____

_____

Figure 10–5

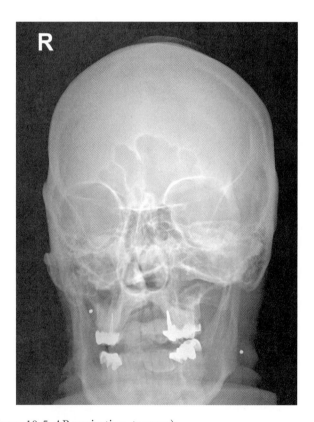

28. (Figure 10-5, AP projection, trauma): _____

_____

_____

_____

Cranium, Facial Bones, and Sinuses: PA Axial Projection (Caldwell Method)

1. Identify the labeled anatomy in Figure 10-6.

Figure 10–6

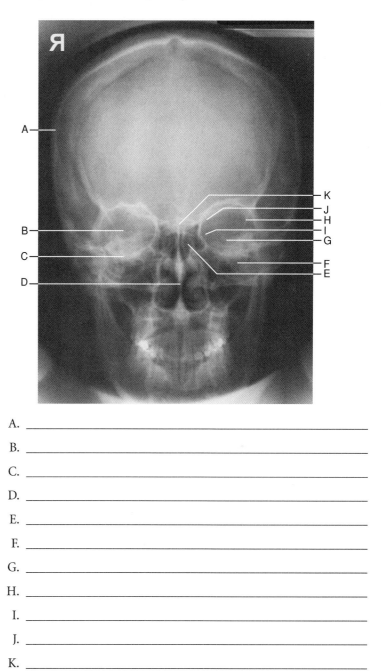

A. _____

B. _____

C. _____

D. _____

E. _____

F. _____

G. _____

H. _____

I. _____

J. _____

K. _____

2. Describe how the patient is positioned to prevent rotation on a PA axial (Caldwell) image.

_____

_____

3. What plane is positioned perpendicular to the IR for a PA axial (Caldwell) image? _____

4. What two cranial distances are equal on a PA axial (Caldwell) image if no rotation is present?

   A. _____

   B. _____

5. Cranial rotation results when the distances stated in question 4 are no longer equal. When rotation is present on a PA axial (Caldwell) image, the patient's face is rotated (A) _____ (toward/away from) the side of the cranium that demonstrates the greater distance. On an AP (Caldwell) image, the patient's face is rotated (B) _____ (toward/away from) the side of the cranium that demonstrates the greater distance.

6. Why are the orbits more magnified on an AP (Caldwell) projection of the cranium than on a PA axial (Caldwell) projection?

   A. _____

   _____

   Which projection demonstrates less parietal magnification?

   B. _____

7. What are the degree and direction of the central ray angulation used on a PA axial (Caldwell) projection of the cranium?

   _____

8. What are the degree and direction of the central ray angulation used on an AP (Caldwell) projection of the cranium when the patient is capable of adequately positioning the head?

   _____

9. On a PA or AP (Caldwell) image with accurate positioning, the (A) _____ are demonstrated horizontally through the lowest third of the orbits and the superior orbital fissures are demonstrated within the (B) _____. This position is obtained by aligning the (C) _____ perpendicular to the IR.

10. How is the central ray angulation determined for a PA axial (Caldwell) cranial image of a patient who is unable to accurately position the head? _____

    _____

11. What is the central ray angulation for a PA axial (Caldwell) projection of the cranium for a patient who can tuck the chin only enough to place the OML at a 10-degree cephalad angle with the IR?

    _____

12. What is the central ray angulation for an AP (Caldwell) projection of the cranium for a patient who can tuck the chin only enough to place the OML at a 5-degree caudal angle with the IR?

    _____

13. How is the patient positioned to align the crista galli and nasal septum with the long axis of the collimated field? _____

    _____

14. On a PA and AP (Caldwell) image with accurate positioning, the
    (A) _____ are centered within the collimated
    field. This is accomplished by centering the central ray to
    (B) _____.

15. Describe the location of the nasion. _____

    _____

16. What anatomical structures are included on a PA or AP (Caldwell)
    image of the cranium with accurate positioning?

    A. _____

    On an image of facial bones or sinuses?

    B. _____

**For the following descriptions of PA axial (Caldwell) cranial images with
poor positioning, state how the patient or central ray would have been
mispositioned for such an image to be obtained.**

17. The distance from the lateral orbital margin to the lateral cranial
    cortex on the left side is greater than that on the right side. Will the
    distance from the left or right side of the crista galli to the lateral
    cranial cortex demonstrate the smaller distance on this image?

    A. _____

    How was the patient mispositioned for this image?

    B. _____

18. The petrous ridges are demonstrated inferior to the inferior orbital
    margins. How was the patient mispositioned for such an image to be
    obtained if the central ray was accurately angled?

    A. _____

    How was the central ray mispositioned for such an image to be
    obtained if the patient was accurately positioned?

    B. _____

19. The petrous ridges and pyramids are superior to the supraorbital
    margins, and the internal auditory canals are distorted. How was the
    patient mispositioned for such an image to be obtained if the central
    ray was accurately angled?

    A. _____

    How was the central ray mispositioned for such an image to be
    obtained if the patient was accurately positioned?

    B. _____

For the following PA axial (Caldwell) cranial images with poor positioning, state what anatomical structures are misaligned and how the patient should be repositioned for an optimal image to be obtained.

Figure 10–7

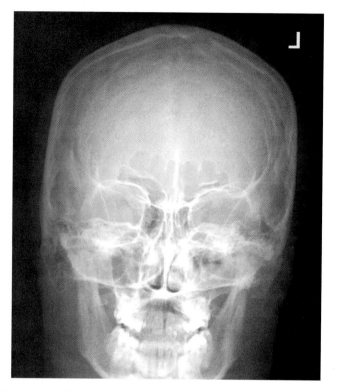

20. (Figure 10-7, PA axial projection): _____

_____

_____

_____

Figure 10–8

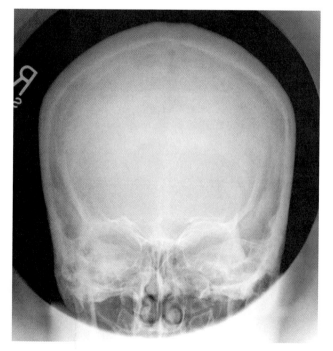

21. (Figure 10-8, PA axial projection): _____

_____

_____

_____

Figure 10–9

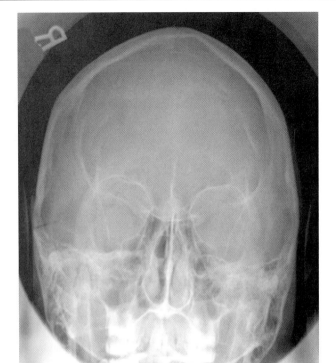

22. (Figure 10-9, PA axial projection): _____

_____

_____

_____

Figure 10–10

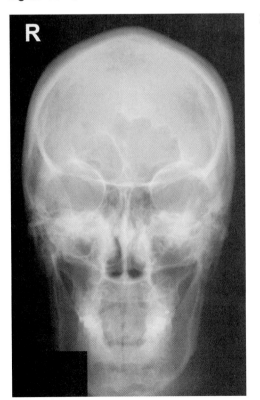

23. (Figure 10-10, AP axial projection, trauma): _____

_____

_____

_____

Cranium, Mandible, and Petromastoid Portion: AP Axial Projection (Towne Method)

1. Identify the labeled anatomy in Figure 10-11.

Figure 10–11

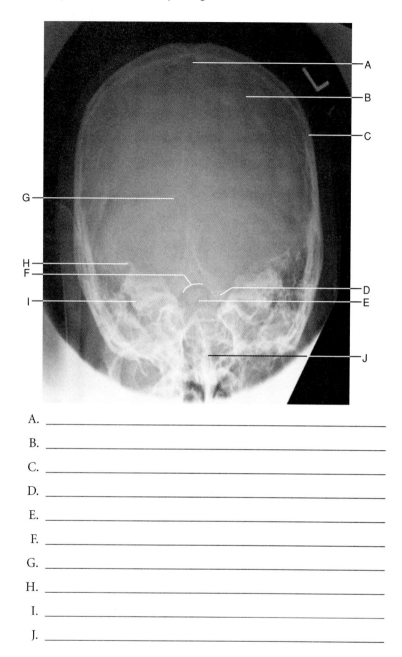

A. _____

B. _____

C. _____

D. _____

E. _____

F. _____

G. _____

H. _____

I. _____

J. _____

2. Identify the labeled anatomy in Figure 10-12.

Figure 10–12

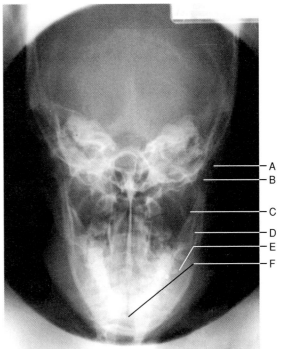

A. _____

B. _____

C. _____

D. _____

E. _____

F. _____

3. Define *infraorbitomeatal line*. _____

_____

4. The cranium is demonstrated without rotation on an AP axial (Towne) image when the distances from the
(A) _____ to the lateral borders of the foramen magnum on both sides are equal and the dorsum sella is centered within the (B) _____.

5. How is the patient positioned to prevent rotation on an AP axial (Towne) cranial image with accurate positioning?

_____

_____

6. State two methods for identifying rotation on an AP axial (Towne) cranial image.

A. _____

_____

B. _____

_____

7. The (A) _____ plane is positioned
   (B) _____ to the IR to prevent rotation on an AP
   axial (Towne) image.

8. When rotation is present on an AP axial (Towne) image, the
   side demonstrating less distance between the posterior clinoid
   process and the lateral border of the foramen magnum is the
   side _____ (toward/away from) which the patient's
   face is rotated.

9. When the correct central ray angulation and head position are used
   on an AP axial (Towne) image, the (A) _____
   and posterior clinoids are demonstrated within the
   (B) _____.

10. What are the degree and direction of the central ray angulation used
    on an AP axial (Towne) projection of the cranium?

    _____

11. What positioning line is aligned perpendicular to the IR for
    an AP axial (Towne) projection of the cranium? _____

12. How is the central ray angulation determined for an AP axial (Towne)
    cranial image in a patient who is unable to accurately position the
    head?

    _____

13. What two anatomical structures are aligned with the long axis of the
    IR if the patient's midsagittal plane is accurately aligned with the
    collimated field on an AP axial (Towne) image?

    A. _____

    B. _____

14. What anatomical structures are included on an AP axial (Towne)
    image with accurate positioning? _____

    _____

**For the following descriptions of AP axial (Towne) cranial images with
accurate positioning, state how the patient or central ray would have been
mispositioned for such an image to be obtained.**

15. The distance from the posterior clinoid process to the lateral foramen
    magnum on the patient's left side is less than that on the patient's
    right side.

    _____

16. The dorsum sellae and anterior clinoids are demonstrated
    superior to the foramen magnum. How would the patient have been
    mispositioned for such an image to be obtained if the central ray was
    accurately angled?

    A. _____

    How would the central ray have been mispositioned for such an image
    to be obtained if the patient was accurately positioned?

    B. _____

17. The dorsum sella is foreshortened and superimposed over the atlas's posterior arch. How would the patient have been mispositioned for such an image to be obtained if the central ray was accurately angled?

A. _____

How would the central ray have been mispositioned for such an image to be obtained if the patient was accurately positioned?

B. _____

For the following AP axial (Towne) cranial and mandible images with poor positioning, state what anatomical structures are misaligned and how the patient should be repositioned for an optimal image to be obtained.

Figure 10–13

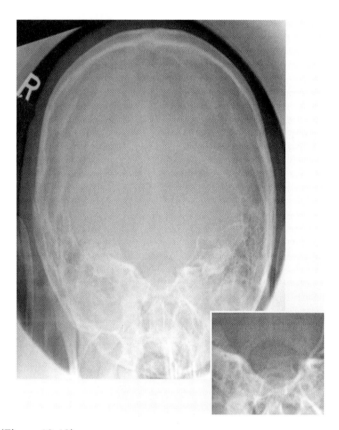

18. (Figure 10-13): _____

_____

_____

_____

Figure 10–14

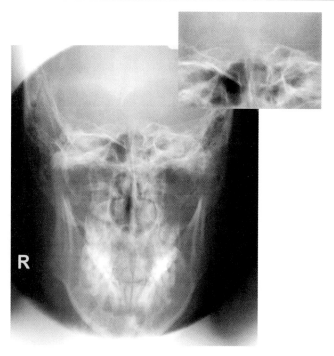

19. (Figure 10-14): _____

_____

_____

_____

Figure 10–15

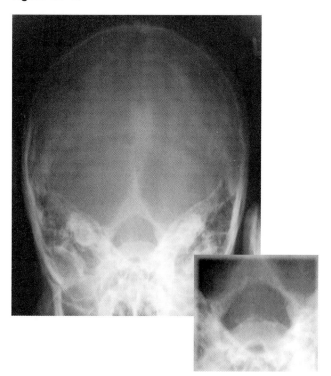

20. (Figure 10-15): _____

_____

_____

_____

Cranium, Facial Bones, Nasal Bones, and Sinuses: Lateral Position

1. Identify the labeled anatomy in Figure 10-16.

Figure 10–16

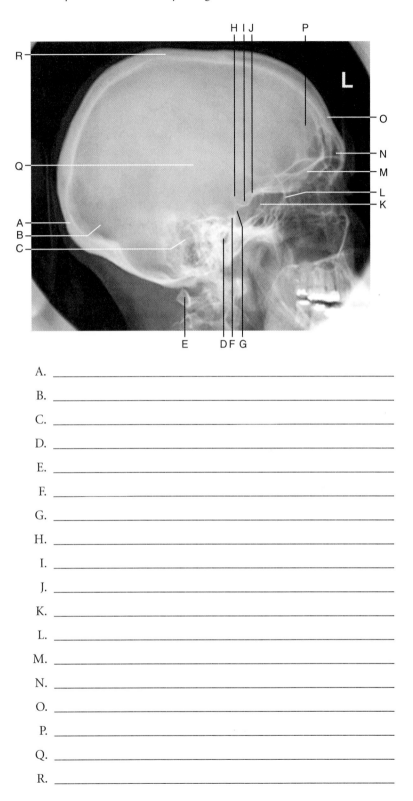

A. _____

B. _____

C. _____

D. _____

E. _____

F. _____

G. _____

H. _____

I. _____

J. _____

K. _____

L. _____

M. _____

N. _____

O. _____

P. _____

Q. _____

R. _____

2. Identify the labeled anatomy in Figure 10-17.

Figure 10–17

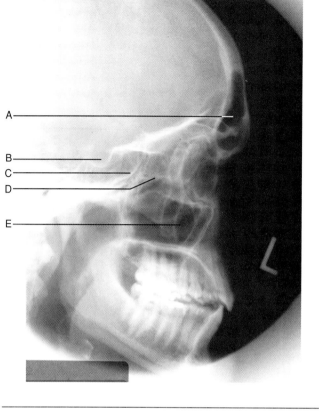

A. _____

B. _____

C. _____

D. _____

E. _____

3. Identify the labeled anatomy in Figure 10-18.

Figure 10–18

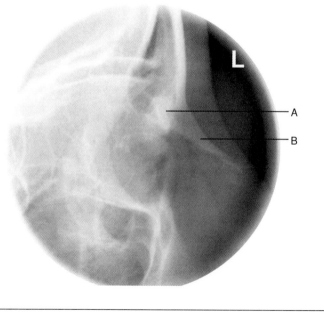

A. _____

B. _____

4. Define the following terms.

   A. Interpupillary line: _____

   _____

   B. Outer canthus: _____

   C. EAM: _____

5. What sinuses are demonstrated on a lateral sinus image when adequate contrast and density have been obtained?

   _____

6. What bilateral structures are superimposed on a lateral cranial image with accurate positioning?

   A. _____

   B. _____

   C. _____

   D. _____

   E. _____

7. Why is it best to take a lateral sinus image with the patient in an upright position?

   _____

8. What plane is used to position the patient to prevent rotation and tilting on a lateral cranial image?

   A. _____

   How is it aligned with the IR?

   B. _____

   How does this positioning align the interpupillary (IP) line with the IR?

   C. _____

9. How is the patient or IR positioned to include the occipital bone for a lateral cranial image of a recumbent patient without cervical trauma?

   A. _____

   Of a recumbent patient with cervical trauma?

   B. _____

10. How can cranial tilting be distinguished from rotation on a lateral cranial image? _____

    _____

    _____

11. How is the patient positioned to ensure that the posteroinferior occipital bone and posterior arch of the atlas are free of superimposition?

    _____

12. On a lateral cranial image with accurate positioning, the central ray is centered 2 inches (5 cm) (A) _____ to the (B) _____.

13. What anatomical structures are included on a lateral cranial image with accurate positioning?

    _____

14. On a lateral sinus image with accurate positioning, the
    (A) _____
    are centered within the collimated field. This is accomplished
    by centering the central ray halfway between the
    (B) _____ and (C) _____.

15. What anatomical structures are included on a lateral sinus image with
    accurate positioning?

    _____

16. On a lateral nasal image with accurate positioning, the
    (A) _____ are centered within the collimated field. This is
    accomplished by centering the central ray ½ inch (1.25 cm)
    (B) _____ to the nasion.

17. What anatomical structures are included on a lateral nasal bone image
    with accurate positioning? _____

    _____

For the following descriptions of lateral cranial images with poor positioning, state how the patient would have been mispositioned for such an image to be obtained.

18. The greater wings of the sphenoid and the anterior cranial cortices are
    demonstrated without superimposition. One of each corresponding
    structure is demonstrated anterior to the other.

    _____

19. The orbital roofs, external auditory meatus, and inferior cranial
    cortices are demonstrated without superimposition. One of each
    corresponding structure is demonstrated superior to the other and the
    posterior arch is seen in profile.

    _____

For the following lateral cranial images with poor positioning, state what anatomical structures are misaligned and how the patient should be repositioned for an optimal image to be obtained.

Figure 10–19

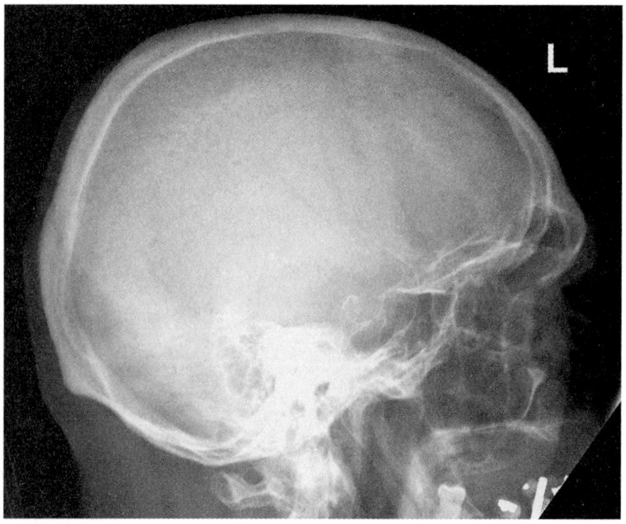

20. (Figure 10-19): _____

    _____

    _____

    _____

Figure 10–20

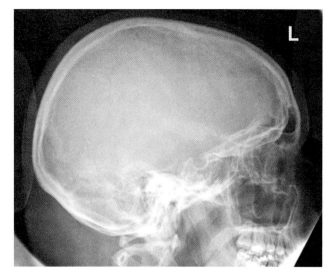

21. (Figure 10-20): _____

_____

_____

_____

Cranium, Mandible, and Sinuses: SMV Projection (Schueller Method)

1. Identify the labeled anatomy in Figure 10-21.

Figure 10–21

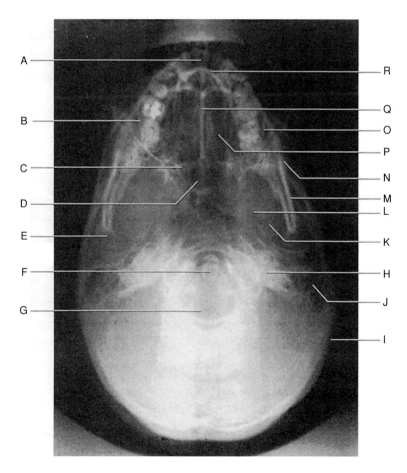

A. _____

B. _____

C. _____

D. _____

E. _____

F. _____

G. _____

H. _____

I. _____

J. _____

K. _____

L. _____

M. _____

N. _____

O. _____

P. _____

Q. _____

R. _____

2. Where are the mandibular mentum and nasal fossae demonstrated on an SMV (Schueller) cranial image with accurate positioning?

A. _____

What anatomical positioning line is used to ensure this centering?

B. _____

How is this line aligned with the IR?

C. _____

3. What structures are obscured on an SMV cranial projection if the patient's neck is not adequately extended?

A. _____

B. _____

C. _____

D. _____

4. How is the positioning setup adjusted for an SMV cranial projection in a patient who is unable to extend the neck as far as needed?

_____

5. How is cranial tilting identified on a tilted SMV cranial image?

A. _____

_____

How is the patient positioned to prevent tilting on an SMV cranial image?

B. _____

6. How is the patient positioned to align the vomer, bony nasal septum, and dens with the long axis of the collimated field on an SMV image?

   A. _____

   Will rotation of the head affect any anatomical relationships on an SMV image?

   B. _____ (Yes/No)

7. On an SMV cranial image with accurate positioning, the (A) _____ is centered within the collimated field. This is accomplished when the central ray is centered to the (B) _____ plane at a level (C) _____ inch anterior to the level of the (D) _____.

8. What anatomical structures are included on an SMV cranial image with accurate positioning? _____

9. On an SMV sinus and mandible image with accurate positioning, the (A) _____ are centered within the collimated field. This is accomplished by centering the central ray to the (B) _____ plane at a level (C) _____ inches inferior to the (D) _____.

10. What anatomical structures are included on an SMV sinus and mandible image with accurate positioning? _____

   _____

For the following descriptions of SMV cranial images with poor positioning, state how the patient or central ray would have been mispositioned for such an image to be obtained.

11. The mandibular mentum is demonstrated too far anterior to the ethmoid sinuses.

   _____

12. The mandibular mentum is demonstrated posterior to the ethmoid sinuses. How would the patient have been mispositioned?

   A. _____

   _____

   How would the central ray have been mispositioned?

   B. _____

13. The distance from the left mandibular ramus and body to its corresponding lateral cranial cortex is greater than the distance from the right mandibular ramus and body to its corresponding lateral cranial cortex.

   _____

For the following SMV cranial, facial bone, and sinus images with poor positioning, state what anatomical structures are misaligned and how the patient should be repositioned for an optimal image to be obtained.

Figure 10–22

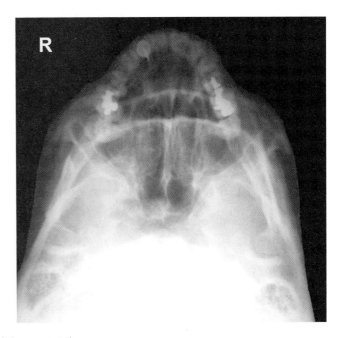

14. (Figure 10-22): _____

_____

_____

_____

Figure 10–23

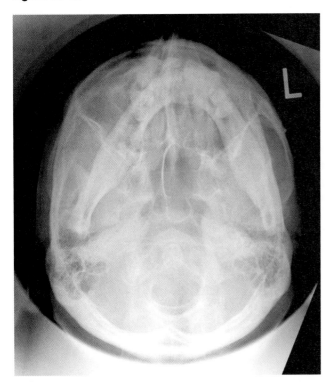

15. (Figure 10-23): _____

_____

_____

_____

_____

_____

Figure 10–24

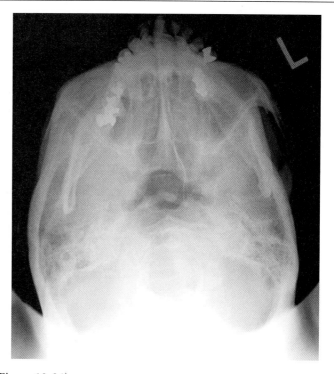

16. (Figure 10-24): _____

_____

_____

_____

Facial Bones and Sinuses: Parietoacanthial and Acanthioparietal Projection (Waters and Open-Mouth Waters Methods)

1. Identify the labeled anatomy in Figure 10-25.

Figure 10–25

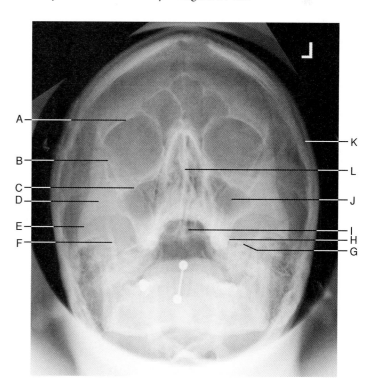

A. _____

B. _____

C. _____

D. _____

E. _____

F. _____

G. _____

H. _____

I. _____

J. _____

K. _____

L. _____

2. Define *mentomeatal line.* _____

_____

3. What sinuses are demonstrated on an open-mouth parietoacanthial (Waters) image that are not demonstrated on a closed-mouth parietoacanthial image? _____

4. Describe how the patient is positioned to prevent rotation on a parietoacanthial sinus image.

_____

_____

5. What two cranial distances are equal on a parietoacanthial sinus image if no rotation is present?

A. _____

B. _____

6. Cranial rotation results when the distances stated in question 5 are no longer equal. When rotation is present on a parietoacanthial image, the patient's face is rotated (A) _____ (toward/away from) the side of the cranium that demonstrates the greatest distance. If an acanthioparietal image is taken, the patient's face is rotated (B) _____ (toward/away from) the side of the cranium that demonstrates the greatest distance.

7. Why are the orbits more magnified on an acanthioparietal projection of the cranium than on a parietoacanthial projection?

A. _____

Which projection demonstrates the least parietal magnification?

B. _____

8. How is the patient positioned to accurately demonstrate the petrous ridges inferior to the maxillary sinuses on a parietoacanthial projection? _____

9. How is the patient positioned for a parietoacanthial image to align the bony nasal septum with the long axis of the collimated field?

_____

10. What are the results of cranial tilting on a parietoacanthial image?

   A. _____

   B. _____

11. On a parietoacanthial image with accurate positioning, the (A) _____ is centered within the collimated field. This is accomplished by centering the central ray to the (B) _____.

12. What anatomical structures are included on a parietoacanthial image with accurate positioning? _____

For the following descriptions of parietoacanthial cranial images with poor positioning, state how the patient would have been mispositioned for such an image to be obtained.

13. The distances from the lateral orbital margin to the lateral cranial cortex and from the bony nasal septum to the lateral cranial cortex on the left side of the patient are greater than the distances on the right side.

---

14. The petrous ridges are demonstrated within the maxillary sinuses and superior to the posterior maxillary alveolar process.

---

15. The petrous ridges are inferior to the maxillary sinuses and posterior maxillary alveolar process.

For the following parietoacanthial images with poor positioning, state what anatomical structures are misaligned and how the patient should be repositioned for an optimal image to be obtained.

Figure 10–26

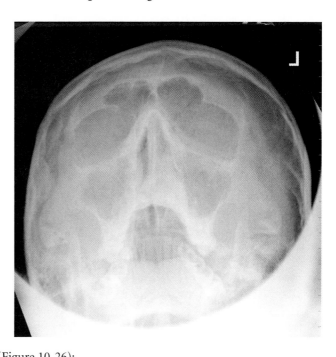

16. (Figure 10-26): _____

_____

_____

Figure 10–27

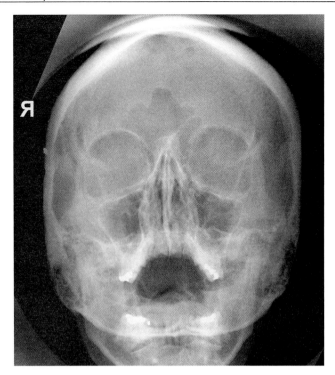

17. (Figure 10-27, parietocanthial): _____

_____

_____

_____

Figure 10–28

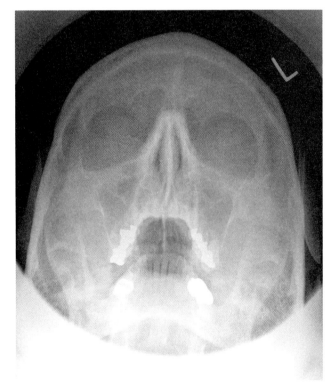

18. (Figure 10-28, parietocanthial): _____

_____

_____

_____

Optic Canal and Foramen: Parietoorbital Oblique Projection (Rhese Method)

1. Identify the labeled anatomy in Figure 10-29.

Figure 10–29

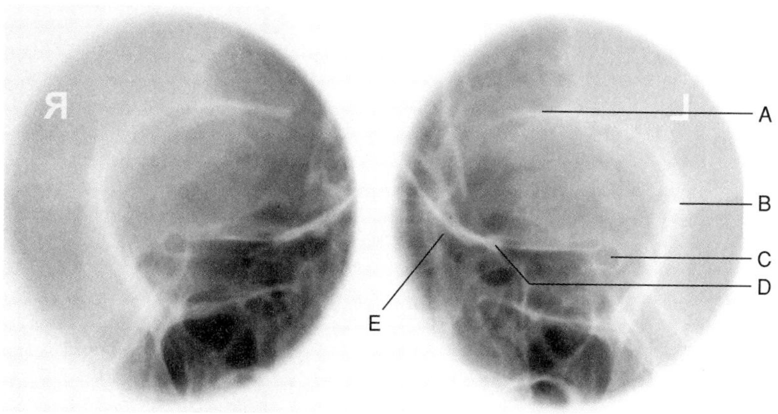

A. _____

B. _____

C. _____

D. _____

E. _____

2. A parietoorbital oblique optic canal and foramen image with accurate positioning demonstrates the optic canal (A) _____ and the optic foramen demonstrated in the (B) _____ of the orbit, adjacent to the (C) _____.

3. Define *acanthiomeatal line.* _____

   _____

4. To obtain accurate parietoorbital oblique optic canal and foramen positioning, tuck the patient's chin until the (A) _____ is perpendicular to the IR and the (B) _____ is level, then rotate the head toward the affected orbit until the (C) _____ plane is at a (D) _____ angle.

5. On a parietoorbital oblique optic canal and foramen image with accurate positioning, the (A) _____ is centered within the collimated field. This is accomplished by centering the central ray to the (B) _____.

6. What anatomical structures are included on a parietoorbital oblique optic canal and foramen image with accurate positioning?

   _____

   _____

For the following descriptions of parietoorbital oblique optic canal and foramen images with poor positioning, state how the patient would have been mispositioned for such an image to be obtained.

7. The optic foramen is situated in the superior half of the orbit.

   _____

8. The optic foramen is situated closer to the center of the orbit.

   _____

Nasal Bones: Tangential Projection (Superoinferior Projection)

1. Identify the labeled anatomy in Figure 10-30.

Figure 10–30

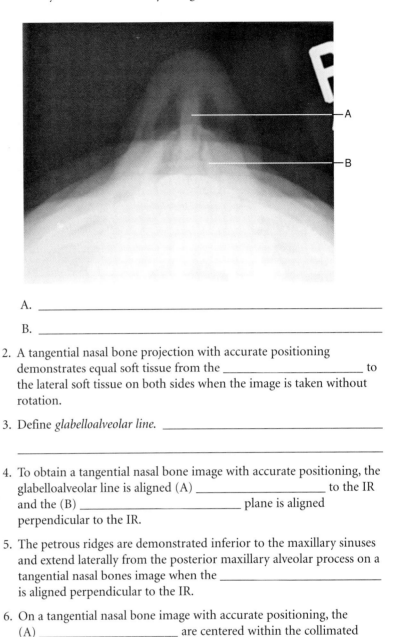

A. _____

B. _____

2. A tangential nasal bone projection with accurate positioning demonstrates equal soft tissue from the _____ to the lateral soft tissue on both sides when the image is taken without rotation.

3. Define *glabelloalveolar line.* _____

_____

4. To obtain a tangential nasal bone image with accurate positioning, the glabelloalveolar line is aligned (A) _____ to the IR and the (B) _____ plane is aligned perpendicular to the IR.

5. The petrous ridges are demonstrated inferior to the maxillary sinuses and extend laterally from the posterior maxillary alveolar process on a tangential nasal bones image when the _____ is aligned perpendicular to the IR.

6. On a tangential nasal bone image with accurate positioning, the (A) _____ are centered within the collimated field. This is accomplished by centering the central ray to the (B) _____.

7. What anatomical structures are included on a tangential nasal bone image with accurate positioning? _____

_____

For the following descriptions of tangential nasal bones images with poor positioning, state how the patient would have been mispositioned for such an image to be obtained.

8. More soft-tissue width is demonstrated from the nasal bones to the lateral soft tissue on right side then on the left side.

_____

9. The posterior nasal bones are superimposed by the glabella.

Petromastoid Portion: Axiolateral Oblique (Modified Law) Projection (Modified Law Method)

1. Identify the labeled anatomy in Figure 10-31.

Figure 10–31

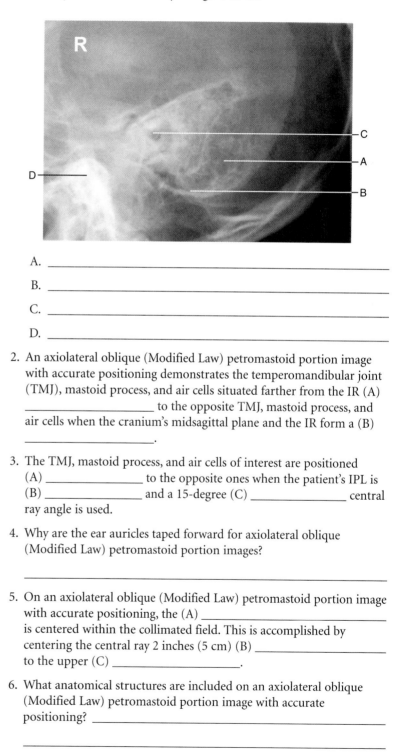

A. _____

B. _____

C. _____

D. _____

2. An axiolateral oblique (Modified Law) petromastoid portion image with accurate positioning demonstrates the temperomandibular joint (TMJ), mastoid process, and air cells situated farther from the IR (A) _____ to the opposite TMJ, mastoid process, and air cells when the cranium's midsagittal plane and the IR form a (B) _____.

3. The TMJ, mastoid process, and air cells of interest are positioned (A) _____ to the opposite ones when the patient's IPL is (B) _____ and a 15-degree (C) _____ central ray angle is used.

4. Why are the ear auricles taped forward for axiolateral oblique (Modified Law) petromastoid portion images?

_____

5. On an axiolateral oblique (Modified Law) petromastoid portion image with accurate positioning, the (A) _____ is centered within the collimated field. This is accomplished by centering the central ray 2 inches (5 cm) (B) _____ to the upper (C) _____.

6. What anatomical structures are included on an axiolateral oblique (Modified Law) petromastoid portion image with accurate positioning? _____

_____

For the following description of an axiolateral oblique (Modified Law) petromastoid portion image with poor positioning, state how the patient would have been mispositioned for such an image to be obtained.

7. The right and left TMJ, mastoid process, and air cells are aligned anteroposteriorly.

_____

Petromastoid Portion: Axiolateral Oblique Projection (Stenvers Method, Posterior Profile)

1. Identify the labeled anatomy in Figure 10-32.

Figure 10–32

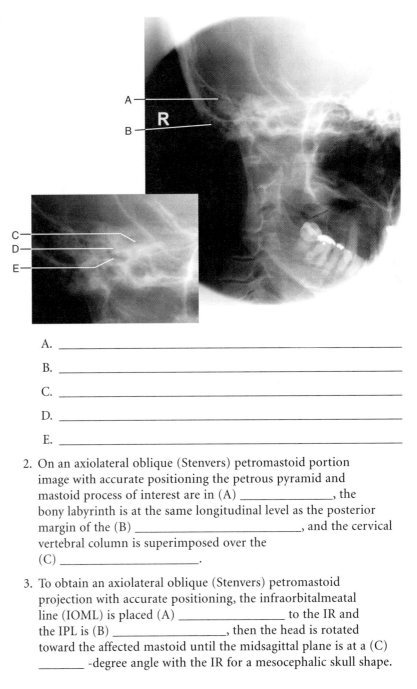

A. _____

B. _____

C. _____

D. _____

E. _____

2. On an axiolateral oblique (Stenvers) petromastoid portion image with accurate positioning the petrous pyramid and mastoid process of interest are in (A) _____, the bony labyrinth is at the same longitudinal level as the posterior margin of the (B) _____, and the cervical vertebral column is superimposed over the (C) _____.

3. To obtain an axiolateral oblique (Stenvers) petromastoid projection with accurate positioning, the infraorbitalmeatal line (IOML) is placed (A) _____ to the IR and the IPL is (B) _____, then the head is rotated toward the affected mastoid until the midsagittal plane is at a (C) _____ -degree angle with the IR for a mesocephalic skull shape.

4. Describe the skull shapes indicated below and state the degree of rotation required to obtain an axiolateral oblique (Stenvers) petromastoid portion image with accurate positioning.

   A. Brachycephalic: _____

   B. Dolichocephalic: _____

5. How is the patient positioned to place the supraorbital margin and the petrous ridge of interest on the same transverse plane on an axiolateral oblique (Stenvers) petromastoid portion image with accurate positioning? _____

   _____

6. On an axiolateral oblique (Stenvers) petromastoid portion image with accurate positioning, the (A) _____ and (B) _____ are centered within the collimated field. This is accomplished by centering a 12-degree (C) _____ angled central ray 3 to 4 inches (7 to 10 cm) (D) _____ and ½ inch (1.25 cm) inferior to the upside (E) _____.

7. What anatomical structures are included on an axiolateral oblique (Stenvers) petromastoid portion image with accurate positioning?

   _____

   _____

For the following descriptions of axiolateral oblique (Stenvers) petromastoid portion images with poor positioning, state how the patient would have been mispositioned for such an image to be obtained.

8. The IAC is foreshortened, the semicircular canals (bony labyrinth) are not in profile and are visible anterior to the posterior margin of the mandibular rami, and the cervical vertebral column is not superimposed over the entire mandibular rami.

   _____

   _____

9. The IAC and semicircular canals (bony labyrinth) are obscured, and the supraorbital margin is demonstrated superior to the petrous ridge.

   _____

   _____

For the following axiolateral oblique (Stenvers) petromastoid portion images with poor positioning, state what anatomical structures are misaligned and how the patient should be repositioned for an optimal image to be obtained.

Figure 10–33

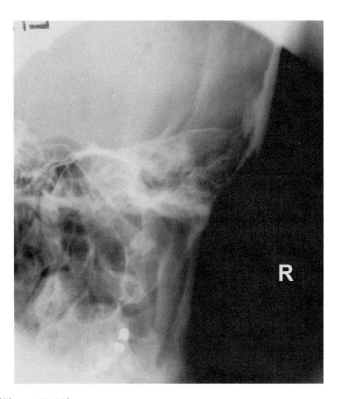

10. (Figure 10-33): _____

_____

_____

_____

Figure 10–34

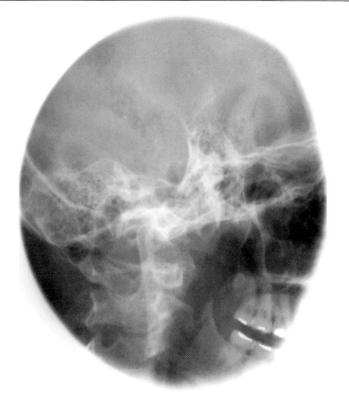

11. (Figure 10-34): _____

_____

_____

_____

Figure 10–35

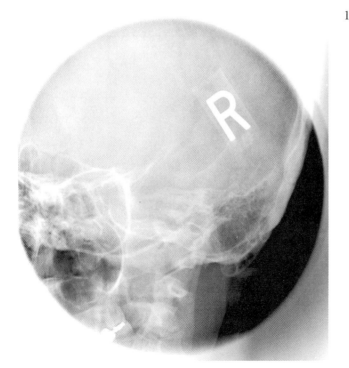

12. (Figure 10-35): _____

_____

_____

_____

Figure 10–36

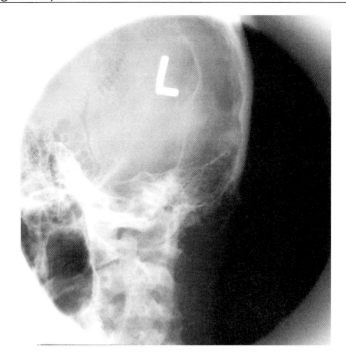

13. (Figure 10-36): _____

_____

_____

_____

CHAPTER 10

STUDY QUESTION ANSWERS

Cranium, Facial Bones, Mandible, Sinuses, and Petromastoid Portion

1. A. As if the patient was in an upright position with the marker correct
   B. As if the patient was in an upright position with the marker reversed
   C. With the anterior mandible facing upward with the marker correct
   D. As if the patient was in an upright position with the marker correct

2. Table 10-1

Position or Projection	Structure	kVp	Grid	AEC Chamber(s)	SID
AP or PA projection	Cranium	70-80	Grid	Center	40-48 inches (100-120 cm)
	Mandible	70-80	Grid		
PA axial (Caldwell) projection	Cranium	70-80	Grid	Center	40-48 inches (100-120 cm)
	Facial bones	70-80	Grid	Center	
	Sinuses	70-80	Grid	Center	
AP axial (Towne) projection	Cranium	70-80	Grid	Center	40-48 inches (100-120 cm)
	Mandible	70-80	Grid		
	Petromastoid portion	70-80	Grid	Center	
Lateral position	Cranium	70-80	Grid	Center	40-48 inches (100-120 cm)
	Facial bones	70-80	Grid	Center	
	Sinuses	50-60	Grid		
	Nasal bones	70-80	Grid		
Submentovertex (Schueller) projection	Cranium	70-80	Grid	Center	40-48 inches (100-120 cm)
	Mandible	70-80	Grid	Center	
	Sinuses	70-80	Grid	Center	
	Zygomatic arches	60-70	Nongrid		
Parietoacanthial (Waters) projection	Facial bones	70-80	Grid	Center	40-48 inches (100-120 cm)
	Sinuses	70-80	Grid	Center	
Parietoorbital oblique (Rhese) projection	Optic canal and foramen	70-80	Grid		40-48 inches (100-120 cm)
Tangential (superoinferior) projection	Nasal bones	50-60			40-48 inches (100-120 cm)
Axiolateral oblique (modified Law) projection	Petromastoid portion	70-80	Grid		40-48 inches (100-120 cm)
Axiolateral oblique (Stenvers) projection	Petromastoid portion	70-80	Grid	Center	40-48 inches (100-120 cm)

AEC, Automatic exposure control; *AP*, anteroposterior; *kVp*, kilovolt-peak; *PA*, posteroanterior; *SID*, source–image receptor distance.

3. Table 10-2

Position or Projection	Structure	IR Size	Placement and Direction
AP or PA projection	Cranium	10 × 12 inches (24 × 30 cm)	Lengthwise
	Mandible	8 × 10 inches (18 × 24 cm)	Lengthwise
PA axial (Caldwell) projection	Cranium	10 × 12 inches (24 × 30 cm)	Lengthwise
	Facial bones	8 × 10 inches (18 × 24 cm)	Lengthwise
	Sinuses	8 × 10 inches (18 × 24 cm)	Lengthwise
AP axial (Towne) projection	Cranium	10 × 12 inches (24 × 30 cm)	Lengthwise
	Mandible	8 × 10 inches (18 × 24 cm)	Lengthwise
	Petromastoid portion	10 × 12 inches (24 × 30 cm)	Lengthwise
Lateral position	Cranium	10 × 12 inches (24 × 30 cm)	Lengthwise
	Facial bones	8 × 10 inches (18 × 24 cm)	Lengthwise
	Sinuses	8 × 10 inches (18 × 24 cm)	Lengthwise
	Nasal bones	8 × 10 inches (18 × 24 cm)	Lengthwise
Submentovertex (Schueller) projection	Cranium	10 × 12 inches (24 × 30 cm)	Lengthwise
	Mandible	8 × 10 inches (24 × 30 cm)	Lengthwise
	Sinuses	8 × 10 inches (18 × 24 cm)	Lengthwise
Parietoacanthial (Waters) projection	Facial bones	8 × 10 inches (18 × 24 cm)	Lengthwise
	Sinuses	8 × 10 inches (18 × 24 cm)	Lengthwise
Parietoorbital oblique (Rhese) projection	Optic canal and foramen	8 × 10 inches (18 × 24 cm)	Lengthwise
Tangential (superoinferior) projection	Nasal bones	8 × 10 inches (18 × 24 cm)	Lengthwise
Axiolateral oblique (modified Law) projection	Petromastoid portion	8 × 10 inches (18 × 24 cm)	Lengthwise
Axiolateral oblique (Stenvers) projection	Petromastoid portion	8 × 10 inches (18 × 24 cm)	Lengthwise

AP, Anteroposterior; *IR*, image receptor; *PA*, posteroanterior.

Cranium and Mandible: PA or AP Projection

4. A. Frontal bone
   B. Anterior clinoid process
   C. Petrous ridge
   D. Oblique orbital line
   E. Nasal septum
   F. Internal auditory canal
   G. Supraorbital margin
   H. Lateral cranial cortex
   I. Dorsum sellae
   J. Crista galli
   K. Frontal sinus
5. A. Imaginary line connecting the outer eye canthus and external auditory opening
   B. Area located on the midsagittal plane at the level of the eyebrows
6. A. Lateral cranial cortices
   B. Lateral cranial cortices
7. A. Perpendicular
   B. Place an extended flat palm next to each parietal bone and adjust the head rotation until your hands are positioned perpendicular to the IR.

8. When the distance from the lateral orbital margin to the lateral cranial cortex or from the crista galli to the lateral cranial cortex on one side is greater than the opposite side
9. The patient's head should not be adjusted. The image should be taken with the head positioned as is.
10. A. AP projection
    B. PA projection
11. A. Ethmoid sinuses
    B. Supraorbital margins
    C. Center of the orbits
    D. OML
    E. Perpendicular
12. Angle the central ray parallel with the OML.
13. Inferiorly
14. Angle the central ray parallel with the OML.
15. They would be demonstrated within the ethmoid sinuses.
16. Increase
17. A. Crista galli
    B. Nasal septum
18. A. Dorsum sellae
    B. Glabella

19. The outer cranial cortex and maxillary sinus
20. A. Midpoint between the mandibular rami
    B. Exit the acanthion
21. Entire mandible
22. The patient's face was rotated toward the right side.
23. A. The patient's chin was not tucked enough.
    B. The central ray was angled too cephalically.
24. A. The patient's chin was tucked too much.
    B. The central ray was angled too caudally.
25. The distance from the lateral orbital margins to the lateral cranial borders and from the crista galli to the lateral cranial cortex on the left side is greater than the same distance on the right side. Rotate the patient's face to the left until the midsagittal plane is aligned perpendicular to the IR.
26. The petrous ridges are demonstrated inferior to the supraorbital margins, and the dorsum sellae and anterior clinoids are demonstrated within the ethmoid sinuses. Tuck the chin until the OML is aligned perpendicular to the IR or move the chin downward half the distance demonstrated between the petrous ridges and supraorbital margins.
27. The petrous ridges are demonstrated superior to the supraorbital margins, and the internal auditory canals are distorted. Extend the chin, moving it away from the thorax until the OML is aligned perpendicular to the IR or move the chin upward half the distance demonstrated between the petrous ridges and supraorbital margin.
28. The petrous ridges are demonstrated inferior to the supraorbital margins, and the dorsum sellae and anterior clinoids are demonstrated within the ethmoid sinuses. The supraorbital margins need to be moved toward the petrous ridges. Tuck the chin until the OML is aligned perpendicular to the IR, or adjust the central ray angulation caudally. The distance from the right lateral orbital margin to the lateral cranial cortex is less than the distance from the left lateral orbital margin to the lateral cranial cortex. If a cervical injury is not suspected and the patient allows, rotate the face toward the left side.

Cranium, Facial Bones, and Sinuses: PA Axial Projection (Caldwell Method)

1. A. Lateral cranial cortex
   B. Greater sphenoidal wing
   C. Inferior orbital margin
   D. Nasal septum
   E. Ethmoid sinus
   F. Petrous pyramid
   G. Petrous ridge
   H. Oblique orbital line
   I. Superior orbital fissure
   J. Lesser sphenoidal wing
   K. Crista galli

2. Place an extended flat palm next to each parietal bone, and adjust the head rotation until your hands are positioned perpendicular to the IR.
3. Midsagittal
4. A. Lateral orbital margins to the lateral cranial cortices on both sides
   B. Crista galli to the lateral cranial cortices on both sides
5. A. Away from
   B. Away from
6. A. Because the orbits are placed at a longer object–image receptor distance (OID) in the AP than in the PA projection
   B. AP projection
7. 15 degrees caudal
8. 15 degrees cephalic
9. A. Petrous ridges
   B. Orbits
   C. OML
10. Position the OML as close as possible to perpendicular to the IR. Angle the central ray parallel with the patient's OML, and adjust it 15 degrees caudally from this angle.
11. 5 degrees caudal
12. 10 degrees cephalic
13. Align the midsagittal plane with the long axis of the IR.
14. A. Ethmoid sinuses
    B. Exit at the nasion
15. The area located on the midsagittal plane at a level ¾ inch (2 cm) inferior to the eyebrows
16. A. The outer cranial cortex and ethmoid sinuses
    B. The frontal and ethmoid sinuses and lateral cranial cortices
17. A. Right
    B. The patient's head was turned toward the right side.
18. A. The patient's chin was not tucked enough.
    B. The central ray was angled too caudally.
19. A. The patient's chin was tucked more than needed.
    B. The central ray was angled too cephalically.
20. The distance from the lateral orbital margin to the lateral cranial cortex and from the crista galli to the lateral cranial cortex on the right side is greater than the distance on the left side. Rotate the patient's face toward the right side.
21. The petrous ridges and pyramids are demonstrated in the superior half of the orbits. Elevate the patient's chin until the OML is aligned perpendicular to the IR, or angle the central ray caudally.
22. The petrous ridges are demonstrated inferior to the inferior orbital margins. Tuck the chin until the OML is aligned perpendicular to the IR, or adjust the central ray angulation cephalically.
23. The petrous ridges are demonstrated too inferior in the orbits. Tuck the chin until the OML is perpendicular to the IR, or adjust the central ray angulation caudally.

Cranium, Mandible, and Petromastoid Portion: AP Axial Projection (Towne Method)

1. A. Sagittal suture
   B. Parietal bone
   C. Lateral cranial cortex
   D. Posterior clinoid process
   E. Dorsum sellae
   F. Foramen magnum
   G. Occipital bone
   H. Petrous ridge
   I. Petrous pyramid
   J. Nasal septum
2. A. Mastoid process
   B. Condyle
   C. Coronoid process
   D. Ramus
   E. Body
   F. Symphysis
3. Imaginary line connecting the lower orbital outline and external auditory meatus
4. A. Posterior clinoid process
   B. Foramen magnum
5. Place an extended flat palm next to each lateral parietal bone, and adjust the patient's head rotation until your hands are positioned perpendicular to the IR.
6. A. By determining that the distance from the posterior clinoid process to the lateral border of the foramen magnum on one side is greater than the distance on the opposite side
   B. By determining that the dorsum sella is demonstrated closer to one side of the foramen magnum than the opposite side
7. A. Midsagittal
   B. Perpendicular
8. Toward
9. A. Dorsum sellae
   B. Foramen magnum
10. 30 degrees caudal
11. OML
12. Angle the central ray until it is parallel with the OML, and adjust it 30 degrees caudally.
13. A. Sagittal suture
    B. Nasal septum
14. The outer cranial cortex, petrous ridges, dorsum sellae, and foramen magnum
15. The patient's face was rotated toward the left side.
16. A. The patient's chin was not tucked enough.
    B. The central ray was angled too cephalically.
17. A. The patient's chin was tucked more than needed.
    B. The central ray was angled too caudally.
18. The distance from the posterior clinoid process to the lateral foramen magnum on the patient's left side is less than the distance on the patient's right side. Rotate the patient's face toward the right side until the midsagittal plane is perpendicular to the IR.

19. The dorsum sellae and anterior clinoids are demonstrated superior to the foramen magnum. Tuck the patient's chin until the OML is perpendicular to the IR, or adjust the central ray caudally. The symphysis is clipped. Lower the central ray and IR by ½ inch (1.25 cm).
20. The dorsum sella is foreshortened and superimposed over the atlas's posterior arch. Elevate the patient's chin or adjust the central ray angulation cephalically.

Cranium, Facial Bones, Nasal Bones, and Sinuses: Lateral Position

1. A. Inion
   B. Occipital bone
   C. Mastoid air cells
   D. External auditory meatus
   E. Posterior arch
   F. Clivus
   G. Dorsum sellae
   H. Posterior clinoid processes
   I. Sella turcica
   J. Anterior clinoid processes
   K. Sphenoidal sinuses
   L. Greater sphenoidal wings
   M. Orbital roofs
   N. Frontal sinuses
   O. Anterior cranial cortex
   P. Frontal bone
   Q. Parietal bone
   R. Superior cranial cortex
2. A. Frontal sinus
   B. Sella turcica
   C. Sphenoid sinuses
   D. Ethmoid air cells
   E. Maxillary sinuses
3. A. Nasofrontal suture
   B. Nasal bone
4. A. Imaginary line connecting the outer corners of each eyelid
   B. Outer corner where eyelids meet
   C. External auditory meatus
5. The sphenoid, ethmoid, frontal, and maxillary sinuses
6. A. Orbital roofs
   B. Mandibular rami
   C. Greater wings of the sphenoid
   D. External auditory canals
   E. Cranial cortices
7. To demonstrate air-fluid levels within the sinus cavities
8. A. Midsagittal
   B. Parallel
   C. Perpendicular
9. A. Elevate the occiput on a radiolucent sponge.
   B. Position the cassette 1 inch (2.5 cm) below the occipital bone.

10. When the patient's cranium is tilted, the inferior cortical outlines of superimposed structures are demonstrated without superimposition. When the cranium is rotated, the posterior and anterior cortices are demonstrated without superimposition.

11. Position the IOML perpendicular to the front edge of the IR.

12. A. Superior
    B. EAM

13. The outer cranial cortex

14. A. Zygoma and greater wings of the sphenoid
    B. Outer canthus
    C. EAM

15. The frontal, ethmoid, sphenoid, and maxillary sinuses and mandible

16. A. Nasal bones
    B. Inferior

17. Nasal bones, surrounding nasal soft tissue, anterior nasal spine of maxilla, anterior cranial cortices, orbital roofs, and zygomatic bones

18. The patient's head was rotated.

19. The patient's head was tilted toward the IR.

20. The greater wings of the sphenoid and the anterior cranial cortices are demonstrated without superimposition. One of each corresponding structure is demonstrated anterior to the other and the posterior arch is in profile. Rotate the patient's head until the midsagittal plane is parallel with the IR. The orbital roofs and inferior cranial cortices are demonstrated without superimposition. One of each corresponding structure is demonstrated superior to the other. Tilt the patient's head away from the IR until the midsagittal plane is parallel and the IP line is perpendicular to the IR.

21. The orbital roofs and inferior cranial cortices are demonstrated without superimposition. One of each corresponding structure is demonstrated superior to the other and the atlas' vertebral foramen is visualized. Tilt the patient's head toward the IR until the midsagittal plane is parallel and the IP line is perpendicular to the IR.

Cranium, Mandible, and Sinuses: SMV Projection (Schueller Method)

1. A. Mandibular mentum
   B. Maxillary sinus
   C. Posterior palatine bone
   D. Sphenoid sinus
   E. Mandibular condyle
   F. Dens
   G. Foramen magnum
   H. Petrous pyramid
   I. Cranial cortex
   J. Mastoid air cells
   K. Foramen spinosum
   L. Foramen ovale
   M. Mandibular ramus
   N. Mandibular coronoid
   O. Mandibular body
   P. Ethmoid sinus
   Q. Vomer and bony nasal septum
   R. Nasal fossae

2. A. Anterior to the ethmoid sinuses
   B. IOML
   C. Parallel

3. A. Nasal fossae
   B. Ethmoid sinus
   C. Foramen ovale
   D. Foramen spinosum

4. Angle the central ray until it is aligned perpendicular to the IOML.

5. A. By comparing the distance from the right mandibular ramus and body to its corresponding lateral cranial cortex with the distance from the left mandibular ramus and body to its corresponding lateral cranial cortex
   B. Align the midsagittal plane perpendicular to the IR.

6. A. Turn the patient's face until the midsagittal plane is aligned with the long axis of the collimator's longitudinal light.
   B. No

7. A. Dens
   B. Midsagittal
   C. ¾ (2 cm)
   D. EAM

8. The mandible and anterior cranial cortices

9. A. Sphenoid sinuses
   B. Midsagittal
   C. 1½ (4 cm)
   D. Mandibular symphysis

10. The mandible, lateral cranial cortices, and mastoid air cells

11. The patient's neck was overextended, preventing the IOML from being positioned parallel with the IR.

12. A. The patient's neck was underextended, preventing the IOML from being positioned parallel with the IR.
    B. The central ray was angled too caudally.

13. The patient's vertex was tilted toward the left side.

14. The mandibular mentum is demonstrated too far anterior to the ethmoid sinuses. Depress the patient's chin until the IOML is aligned parallel with the IR, or adjust the central ray angulation caudally.

15. The mandibular mentum is demonstrated posterior to the ethmoid sinuses. Elevate the patient's chin, or adjust the central ray angulation cephalically. The distance from the right mandibular ramus and body to its corresponding lateral cranial cortex is greater than the distance from the left mandibular ramus and body to its

corresponding lateral cranial cortex. Tilt the patient's cranial vertex toward the left side.

16. The distance from the right mandibular ramus and body to its corresponding lateral cranial cortex is greater than the distance from the left mandibular ramus and body to its corresponding lateral cranial cortex. Tilt the patient's cranial vertex toward the left side.

Facial Bones and Sinuses: Parietoacanthial and Acanthioparietal Projection (Waters and Open-Mouth Waters Methods)

1. A. Supraorbital margin
   B. Lateral orbital margin
   C. Inferior orbital margin
   D. Zygomatic bone
   E. Zygomatic arch
   F. Coronoid process
   G. Petrous ridge
   H. Posterior maxillary process
   I. Sphenoid sinus
   J. Maxillary sinus
   K. Lateral cranial cortex
   L. Nasal septum
2. Imaginary line connecting the chin with the external ear opening
3. Sphenoid sinuses
4. Position an extended flat palm next to each lateral parietal bone, and adjust the head rotation until your hands are positioned perpendicular to the IR.
5. A. Distance from the lateral orbital margins to the lateral cranial cortices
   B. Distance from the bony nasal septum to the lateral cranial cortices
6. A. Away from
   B. Away from
7. A. Because they are placed at a longer OID for the acanthioparietal projection
   B. Acanthioparietal
8. Align the mentomeatal line perpendicular to the IR.
9. Align the cranium's midsagittal plane with the collimator's longitudinal light line.
10. A. It prevents tight collimation.
    B. It makes viewing the image more awkward.
11. A. Anterior nasal spine
    B. Acanthion
12. The frontal and maxillary (and sphenoidal with the open-mouth position) sinuses and lateral cranial cortices.
13. The patient's face was rotated toward the right side.
14. The patient's chin was not elevated enough to position the mentomeatal line perpendicular to the IR.

15. The patient's chin was elevated more than needed to align the mentomeatal line perpendicular to the IR.
16. The petrous ridges are inferior to the maxillary sinuses and posterior maxillary alveolar process, and the distance from the lateral orbital margin to the lateral cranial cortex on the left side is greater than on the right side. Tuck the patient's chin until the mentomeatal line (MML) is perpendicular to the IR, and rotate the face toward the left side until the midsagittal plane is perpendicular to the IR.
17. The petrous ridges are demonstrated within the maxillary sinuses and superior to the posterior maxillary alveolar process. Elevate the patient's chin until the MML is perpendicular to the IR or adjust the central ray angulation caudally if air-fluid levels are not being evaluated.
18. The petrous ridges are inferior to the maxillary sinuses and posterior maxillary alveolar process. Depress the patient's chin until the MML is perpendicular to the IR or adjust the central ray angulation cephalically if air-fluid levels are not being evaluated.

Optic Canal and Foramen: Parietoorbital Oblique Projection (Rhese Method)

1. A. Superior orbital margin
   B. Lateral orbital margin
   C. Optic canal and foramen
   D. Lesser sphenoid wing
   E. Medial orbital margin
2. A. On end
   B. Lower half of the orbit
   C. Lateral orbital margin
3. Imaginary line connecting the acanthion and external acoustic meatus
4. A. Acanthiomeatal line
   B. IPL
   C. Midsagittal
   D. 53-degree
5. A. Optic canal
   B. Downside orbit
6. Optic canal and foramen, lesser wing of sphenoid, and orbital margins
7. The chin is tucked more then needed to bring the AML perpendicular to the IR.
8. The patient's head was rotated less than 53 degrees.

Nasal Bones: Tangential Projection (Superoinferior Projection)

1. A. Septal cartilage
   B. Nasal bone
2. Anterior nasal spine
3. Imaginary line connecting the glabella and maxillary alveolar

4. A. Perpendicular
   B. Midsagittal
5. Glabelloalveolar line (GAL)
6. A. Nasal bones
   B. Nasion
7. Nasal bones and surrounding nasal soft tissue.
8. The patient's chin was rotated toward the right side and cranium toward the left side.
9. The patient's chin was not elevated enough to position the GAL perpendicular to the IR.

Petromastoid Portion: Axiolateral Oblique (Modified Law) Projection (Modified Law Method)

1. A. Mastoid air cell
   B. Mastoid process
   C. Internal and external acoustic meatus
   D. Mandibular condyle
2. A. Anterior
   B. 15-degree angle
3. A. Inferior
   B. Leveled
   C. Caudal
4. To prevent them from being superimposed over the mastoid air cells
5. A. Mastoid process
   B. Posterior
   C. Superior
6. Mastoid air cells, lateral portion of the petrous pyramid, and internal and external acoustic meatus
7. The face was not rotated toward the IR until the midsagittal plane was positioned at a 15-degree angle with the IR.

Petromastoid Portion: Axiolateral Oblique Projection (Stenvers Method, Posterior Profile)

1. A. Mastoid air cells
   B. Mastoid process
   C. Internal acoustic canal
   D. External acoustic canal
   E. Semicircular canal (bony labyrinth)

2. A. Profile
   B. Mandibular rami
   C. Mandibular rami
3. A. Perpendicular
   B. Leveled
   C. 45
4. A. Short, broad skull; 54 degrees
   B. Long, narrow; 40 degrees
5. Position the IOML perpendicular to the IR and place the IPL level.
6. A. IAC
   B. Bony labyrinth
   C. Cephalically
   D. Posterior
   E. External acoustic meatus
7. Mastoid air cells, petrous pyramid and ridge, bony labyrinth, tympanic cavity, and IAC
8. The patient's head was rotated more than the required amount to place the petrous pyramid parallel with the IR.
9. The patient's chin was not tucked enough to position the IOML perpendicular to the IR, or the image was obtained without the required 12-degree cephalic central ray angulation.
10. The IAC is foreshortened, the semicircular canals are not in profile and are visible anterior to the posterior margin of the mandibular rami, and the cervical vertebral column is not superimposed over the entire mandibular rami. Increase the degree of head rotation.
11. The IAC is foreshortened, the semicircular canals are not in profile and are visible posterior to the posterior margin of the mandibular rami, and the cervical column is not superimposed over the entire mandibular rami. Decrease the degree of patient head rotation.
12. The IAC and semicircular canals are obscured, and the supraorbital margin is demonstrated superior to the petrous ridge. Tuck the patient's chin toward the chest until the IOML is aligned perpendicular to the IR.
13. The IAC and semicircular canals are obscured, and the supraorbital margin is demonstrated inferior to the petrous ridge. Elevate the patient's chin away from the chest until the IOML is aligned perpendicular to the IR.

Image Analysis of the Digestive System

LEARNING OBJECTIVES   After completion of this chapter you should be able to:

_____ 1. Identify the required anatomy on upper and lower gastrointestinal images.

_____ 2. Describe how to properly position the patient, image receptor (IR), and central ray for upper and lower gastrointestinal images.

_____ 3. State how to properly mark and display upper and lower gastrointestinal images.

_____ 4. Explain the patient preparation procedure used before upper and lower gastrointestinal examinations to prevent residual debris and fluid from obscuring areas of interest.

_____ 5. List the analysis requirements for upper and lower gastrointestinal images with accurate positioning.

_____ 6. State when proper density, contrast, and penetration have been achieved for upper and lower gastrointestinal images.

_____ 7. State how to properly reposition the patient when upper and lower gastrointestinal images with poor positioning are produced.

_____ 8. Describe the differences in size, shape, and position of the stomach and abdominal cavity placement of the small and large intestinal structures among the different habitus.

_____ 9. Define the difference in the barium suspension that is ingested for upper and for lower gastrointestinal images.

_____ 10. State how a woman who has had one breast removed may have to be positioned at a greater object–image receptor distance (OID) for posteroanterior (PA) projection images.

_____ 11. Describe the differences in the appearance of the stomach on images of patients with different body habitus.

_____ 12. State where the barium and air will be situated for the different upper and lower gastrointestinal double-contrast images.

_____ 13. Explain why the small intestine is imaged at set time intervals for a small intestine study.

_____ 14. Discuss how to determine the amount of patient or central ray adjustment that is required to improve upper and lower gastrointestinal images with poor positioning.

_____ 15. State the kilovoltage, automatic exposure control (AEC) chamber, and source–image receptor distance (SID) routinely used for upper and lower gastrointestinal images, and describe what anatomical structures are visible when the correct technical factors are used.

STUDY QUESTIONS

Digestive System

1. How is the patient instructed to dress before upper and lower gastrointestinal examinations?

   _____

   _____

2. List the patient preparation procedure for the following examinations.

   A. Esophagus: _____

   _____

   B. Stomach: _____

   _____

   C. Small intestine: _____

   _____

   _____

   D. Large intestine: _____

   _____

   _____

3. Why are short exposure times needed when imaging the digestive system? _____

   _____

4. Define *peristalsis,* and state how it is recognized on stomach and large and small intestine images. _____

   _____

   _____

   _____

   _____

5. Complete Table 11-1.

TABLE 11-1   Digestive System Technical Data

Position or Projection	kVp	Grid	AEC Chamber(s)	SID
UPPER GASTROINTESTINAL SYSTEM				
PA oblique (RAO) projection, esophagus	SC=			
Lateral position, esophagus	SC=			
AP or PA projection, esophagus	SC=			
PA oblique (RAO) projection, stomach	SC= DC=			
PA projection, stomach	SC= DC=			
Right lateral position, stomach	SC= DC=			
AP oblique (LPO) projection, stomach	SC= DC=			
AP projection, stomach	SC= DC=			
SMALL INTESTINE				
PA or AP projection	SC=			
LARGE INTESTINE				
PA or AP projection	SC= DC=			
Lateral (rectum) position	SC= DC=			
AP or PA (lateral) decubitus projection	DC=			
PA oblique (RAO) projection	SC= DC=			
PA oblique (LAO) projection	SC= DC=			
PA or AP axial projection	SC= DC=			

AEC, Automatic exposure control; AP, anteroposterior; DC, double contrast; kVp, kilovolt-peak; LAO, left anterior oblique; LPO, left posterior oblique; PA, posteroanterior; RAO, right anterior oblique; SC, single contrast; SID, source–image receptor distance.

6. Complete Table 11-2.

TABLE 11-2	Image Receptor Size, Placement, and Direction	
Position or Projection	**IR Size**	**Placement and Direction**
UPPER GASTROINTESTINAL SYSTEM		
PA oblique (RAO) projection, esophagus		
Lateral position, esophagus		
AP or PA projection, esophagus		
PA oblique (RAO) projection, stomach		
PA projection, stomach		
Right lateral position, stomach		
AP oblique (LPO) projection, stomach		
AP projection, stomach		
SMALL INTESTINE		
PA or AP projection		
LARGE INTESTINE		
PA or AP projection		
Lateral (rectum) position		
AP or PA (lateral) decubitus projection		
PA oblique (RAO) projection		
PA oblique (LAO) projection		
PA or AP axial oblique (RAO) projection		

AP, Anteroposterior; *IR*, image receptor; *LAO*, left anterior oblique; *LPO*, left posterior oblique; *PA*, posteroanterior; *RAO*, right anterior oblique.

7. State the size, shape, and placement in the abdominal cavity of the stomach for the following habitus.

  A. Hypersthenic: _____

  _____

  _____

  B. Asthenic: _____

  _____

  _____

  C. Sthenic: _____

  _____

  _____

8. State the position of the lower intestine within the abdominal cavity for the following habitus.

  A. Hypersthenic: _____

  _____

  _____

B. Asthenic: _____

_____

_____

C. Sthenic: _____

_____

_____

9. How many posterior ribs are demonstrated superior to the diaphragm dome when an upper or lower gastrointestinal image is obtained after full expiration, and why is this important?

_____

UPPER GASTROINTESTINAL SYSTEM

Esophagram

1. What barium weight or volume suspension is used for esophagus images? _____

2. When might the patient be asked to swallow cotton balls soaked in barium, barium-filled gelatin capsules, or barium tablets for an esophagram?

_____

Esophagram: PA Oblique Projection (RAO Position)

3. Identify the labeled anatomy in Figure 11-1.

Figure 11–1

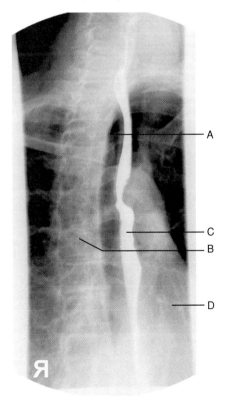

A. _____

B. _____

C. _____

D. _____

4. An adequately rotated PA oblique (RAO) esophagram image will demonstrate the esophagus between the (A) _____ and (B) _____ and approximately (C) _____ inch of the right sternal clavicular end to the left of the vertebrae and is accomplished by rotating the patient (D) _____ degrees.

5. On a PA oblique (RAO) esophagram image with accurate positioning the (A) _____ is centered within the collimated field. This centering is obtained when a perpendicular central ray is centered 3 inches to the left of the (B) _____ and (C) _____ inches inferior to the jugular notch.

6. What anatomical structures are included on a PA oblique (RAO) esophagram image with accurate positioning?

_____

For the following descriptions of PA oblique (RAO) esophagram images with poor positioning, state how the patient or central ray would have been mispositioned for such an image to be obtained.

7. The superior and inferior ends of the esophagus are not filled with barium.

_____

8. The vertebrae are superimposed over the right sternal clavicular end and a portion of the esophagus.

_____

For the following PA oblique (RAO) esophagram images with poor positioning, state what anatomical structures are misaligned and how the patient should be repositioned for an optimal image to be obtained.

Figure 11–2

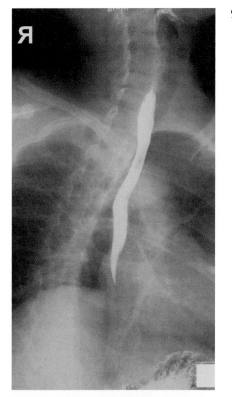

9. (Figure 11-2): _____

_____

_____

_____

Figure 11–3

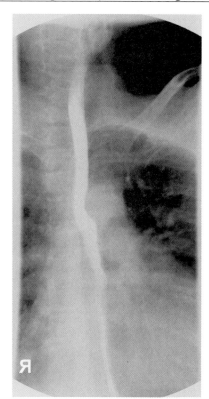

10. (Figure 11-3): _____

    _____

    _____

    _____

Esophagram: Lateral Position

1. Identify the labeled anatomy in Figure 11-4.

Figure 11–4

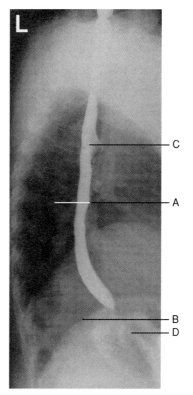

A. _____

B. _____

C. _____

D. _____

2. A lateral image of the esophagus is obtained when the esophagus is demonstrated anterior to the thoracic vertebrae, the (A) _____ surfaces of each vertebral body are superimposed and no more than (B) _____ inch of space is seen between the (C) _____.

3. How should the patient be positioned to prevent rotation on a lateral esophagram image? _____

_____

4. How are the patient's shoulders and humeri positioned to place them away from the esophagus on a lateral image? _____

_____

_____

5. On a lateral esophagram image with accurate positioning the (A) _____, at the level of (B) _____, is centered within the collimated field. This centering is obtained when a perpendicular central ray is centered 2 to 3 inches inferior to the (C) _____.

6. What anatomical structures are included on a lateral esophagram image with accurate positioning? _____

_____

For the following description of a lateral esophagram image with poor positioning, state how the patient or central ray would have been mispositioned for such an image to be obtained.

7. The posterior ribs demonstrate more than ½ inch (1.25 cm) of space between them.

_____

Esophagram: PA Projection

1. Identify the labeled anatomy in Figure 11-5.

Figure 11–5

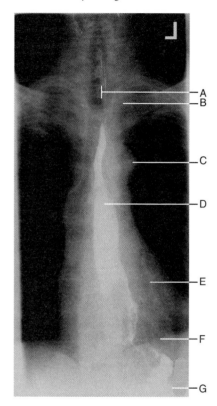

A. _____

B. _____

C. _____

D. _____

E. _____

F. _____

G. _____

2. The distances from the (A) _____ to the (B) _____ are equal, and the vertebrae are superimposed over the esophagus on a nonrotated PA esophagram image.

3. How is the patient positioned to obtain a nonrotated PA esophagram image? _____

_____

4. How should a patient who has had one breast removed be positioned differently? _____

5. On a PA esophagram image with accurate positioning the (A) _____, at the level of (B) _____, is centered within the collimated field. This centering is obtained when a perpendicular central ray is centered 2 to 3 inches superior to the (C) _____.

6. What anatomical structures are included on a lateral esophagram image with accurate positioning? _____

For the following description of a PA esophagram image with poor positioning, state how the patient or central ray would have been mispositioned for such an image to be obtained.

7. The esophagus is to the right of the vertebrae, and the right sternal clavicular end is demonstrated without vertebral column superimposition.

_____

For the following PA esophagram image with poor positioning, state what anatomical structures are misaligned and how the patient should be repositioned for an optimal image to be obtained.

Figure 11–6

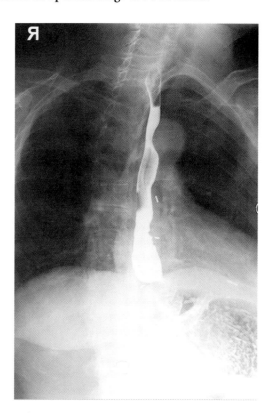

8. (Figure 11-6): _____

_____

_____

_____

STOMACH AND DUODENUM

1. What is the goal of the following upper gastrointestinal studies.

   A. Single contrast: _____

   _____

   B. Double contrast: _____

   _____

2. What barium weight or volume suspension is used for single- and double-contrast upper gastrointestinal images?

   A. Single contrast: _____

   B. Double contrast: _____

3. The negative contrast used in a double-contrast study is mostly commonly (A) _____ and is used to provide (B) _____

   _____

4. The barium in a double contrast study provides the thin coating that covers the (A) _____. How is adequate barium coating of the stomach and duodenum achieved? _____

   _____

   _____

5. List the stomach and duodenum structures that are barium filled and air filled for a double-contrast study when the patient is placed in the following positions (Table 11-3).

Stomach	Barium-Filled Structure	Air-Filled Structure
RAO position		
PA projection		
Right lateral position		
LPO position		
AP projection		

AP, Anteroposterior; LPO, left posterior oblique; PA, posteroanterior; RAO, right anterior oblique.

6. The quality of the mucosal coating depends on:

   A. _____

   B. _____

   C. _____

   D. _____

   _____

Stomach and Duodenum: PA Oblique Projection (RAO Position)

1. Identify the labeled anatomy in Figure 11-7.

Figure 11–7

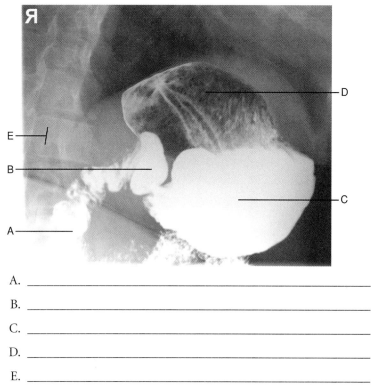

A. _____

B. _____

C. _____

D. _____

E. _____

2. Identify what body type is being represented in the PA oblique (RAO) stomach and duodenal images indicated below, and state the degree of patient obliquity required to obtain the image.

A. (Figure 11-7): _____

Figure 11–8

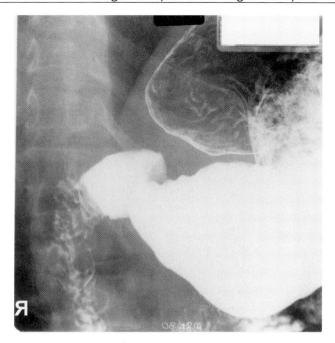

B. (Figure 11-8): _____

Figure 11–9

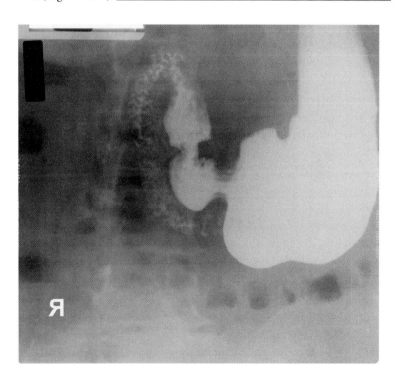

C. (Figure 11-9): _____

3. An adequately rotated hypersthenic PA oblique (RAO) stomach and duodenal image will demonstrate the left zygapophyseal joints in the (A) _____ of the vertebral body, the duodenal bulb and (B) _____ duodenum in profile, and the long axis of the stomach demonstrating foreshortening with a (C) _____ lesser curvature.

4. An adequately rotated sthenic PA oblique (RAO) stomach and duodenal image demonstrates the left zygapophyseal joints at the (A) _____ of the vertebral body, the duodenal bulb and (B) _____ duodenum in profile, and the long axis of the stomach demonstrating partial foreshortening with a closed (C) _____.

5. An adequately rotated asthenic PA oblique (RAO) stomach and duodenal image demonstrates the left zygapophyseal joints in the (A) _____ of the vertebral bodies, the duodenal bulb and (B) _____ duodenum in profile, and the long axis of the stomach demonstrated without foreshortening; the (C) _____ is open.

6. Explain why it is necessary to rotate the patient differing amounts for a PA oblique (RAO) stomach and duodenal image to demonstrate the duodenal bulb and descending duodenum in profile.

_____

_____

7. On a PA oblique (RAO) stomach and duodenal image with accurate positioning the (A) _____ is centered within the collimated field. This centering is obtained on the sthenic patient when a perpendicular central ray is centered halfway between the (B) _____ and (C) _____ of the elevated side, at a level 1 to 2 inches (2.5 to 5 cm) (D) _____ to the inferior rib margin.

8. State how the central ray position is adjusted from the sthenic patient for a PA oblique (RAO) stomach and duodenal image for the following habitus.

   A. Hypersthenic: _____

   _____

   B. Asthenic: _____

   _____

9. What anatomical structures are included on a PA oblique (RAO) stomach and duodenal image with accurate positioning?

_____

Stomach and Duodenum: PA Projection

1. Identify the labeled anatomy in Figure 11-10.

Figure 11–10

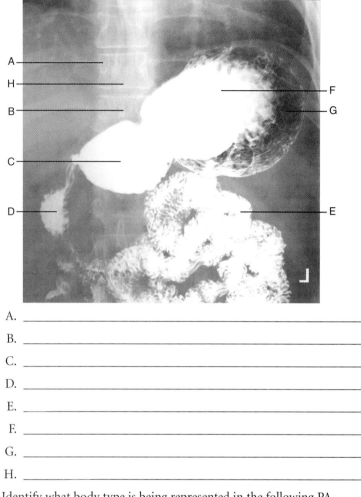

A. _____

B. _____

C. _____

D. _____

E. _____

F. _____

G. _____

H. _____

2. Identify what body type is being represented in the following PA stomach and duodenal images.

A. (Figure 11-10): _____

Figure 11–11

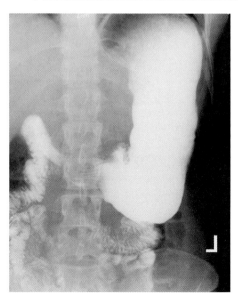

B. (Figure 11-11): _____

Figure 11–12

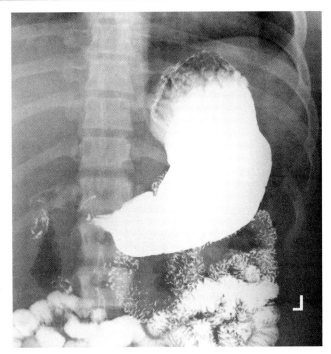

C. (Figure 11-12): _____

3. An optimal PA stomach and duodenal image has been obtained when the spinous processes are aligned with the (A) _____ of the vertebral bodies and the distances from the pedicles to the (B) _____ are equal on both sides.

4. A hypersthenic PA stomach and duodenal image will demonstrate the stomach aligned nearly (A) _____ with the duodenal bulb at the level of the (B) _____ thoracic vertebrae. The lesser and greater curvatures are demonstrated nearly on end with the greater curvature being more (C) _____ situated and the (D) _____ nearly on end.

5. A sthenic PA stomach and duodenal image will demonstrate the stomach aligned nearly (A) _____, with the duodenal bulb at the level of the (B) _____ lumbar vertebrae. The lesser and greater curvature, esophagogastric junction, pylorus, and duodenal bulb are in (C) _____.

6. An asthenic PA stomach and duodenal image will demonstrate the stomach aligned (A) _____, with the duodenal bulb at the level of the (B) _____ lumbar vertebrae. The stomach is (C) _____-shaped, and its long axis is demonstrated without foreshortening; the (D) _____, _____, _____, and _____ are in profile.

7. On a PA stomach and duodenal image with accurate positioning the (A) _____ is centered within the collimated field. For the sthenic patient this centering is obtained when a perpendicular central ray is centered halfway between the (B) _____ and (C) _____ at a point approximately 1 to 2 inches (2.5 to 5 cm) (D) _____ to the lower rib margin.

8. State how the central ray position is adjusted from the sthenic patient for a PA stomach and duodenal image for the following habitus.

   A. Hypersthenic: _____

   _____

   B. Asthenic: _____

   _____

9. What anatomical structures are included on a PA stomach and duodenal image with accurate positioning? _____

   _____

For the following descriptions of PA stomach and duodenal images with poor positioning, state how the patient or central ray would have been mispositioned for such an image to be obtained.

10. The stomach demonstrates a blotchy appearance within the barium. The stomach contains residual food particles.

   _____

11. The distance from the right pedicles to the spinous processes is greater than the distance from the left pedicles to the spinous processes.

   _____

Stomach and Duodenum: Lateral Projection (Right Lateral Position)

1. Identify the labeled anatomy in Figure 11-13.

Figure 11–13

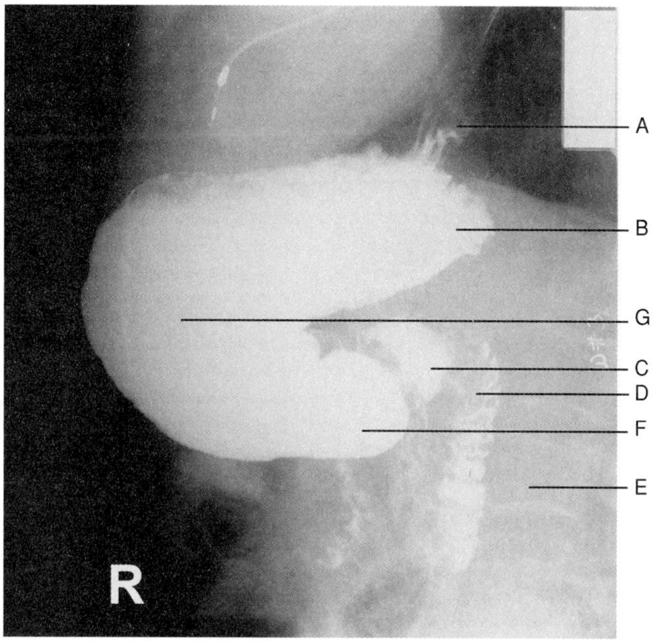

A. _____

B. _____

C. _____

D. _____

E. _____

F. _____

G. _____

2. Identify what body type is being represented in the lateral stomach and duodenal images indicated below.

A. (Figure 11-13): _____

Figure 11–14

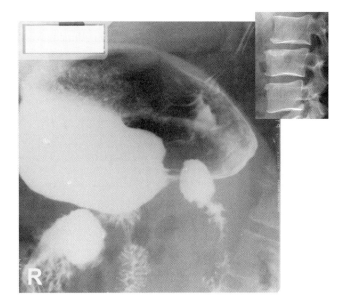

B. (Figure 11-14): _____

Figure 11–15

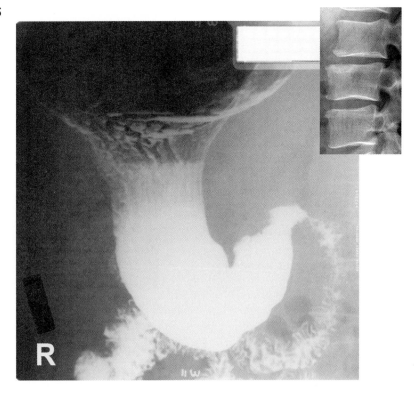

C. (Figure 11-15): _____

3. An optimal right lateral stomach and duodenal image has been obtained when the (A) _____ surfaces of the thoracic and lumbar vertebrae are superimposed and the (B) _____ space is demonstrated.

4. A hypersthenic lateral stomach and duodenal image demonstrates the (A) _____ and (B) _____ in profile, and the long axis of the stomach demonstrates foreshortening with a (C) _____ lesser curvature.

5. A sthenic lateral stomach and duodenal image demonstrates the (A) _____ and (B) _____ in profile, and the long axis of the stomach is (C) _____ foreshortened with a (D) _____ lesser curvature.

6. An asthenic lateral stomach and duodenal image demonstrates the (A) _____ and (B) _____ in profile, and the long axis of the stomach is demonstrated (C) _____ foreshortening, with an (D) _____ lesser curvature.

7. On a lateral stomach and duodenal image with accurate positioning the (A) _____ is centered within the collimated field. For the sthenic patient, this centering is obtained when a perpendicular central ray is centered halfway between the (B) _____ and (C) _____ at the level of the (D) _____.

8. State how the central ray position is adjusted from the sthenic patient for a lateral stomach and duodenal image for the following habitus.

   A. Hypersthenic: _____

   _____

   B. Asthenic: _____

   _____

9. What anatomical structures are included on a lateral stomach and duodenal image with accurate positioning? _____

   _____

For the following description of a lateral stomach and duodenal image with poor positioning, state how the patient or central ray would have been mispositioned for such an image to be obtained.

10. The descending duodenum is partially superimposed over the duodenal bulb and vertebrae, and the posterior surfaces of the thoracic and lumbar vertebrae are not superimposed.

   _____

Stomach and Duodenum: AP Oblique Projection (LPO Position)

1. Identify the labeled anatomy in Figure 11-16.

Figure 11–16

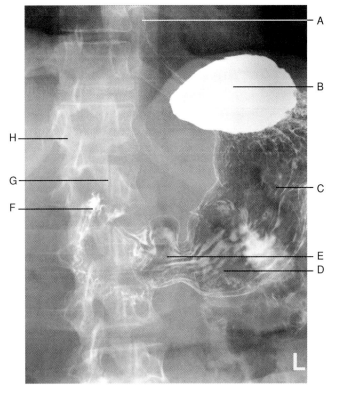

A. _____

B. _____

C. _____

D. _____

E. _____

F. _____

G. _____

H. _____

2. Identify what body type is being represented in the following AP oblique (LPO) stomach and duodenal images, and state the degree of patient obliquity required to obtain the image.

A. (Figure 11-16): _____

Figure 11–17

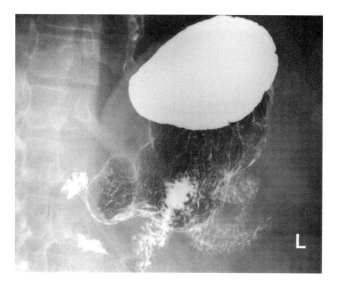

B. (Figure 11-17): _____

Figure 11–18

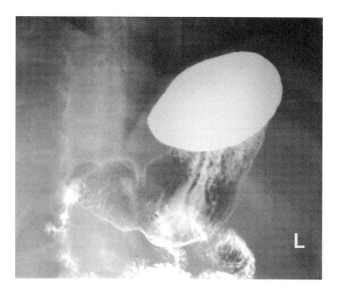

C. (Figure 11-18): _____

3. An adequately rotated hypersthenic AP oblique (LPO) stomach and duodenal image will demonstrate the left zygapophyseal joints in the (A) _____ of the vertebral body, the duodenal bulb and (B) _____ duodenum in profile, and the pylorus superimposed over the (C) _____.

4. An adequately rotated sthenic AP oblique (LPO) stomach and duodenal image demonstrates the left zygapophyseal joints at the (A) _____ of the vertebral body, the duodenal bulb and

(B) _____ duodenum in profile, and the pylorus with
(C) _____ vertebral superimposition.

5. An adequately rotated asthenic AP oblique (LPO) stomach and duodenal image demonstrates the left zygapophyseal joints in the (A) _____ of the vertebral bodies, the duodenal bulb and (B) _____ duodenum in profile, and the pylorus with (C) _____ vertebral superimposition.

6. On an AP oblique (LPO) stomach and duodenal image with accurate positioning the (A) _____ is centered within the collimated field. This centering is obtained on the sthenic patient when a perpendicular central ray is centered halfway between the (B) _____ and (C) _____, at a level (D) _____ between the xiphoid process and inferior rib margin.

7. State how the central ray position is adjusted from the sthenic patient for an AP oblique (LPO) stomach and duodenal image for the following habitus.

   A. Hypersthenic: _____

   _____

   B. Asthenic: _____

   _____

8. What anatomical structures are included on an AP oblique (LPO) stomach and duodenal image with accurate positioning?

   _____

Stomach and Duodenum: AP Projection

1. Identify the labeled anatomy in Figure 11-19.

Figure 11–19

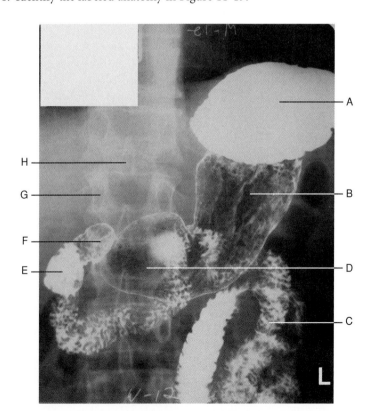

A. _____

B. _____

C. _____

D. _____

E. _____

F. _____

G. _____

H. _____

2. Identify what body type is being represented in the following AP stomach and duodenal images.

A. (Figure 11-19): _____

Figure 11–20

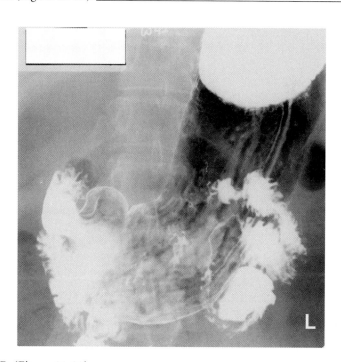

B. (Figure 11-20): _____

Figure 11-21

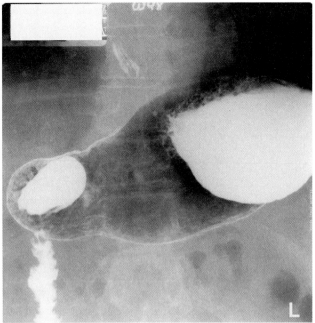

C. (Figure 11-21): _____

3. An optimal AP stomach and duodenal image has been obtained when the spinous processes are aligned with the (A) _____ of the vertebral bodies and the distances from the pedicles to the (B) _____ are equal on each side.

4. A hypersthenic AP stomach and duodenal image will demonstrate the stomach aligned nearly (A) _____ with the duodenal bulb at the level of the (B) _____ thoracic vertebrae. The lesser and greater curvatures are demonstrated nearly on end, with the greater curvature being more (C) _____ situated and the (D) _____ nearly on end.

5. A sthenic AP stomach and duodenal image will demonstrate the stomach aligned nearly (A) _____, with the duodenal bulb at the level of the (B) _____ lumbar vertebrae. The lesser and greater curvature, esophagogastric junction, pylorus, and duodenal bulb are in (C) _____.

6. An asthenic AP stomach and duodenal image will demonstrate the stomach aligned (A) _____, with the duodenal bulb at the level of the (B) _____ lumbar vertebrae. The stomach is (C) _____-shaped, and its long axis is demonstrated without foreshortening; the (D) _____ _____, _____, and _____ are in profile.

7. On an AP stomach and duodenal image with accurate positioning the (A) _____ is centered within the collimated field. For the sthenic patient this centering is obtained when a perpendicular central ray is centered halfway between the (B) _____ and (C) _____ at a level (D) _____ between the xiphoid process and inferior rib margin.

8. State how the central ray position is adjusted from the sthenic patient for an AP stomach and duodenal image for the following habitus.

A. Hypersthenic: _____

_____

B. Asthenic: _____

_____

9. What anatomical structures are included on an AP stomach and duodenal image with accurate positioning? _____

_____

For the following description of an AP stomach and duodenal image with poor positioning, state how the patient or central ray would have been mispositioned for such an image to be obtained.

10. The distance from the left pedicles to the spinous processes is greater than the distance from the right pedicles to the spinous processes.

_____

_____

SMALL INTESTINE

Small Intestine: PA Projection

1. Identify the labeled anatomy in Figure 11-22.

Figure 11–22

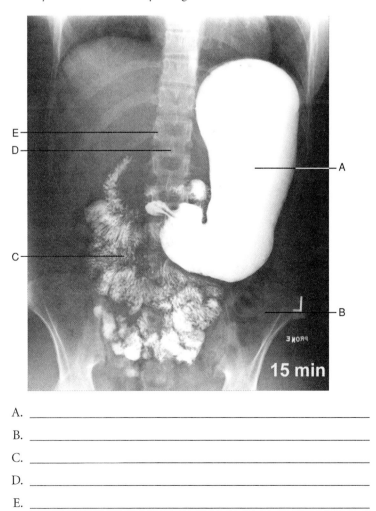

A. _____

B. _____

C. _____

D. _____

E. _____

2. How are PA small intestine images marked?

_____

_____

3. What is the typical timing sequence for a small intestine series?

_____

4. A nonrotated PA small intestine image demonstrates the spinous processes aligned with the (A) _____ and symmetrical (B) _____.

5. Why is the prone position chosen over the supine position for the small intestine series?

_____

6. Compare Figures 11-23 and 11-24. State which image was taken earlier in the series, and explain how you know this.

Figure 11–23

Figure 11–24

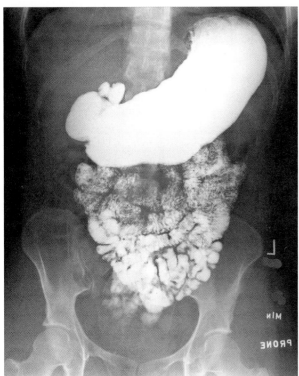

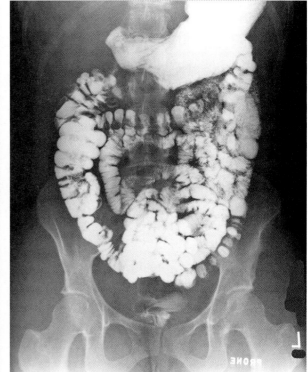

_____

_____

_____

_____

7. Figure 11-25 demonstrates the latest image that was taken in a small bowel series. Based on this image, should the patient wait longer and have another image obtained? Why or why not?

Figure 11–25

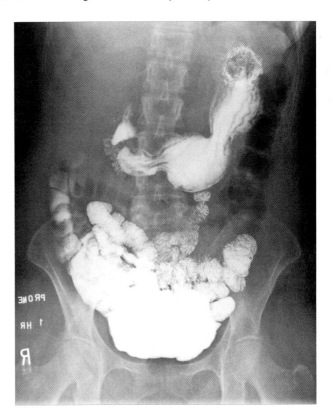

_____

_____

_____

_____

8. On a PA small intestine image with accurate positioning the (A) _____ is centered within the collimated field. Early in the series a perpendicular central ray is centered to the (B) _____ at a level 2 inches (5 cm) (C) _____ to the iliac crest. Later in the series the central ray is centered at the level of the (D) _____.

9. State why the central ray is centered in different locations when an image is obtained early versus late in the series.

_____

_____

10. What anatomical structures are included on an AP stomach and duodenal image with accurate positioning? _____

_____

_____

LARGE INTESTINE

1. Optimal double-contrast coating has been obtained when the lumina are distended, without (A) _____, the mucosal surface demonstrates a thin coating of barium, and barium pooling is limited to (B) _____.

2. What is the purpose of the barium pool? _____

_____

3. State whether air or barium will be within the indicated structure for the positions listed in Table 11-4.

Table 11-4

Large Intestine	Supine Position	Prone Position
Cecum		
Ascending colon		
Ascending limb right colic (hepatic) flexure		
Descending limb right colic (hepatic) flexure		
Transverse colon		
Ascending limb left colic (splenic) flexure		
Descending limb left colic (splenic) flexure		
Descending colon		
Sigmoid colon		
Rectum		

4. How is poor gaseous distension identified on a large intestine image?

_____

_____

5. How is poor barium coating identified on a large intestine image?

_____

_____

Large Intestine: PA or AP Projection

6. Identify the labeled anatomy in Figure 11-26.

Figure 11–26

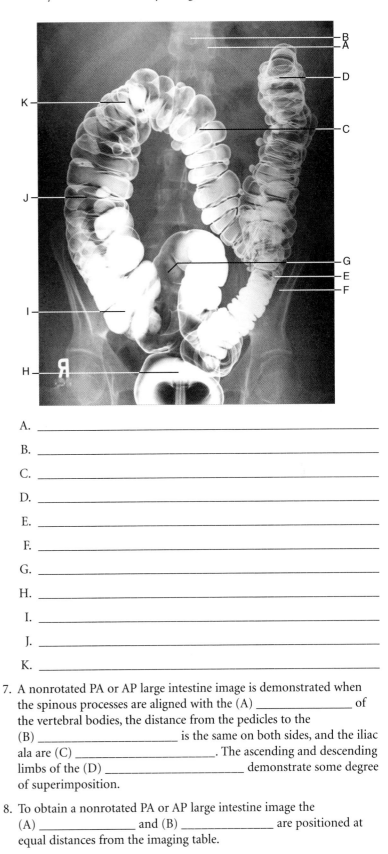

A. _____

B. _____

C. _____

D. _____

E. _____

F. _____

G. _____

H. _____

I. _____

J. _____

K. _____

7. A nonrotated PA or AP large intestine image is demonstrated when the spinous processes are aligned with the (A) _____ of the vertebral bodies, the distance from the pedicles to the (B) _____ is the same on both sides, and the iliac ala are (C) _____. The ascending and descending limbs of the (D) _____ demonstrate some degree of superimposition.

8. To obtain a nonrotated PA or AP large intestine image the (A) _____ and (B) _____ are positioned at equal distances from the imaging table.

9. The side demonstrating the greater distance from the pedicles to the spinous processes, wider iliac ala, and colic flexure with the greater ascending and descending limb superimposition is the side positioned _____ from the IR on a rotated PA large intestine image.

10. The iliac ala on an AP large intestine image are _____ (wider/narrower) than on a PA image.

11. On an AP or PA large intestine image with accurate positioning the (A) _____ is centered within the collimated field. This centering is obtained by centering a perpendicular central ray with the patient's (B) _____ plane at the level of the (C) _____ for a PA large intestine image obtained with a 14-× 17-inch lengthwise IR.

12. For an AP or PA large intestine image obtained on a hypersthenic patient when two 14-× 17-inch IRs are used, the first image is obtained with the central ray centered to the (A) _____ at a level halfway between the (B) _____ and (C) _____ for the lower image.

13. What anatomical structures are included on an AP or PA large intestine image with accurate positioning? _____ _____

14. Compare the images in Figures 11-27 and 11-28. State the projection used to obtain each image, and explain how you know this.

Figure 11–27

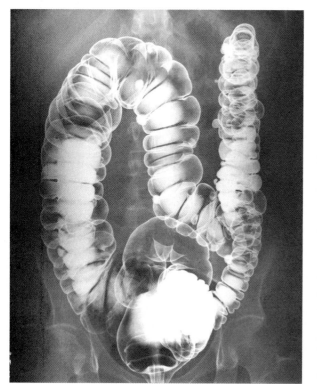

Figure 11–28

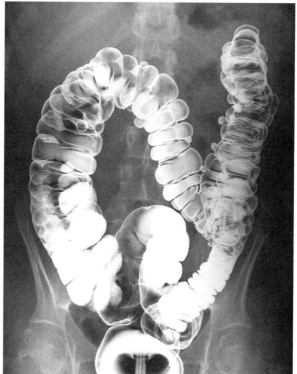

_____
_____
_____
_____

For the following descriptions of AP or PA large intestine images with poor positioning, state how the patient or central ray would have been mispositioned for such an image to be obtained.

15. AP projection: The right iliac ala is narrow and the left wide, the distance from the right pedicles to the spinous processes is narrower than the same distance on the left side, and the left colic (splenic) flexure demonstrates greater ascending and descending limb superimposition.

_____

16. PA projection: The left colic (splenic) flexure and part of the transverse colon are not included on the image.

_____

_____

_____

For the following AP or PA large intestine images with poor positioning, state what anatomical structures are misaligned and how the patient should be repositioned for an optimal image to be obtained.

Figure 11–29

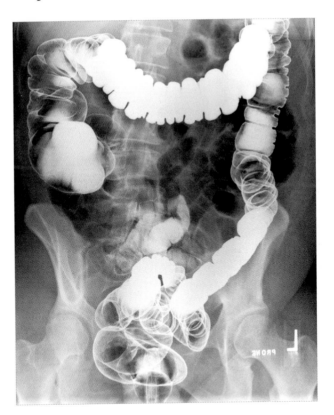

17. (Figure 11-29): _____

_____

_____

_____

Figure 11–30

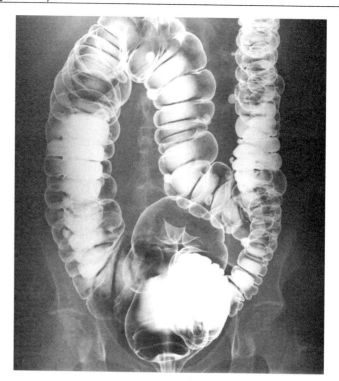

18. (Figure 11-30): _____

_____

_____

_____

Large Intestine (Rectum): Lateral Position

1. Identify the labeled anatomy in Figure 11-31.

Figure 11–31

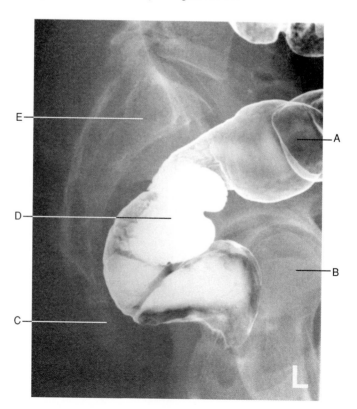

A. _____

B. _____

C. _____

D. _____

E. _____

2. How is scatter radiation controlled for a lateral large intestine (rectum) image?

_____

3. A lateral rectum image with accurate positioning is demonstrated when the sacral medium sacral crest is in (A) _____ and the (B) _____ are superimposed.

4. On a lateral rectum image with accurate positioning the (A) _____ is centered within the collimated field. This centering is obtained by centering a perpendicular central ray with the patient's (B) _____ plane at the level of the (C) _____.

5. What anatomical structures are included on a lateral rectum image with accurate positioning? _____

_____

For the following description of a lateral rectum image with poor positioning, state how the patient or central ray would have been mispositioned for such an image to be obtained.

6. The femoral heads are not superimposed; the right femoral head is rotated anterior to the left femoral head.

_____

For the following lateral rectum images with poor positioning, state what anatomical structures are misaligned and how the patient should be repositioned for an optimal image to be obtained.

Figure 11–32

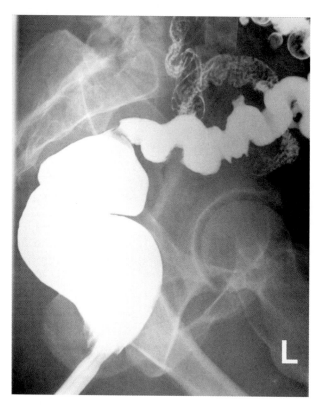

7. (Figure 11-32): _____

_____

_____

_____

Figure 11–33

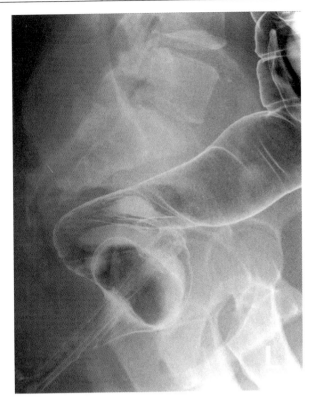

8. (Figure 11-33): _____

_____

_____

_____

Large Intestine: Lateral Decubitus Position (AP or PA Projection)

1. Identify the labeled anatomy in Figure 11-34.

Figure 11–34

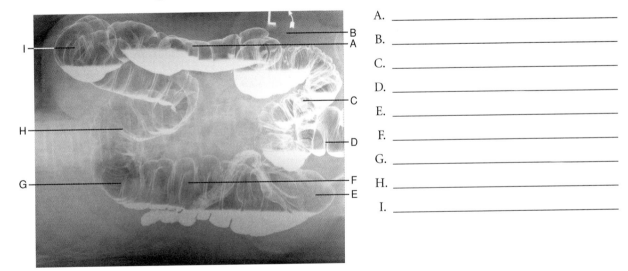

A. _____

B. _____

C. _____

D. _____

E. _____

F. _____

G. _____

H. _____

I. _____

2. How is uniform density obtained across the abdomen when imaging a patient with excessive abdominal soft tissue that drops toward the imaging table for a decubitus large intestine image?

_____

_____

_____

3. A nonrotated AP decubitus image is obtained when the spinous processes are aligned with the midline of the (A) _____, the distances from the pedicles to the (B) _____ are the same on both sides, and the (C) _____ are symmetrical.

4. The side demonstrating the smaller distance from the pedicles to the spinous processes, narrower iliac ala, and colic flexure with less ascending and descending limb superimposition is the side positioned _____ from the IR on a rotated AP decubitus large intestine image.

5. The iliac ala on a PA large intestine image are _____ (wider/narrower) than on an AP image.

6. Why is the patient elevated on a radiolucent sponge or hard surface for a decubitus large intestine image? _____

_____

7. On a decubitus large intestine image with accurate positioning the (A) _____ is centered within the collimated field. This centering is obtained by centering a perpendicular central ray with the patient's (B) _____ plane at the level of the (C) _____.

8. For a decubitus large intestine image of a hypersthenic patient in which two 14-× 17-inch IRs are used, the first image is obtained with the central ray centered to the (A) _____ plane at a level halfway between the (B) _____ and (C) _____ for the lower image.

9. What anatomical structures are included on a decubitus large intestine image with accurate positioning? _____

_____

For the following descriptions of decubitus large intestine images with poor positioning, state how the patient or central ray would have been mispositioned for such an image to be obtained.

10. Artifact lines are superimposed over the left lateral abdominal region.

_____

11. The distances from the right pedicles to the spinous processes are less than the distances from the left pedicles to the spinous processes, the right iliac ala is narrower than the left, and the ascending and descending limbs of the left colic (splenic) flexure demonstrates increased superimposition.

_____

For the following decubitus large intestine images with poor positioning, state what anatomical structures are misaligned and how the patient should be repositioned for an optimal image to be obtained.

Figure 11–35

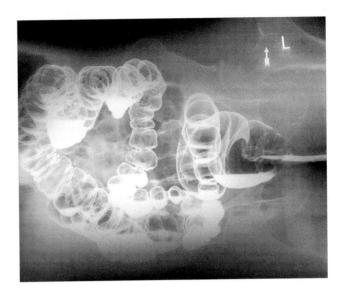

12. (Figure 11-35, AP projection): _____

_____

_____

_____

Figure 11–36

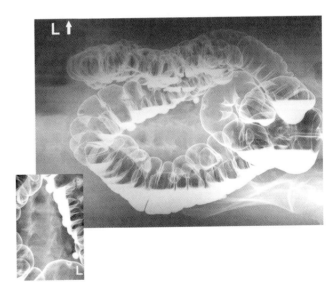

13. (Figure 11-36, AP projection): _____

_____

_____

_____

Figure 11–37

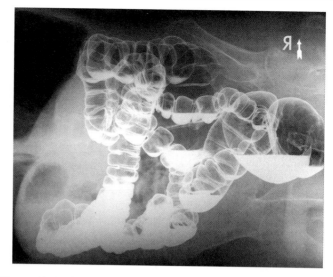

14. (Figure 11-37, PA projection): _____

_____

_____

_____

Large Intestine: PA Oblique Projection (RAO Position)

1. Identify the labeled anatomy in Figure 11-38.

Figure 11–38

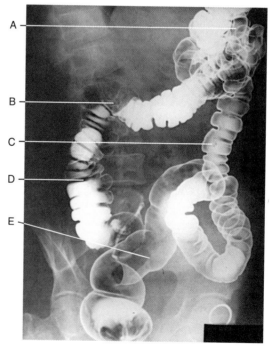

A. _____

B. _____

C. _____

D. _____

E. _____

2. A PA oblique (RAO) large intestine image with accurate positioning demonstrates decreased ascending and descending limb superimposition of the (A) _____ when compared with the PA projection, whereas the limbs of the (B) _____ demonstrate increased superimposition. The (C) _____ (right/left) iliac ala is narrower than the opposite ala.

3. To obtain an accurate PA oblique (RAO) large intestine image, position the midcoronal plane (A) _____ degrees with the IR. Rotating the patient toward the right side moves the (B) _____ (ascending/descending) right colic (hepatic) flexure from beneath the (C) _____ (ascending/descending) right colic flexure and the distal sigmoid from beneath the (D) _____.

4. On a PA oblique (RAO) large intestine image with accurate positioning the (A) _____ is centered within the collimated field. This centering is obtained by centering a perpendicular central ray approximately 1 to 2 inches (2.5 to 5 cm) to the (B) _____ (right/left) of the midsagittal plane at the level of the (C) _____.

5. What anatomical structures are included on a PA oblique (RAO) large intestine image with accurate positioning?

_____

For the following description of a PA oblique (RAO) large intestine image with poor positioning, state how the patient or central ray would have been mispositioned for such an image to be obtained.

6. The ascending and descending limbs of the right colic (hepatic) flexure and the rectum and distal sigmoid, respectively, demonstrate increased superimposition. The iliac ala are uniform in width.

_____

Large Intestine: PA Oblique Projection (LAO Position)

1. Identify the labeled anatomy in Figure 11-39.

Figure 11–39

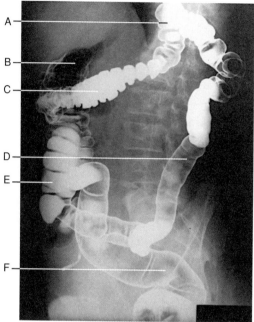

A. _____

B. _____

C. _____

D. _____

E. _____

F. _____

2. The ascending and descending limbs of the (A) _____ (right/left) colic flexure are demonstrated with decreased superimposition when compared with the PA projection and the (B) _____ (right/left) iliac ala is narrower on a PA oblique (LAO) large intestine image with accurate positioning.

3. To obtain an accurate PA oblique (LAO) large intestine image position the midcoronal plane (A) _____ degrees with the IR. Rotating the patient toward the left side moves the (B) _____ (ascending/descending) left colic (hepatic) flexure from beneath the (C) _____ (ascending/descending) left colic flexure.

4. On a PA oblique (LAO) large intestine image with accurate positioning the (A) _____ is centered within the collimated field. This centering is obtained by centering a perpendicular central ray approximately 1 to 2 inches (2.5 to 5 cm) to the (B) _____ (right/left) of the midsagittal plane at the level 1 to 2 inches (2.5 to 5 cm) superior to the (C) _____.

5. What anatomical structures are included on a PA oblique (LAO) large intestine image with accurate positioning?

_____

Large Intestine: PA Axial Oblique (RAO) or PA Axial Projections (Butterfly Positions)

1. Identify the labeled anatomy in Figure 11-40.

Figure 11-40

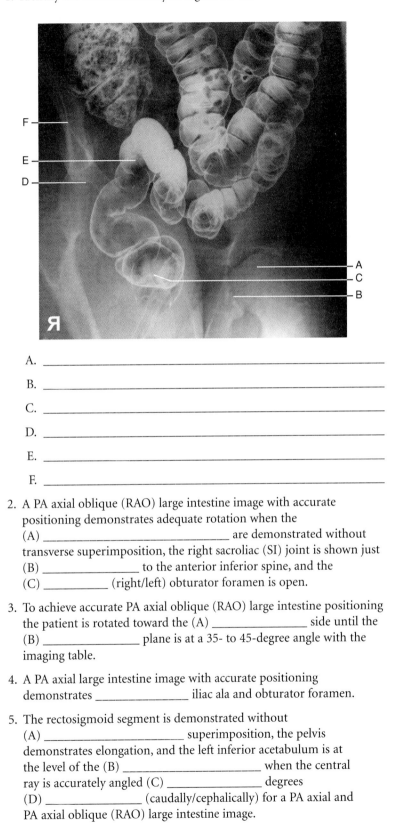

A. _____

B. _____

C. _____

D. _____

E. _____

F. _____

2. A PA axial oblique (RAO) large intestine image with accurate positioning demonstrates adequate rotation when the (A) _____ are demonstrated without transverse superimposition, the right sacroliac (SI) joint is shown just (B) _____ to the anterior inferior spine, and the (C) _____ (right/left) obturator foramen is open.

3. To achieve accurate PA axial oblique (RAO) large intestine positioning the patient is rotated toward the (A) _____ side until the (B) _____ plane is at a 35- to 45-degree angle with the imaging table.

4. A PA axial large intestine image with accurate positioning demonstrates _____ iliac ala and obturator foramen.

5. The rectosigmoid segment is demonstrated without (A) _____ superimposition, the pelvis demonstrates elongation, and the left inferior acetabulum is at the level of the (B) _____ when the central ray is accurately angled (C) _____ degrees (D) _____ (caudally/cephalically) for a PA axial and PA axial oblique (RAO) large intestine image.

6. On a PA axial and PA axial oblique (RAO) large intestine image with accurate positioning the (A) _____ is centered within the collimated field. This centering is obtained for a PA axial image by centering to exit at the level of the (B) _____ and midsagittal plane. This centering is obtained for a PA axial oblique (RAO) image by centering the central ray to exit at the (C) _____ and 2 inches (5 cm) to the (D) _____ (right/left) of the spinous processes.

7. What anatomical structures are included on a PA axial and PA axial oblique large intestine image with accurate positioning?

_____

For the following descriptions of PA axial oblique (RAO) large intestine images with poor positioning, state how the patient or central ray would have been mispositioned for such an image to be obtained.

8. The right SI joint is obscured, and the left obturator foramen is closed.

_____

9. The inferior aspect of the left acetabulum is demonstrated superior to the distal rectum.

_____

For the following PA axial oblique (RAO) large intestine images with poor positioning, state what anatomical structures are misaligned and how the patient should be repositioned for an optimal image to be obtained.

Figure 11–41

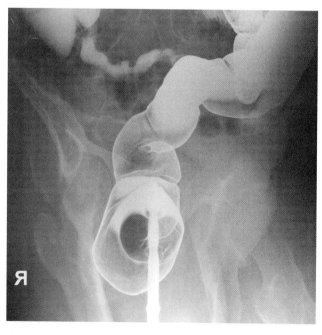

10. (Figure 11-41): _____

_____

_____

_____

Figure 11–42

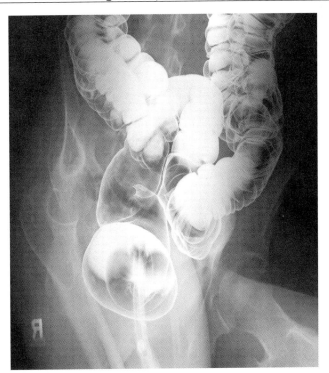

11. (Figure 11-42): _____

_____

_____

_____

CHAPTER 11

STUDY QUESTION ANSWERS

1. The patient is instructed to remove outer clothing and any underclothes containing artifacts, then to change into a snapless hospital gown.
2. A. No preparation procedure is required
   B. Nothing by mouth (NPO) after midnight or at least 8 hours before the examination, and avoid gum and tobacco products before procedure
   C. Low-residue diet for 1 to 2 days before the examination, NPO after midnight or at least 8 hours before the examination, and avoid gum and tobacco products before the examination
   D. Low residue diet for 2 to 3 days before the examination, followed by a clear liquid diet 1 day before the examination, laxatives the afternoon before the examination, and a suppository or cleaning enema the morning of the examination
3. Short exposure times are needed to control the image blur that may result from peristaltic activity within the system.
4. Peristalsis is the contraction and relaxation movement of the smooth muscles in the walls of the digestive system that mixes food and secretions and moves the materials through the system. Peristalsis is identified on an image by sharp bony cortices and blurry gastric and intestine gases or barium.

5. Table 11-1

Position or Projection	kVp	Grid	AEC Chamber(s)	SID
UPPER GASTROINTESTINAL SYSTEM				
PA oblique (RAO) projection, esophagus	SC=100-110	Grid	Center	40-48 inches (100-120 cm)
Lateral position, esophagus	SC=100-110	Grid	Center	40-48 inches (100-120 cm)
AP or PA projection, esophagus	SC=100-110	Grid	Center	40-48 inches (100-120 cm)
PA oblique (RAO) projection, stomach	SC=100-110 DC=80-90	Grid	Center	40-48 inches (100-120 cm)
PA projection, stomach	SC=100-110 DC=80-90	Grid	Center	40-48 inches (100-120 cm)
Right lateral position, stomach	SC=100-110 DC=80-90	Grid	Center	40-48 inches (100-120 cm)
AP oblique (LPO) projection, stomach	SC=100-110 DC=80-90	Grid	Center	40-48 inches (100-120 cm)
AP projection, stomach	SC=100-110 DC=80-90	Grid	Center	40-48 inches (100-120 cm)
SMALL INTESTINE				
PA or AP projection	SC=100-125	Grid	All three	40-48 inches (100-120 cm)
LARGE INTESTINE				
PA or AP projection	SC=100-125 DC=80-90	Grid	All three	40-48 inches (100-120 cm)
Lateral (rectum) position	SC=100-125 DC=80-90	Grid	Center	40-48 inches (100-120 cm)
AP or PA (lateral) decubitus projection	DC=80-90	Grid	All three	40-48 inches (100-120 cm)
PA oblique (RAO) projection	SC=100-125 DC=80-90	Grid	All three	40-48 inches (100-120 cm)
PA oblique (LAO) projection	SC=100-125 DC=80-90	Grid	All three	40-48 inches (100-120 cm)
PA or AP axial projection	SC=100-125 DC=80-90	Grid	All three	40-48 inches (100-120 cm)

AEC, Automatic; *AP,* anteroposterior; *DC,* double contrast, *kVp,* kilovolt-peak; *LAO,* left anterior oblique; *LPO,* left posterior oblique; *PA,* posteroanterior; *RAO,* right anterior oblique; *SC,* single contrast, *SID,* source–image receptor distance.

6. Table 11-2

Position or Projection	IR Size	Placement and Direction
UPPER GASTROINTESTINAL SYSTEM		
PA oblique (RAO) projection, esophagus	14 × 17 inches (35 × 43 cm)	Lengthwise
Lateral position, esophagus	14 × 17 inches (35 × 43 cm)	Lengthwise
AP or PA projection, esophagus	14 × 17 inches (35 × 43 cm)	Lengthwise
PA oblique (RAO) projection, stomach	11 × 14 inches (28 × 35 cm)	Lengthwise
PA projection, stomach	11 × 14 inches (28 × 35 cm)	Lengthwise
Right lateral position, stomach	11 × 14 inches (28 × 35 cm)	Lengthwise
AP oblique (LPO) projection, stomach	11 × 14 inches (28 × 35 cm)	Lengthwise
AP projection, stomach	11 × 14 inches (28 × 35 cm)	Lengthwise
SMALL INTESTINE		
PA or AP projection	14 × 17 inches (35 × 43 cm)	Lengthwise (to patient)—sthenic and asthenic (up to 14 cm width) Crosswise—Hypersthenic, sthenic, and asthenic (over 14 cm width)
LARGE INTESTINE		
PA or AP projection	14 × 17 inches (35 × 43 cm)	Lengthwise (to patient)—sthenic and asthenic (up to 14 cm width) Crosswise—Hypersthenic, sthenic, and asthenic (over 14 cm width)
Lateral (rectum) position	10 × 12 inches (24 × 30 cm)	Lengthwise
AP or PA (lateral) decubitus projection	14 × 17 inches (35 × 43 cm)	Lengthwise (to patient)—sthenic and asthenic (up to 14 cm width) Crosswise—Hypersthenic, sthenic, and asthenic (over 14 cm width)
PA oblique (RAO) projection	14 × 17 inches (35 × 43 cm)	Lengthwise
PA oblique (LAO) projection	14 × 17 inches (35 × 43 cm)	Lengthwise
PA or AP axial oblique (RAO) projection	11 × 14 inches (28 × 35 cm) or 14 × 17 inches (35 × 43 cm)	Lengthwise

AP, Anteroposterior; *IR,* image receptor; *LAO,* left anterior oblique; *LPO,* left posterior oblique; *PA,* posteroanterior; *RAO,* right anterior oblique.

7. A. Hypersthenic: Abdomen is broad and deep from anterior to posterior, the stomach is positioned high in the abdomen and lies transversely at the level of T9 to T12, and the duodenal bulb is demonstrated at the level of T11 to T12.
   B. Asthenic: Abdomen is narrow, and the stomach is positioned low in the abdomen and runs vertically along the left side of the vertebral column, typically extending from T11 to L5, with the duodenal bulb at the level of L3 to L4.
   C. Sthenic: Abdomen is less broad than in the hypersthenic habitus and less narrow than in the asthenic habitus. The stomach also rests at a position between that in the hypersthenic and asthenic habitus and typically extends from T10 to L2, with the duodenal bulb at the level of L1 to L2.
8. A. Hypersthenic: The colic flexures and transverse colon tend to be high in the abdomen.
   B. Asthenic: The small and large intestine structures tend to be positioned low in the abdomen.
   C. Sthenic: The small and large intestine structures tend to be centered within the abdomen.
9. Ninth posterior rib. Full expiration allows increased abdominal space for the structures to be visualized without segment overlapping or foreshortening.

UPPER GASTROINTESTINAL SYSTEM

Esophagram

1. 30% to 50%
2. When foreign bodies and strictures of the esophagus are suspected

Esophagram: PA Oblique Projection (RAO Position)

3. A. Left sternal clavicular end
   B. Vertebrae

C. Esophagus
D. Heart
4. A. Vertebrae
   B. Heart shadow
   C. ½
   D. 35 to 40
5. A. Midesophagus
   B. Spinous process
   C. 2 to 3
6. Entire esophagus
7. The patient did not swallow enough barium before and/or during the examination.
8. The patient was rotated less than the required 35 to 40 degrees.
9. The superior and inferior ends of the esophagus are not filled with barium. The patient should drink barium continuously during the exposure or should swallow two spoonfuls of thick barium and then given a third spoonful that is swallowed directly before the exposure is taken.
10. The vertebrae are superimposed over the right sternal clavicular end and a portion of the esophagus. Increase the degree of patient obliquity until the midcoronal plane is at a 35- to 40-degree angle with the imaging table.

Esophagram: Lateral Position

1. A. Vertebrae
   B. Left hemidiaphragm
   C. Esophagus
   D. Stomach
2. A. Posterior
   B. ½
   C. Posterior ribs
3. Align the posterior shoulders, ribs, and pelvis perpendicular to the imaging table.
4. Place the humeri at a 90-degree angle with the torso, or separate the shoulders by positioning the arm and shoulder placed closer to the imaging table back while maintaining a lateral thorax.
5. A. Midesophagus
   B. T5 to T6
   C. Jugular notch
6. Entire esophagus
7. The patient's elevated side was rotated posteriorly.

Esophagram: PA Projection

1. A. Vertebrae
   B. Left sternal clavicular end
   C. Aortic arch
   D. Esophagus
   E. Heart
   F. Left hemidiaphragm
   G. Stomach

2. A. Vertebral column
   B. Sternal ends
3. Position the shoulders and anterosuperior iliac spines (ASISs) at equal distances from the imaging table.
4. Position the side of the patient with the breast removed at a greater OID than the opposite side.
5. A. Midesophagus
   B. T5 to T6
   C. Inferior scapular angle
6. Entire esophagus
7. The patient was rotated toward the left side.
8. The esophagus is to the left of the vertebrae, and the left sternal clavicular end is demonstrated without vertebral column superimposition. Position the left shoulder toward the imaging table until the shoulders are at equal distances from the IR.

STOMACH AND DUODENUM

1. A. To demonstrate abnormalities of the stomach and lumen contour
   B. To visualize abnormalities in the mucosal details, and contour and lumen of stomach and duodenum
2. A. 30% to 50 %
   B. 250%
3. A. Carbon dioxide
   B. Gastric distention and a smoothing of the rugae.
4. A. Mucosal surface
   B. Barium is washed over the gastric surface by having the patient turn 360 degrees and then positioning the patient so the barium pool will be positioned away from the area of interest.
5. Table 11-3

Stomach	Barium-Filled Structure	Air-Filled Structure
RAO position	Pylorus, duodenum	Fundus
PA projection	Pylorus, duodenum	Fundus
Right lateral position	Pylorus, duodenum, body	Fundus
LPO position	Fundus	Pylorus, duodenum
AP projection	Fundus	Pylorus, duodenum, body

AP, Anteroposterior; LPO, left posterior oblique; PA, posteroanterior; RAO, right anterior oblique.

6. A. Properties of the barium suspension
   B. Volume of barium and gas
   C. Frequency of washing
   D. Amount of fluid or secretions and viscosity of mucus in the stomach

Stomach and Duodenum: PA Oblique Projection (RAO Position)

1. A. Descending duodenum
   B. Duodenal bulb
   C. Pylorus
   D. Fundus
   E. Zygapophyseal joint
2. A. Hypersthenic; 70 degrees
   B. Sthenic; 45 degree
   C. Asthenic; 40 degrees
3. A. Posterior third
   B. Descending
   C. Closed
4. A. Midline
   B. Descending
   C. Lesser curvature
5. A. Anterior third
   B. Descending
   C. Lesser curvature
6. Because of the difference in the amount of superimposition of the pylorus and duodenal bulb that exists among the patients with different habitus.
7. A. Pylorus
   B. Vertebrae
   C. Lateral rib margin
   D. Superior
8. A. Center the central ray at a level 1 inch superior to the sthenic centering.
   B. Center the central ray at a level 2 inches inferior to the sthenic centering.
9. Stomach and duodenal loop

Stomach and Duodenum: PA Projection

1. A. Pedicle
   B. Spinous process
   C. Pylorus
   D. Descending duodenum
   E. Small intestine
   F. Body
   G. Fundus
   H. Tenth
2. A. Hypersthenic
   B. Asthenic
   C. Sthenic
3. A. Midline
   B. Spinous processes
4. A. Horizontally
   B. Eleventh to twelfth
   C. Anteriorly
   D. Esophagogastric junction
5. A. Horizontally
   B. First two second
   C. Partial profile

6. A. Vertically
   B. Third to fourth
   C. J
   D. Lesser and greater curvatures, esophagogastric junction, pylorus, and duodenal bulb
7. A. Pylorus
   B. Vertebrae
   C. Left lateral rib border
   D. Superior
8. A. Direct the central ray just to the left of the vertebrae at a level 2 inches superior to the sthenic centering point.
   B. Direct the central ray 2 inches inferior to the sthenic habitus centering point.
9. Stomach and descending duodenum
10. The patient was did not follow adequate preparation procedures.
11. The patient was rotated toward the left side.

Stomach and Duodenum: Lateral Projection (Right Lateral Position)

1. A. Esophagus
   B. Fundus
   C. Duodenal bulb
   D. Descending duodenum
   E. Lumbar vertebra
   F. Pylorus
   G. Body
2. A. Sthenic
   B. Hypersthenic
   C. Asthenic
3. A. Posterior
   B. Retrogastric space
4. A. Duodenal bulb
   B. Descending duodenum
   C. Closed
5. A. Duodenal bulb
   B. Descending duodenum
   C. Partially
   D. Partially closed
6. A. Duodenal bulb
   B. Descending duodenum
   C. Without
   D. Open
7. A. Pylorus
   B. Midcoronal plane
   C. Anterior abdomen
   D. Inferior rib margin
8. A. Direct the central ray at a level 2 inches superior to the sthenic habitus centering point.
   B. Direct the central ray at a level 2 inches inferior to the sthenic habitus centering point.
9. Stomach and duodenal loop.
10. The patient was not in a lateral position but was rotated.

Stomach and Duodenum: AP Oblique Projection (LPO Position)

1. A. Esophagus
   B. Fundus
   C. Body
   D. Pylorus
   E. Duodenal bulb
   F. Descending duodenum
   G. Zygapophyseal joint
   H. Twelfth thoracic vortebra
2. A. Asthenic; 30 degrees
   B. Sthenic; 45 degrees
   C. Hypersthenic; 60 degrees
3. A. Posterior third
   B. Descending
   C. Vertebrae
4. A. Midline
   B. Descending
   C. Little if any
5. A. Anterior third
   B. Descending
   C. Little if any
6. A. Pylorus
   B. Vertebrae
   C. Left abdominal margin
   D. Midway
7. A. Center the central ray at a level 2 inches superior to the sthenic habitus central ray centering.
   B. Center the central ray at a level 2 inches inferior to the sthenic habitus central ray centering.
8. Stomach and duodenal loop

Stomach and Duodenum: AP Projection

1. A. Fundus
   B. Body
   C. Small intestine
   D. Pylorus
   E. Descending duodenum
   F. Duodenal bulb
   G. Pedicle
   H. Spinous process
2. A. Sthenic
   B. Asthenic
   C. Hypersthenic
3. A. Midline
   B. Spinous processes
4. A. Horizontally
   B. Eleventh to twelfth
   C. Anteriorly
   D. Esophagogastric junction

5. A. Vertically
   B. First to second
   C. Profile
6. A. Vertically
   B. Third to fourth
   C. J
   D. Lesser and greater curvatures, esophagogastric junction, pylorus, duodenal bulb
7. A. Pylorus
   B. Vertebrae
   C. Left abdominal margin
   D. Midway
8. A. Center just to the left side of the vertebrae at a level 2 inches superior to the sthenic central ray centering.
   B. Center at a level 2 inches inferior to the sthenic central ray centering.
9. Stomach and duodenal loop

SMALL INTESTINE

Small Intestine: PA Projection

1. A. Stomach
   B. Left iliac ala
   C. Small intestine
   D. Spinous process
   E. Pedicle
2. With a right or left marker positioned laterally on the correct side and a time marker indicating the amount of time that has elapsed since the patient ingested the contrast.
3. First overhead is taken at 15 minutes, then 30 minutes, then hourly until barium is demonstrated in the cecum.
4. A. Midline of the vertebral bodies
   B. Iliac ala
5. It will cause compression of the abdominal structures, increasing image quality.
6. The image in Figure 11-23 was taken earlier in the series than Figure 11-24. Figure 11-23 demonstrates more barium in the stomach, the central ray was centered above crest, and the barium has not reached as far into the colon when compared with Figure 11-24.
7. Barium is demonstrated in the cecum, which typically indicates the series is complete.
8. A. Small intestine
   B. Midsagittal plane
   C. Superior
   D. Iliac crest
9. The barium is in the stomach and upper small intestine directly after ingestion but moves to the lower small intestine later.
10. The stomach and proximal aspects of the small intestine on images taken early in the series, and

the small intestine and cecum on images taken late in the series

2. To wash away residual fecal material from the dependent surface, coat the mucosal surface, and fill any depressed lesions as the patient is rotated

LARGE INTESTINE

1. A. Mucosal folds
   B. One third of the intestinal diameter
3. Table 11-4

Large Intestine	Supine Position	Prone Position
Cecum	Air	Barium
Ascending colon	Barium	Air
Ascending limb right colic (hepatic) flexure	Barium	Air
Descending limb right colic (hepatic) flexure	Barium	Air
Transverse colon	Air	Barium
Ascending limb left colic (splenic) flexure	Air	Barium
Descending limb left colic (splenic) flexure	Barium	Air
Descending colon	Barium	Air
Sigmoid colon	Air	Barium
Rectum	Barium	Air

4. Poor gaseous distension results in pockets of large barium pools and compacted intestinal segments with tight mucosal folds.
5. Poor mucosal coating is demonstrated by thin, irregular, or interrupted barium coating or excessive barium pooling.

Large Intestine: PA or AP Projection

6. A. Pedicle
   B. Spinous process
   C. Transverse colon
   D. Left colic flexion
   E. Descending colon
   F. Iliac ala
   G. Sigmoid colon
   H. Rectum
   I. Cecum
   J. Ascending colon
   K. Right colic flexure
7. A. Midline
   B. Spinous processes
   C. Symmetrical
   D. Colic flexures
8. A. Shoulders
   B. ASISs
9. Farther
10. Wider
11. A. Fourth lumbar vertebra
    B. Midsagittal
    C. Iliac crest
12. A. Midsagittal plane
    B. Symphysis pubis
    C. ASIS

13. Entire large intestine, to include left colic (splenic) flexure and rectum
14. Figure 11-27 is an AP projection, and Figure 11-28 is a PA projection. The iliac alae are wider in Figure 11-27 than in Figure 11-28.
15. The patient was rotated toward the left side.
16. The central ray and IR were centered too low, or two crosswise IRs should have been used to include all of the structures.
17. The right iliac ala is narrow and the left wide, the distance from the right pedicles to the spinous processes is narrower than the corresponding distance on the left side, and the left colic (splenic) flexure demonstrates more ascending and descending limb superimposition. Rotate the patient toward the left side until the shoulders and iliac alae are equal distances to the imaging table.
18. The left colic (splenic) flexure and part of the transverse colon are not included on the image. Use two crosswise IRs with 2 to 3 inches of overlap.

Large Intestine (Rectum): Lateral Position

1. A. Sigmoid
   B. Femoral heads
   C. Coccyx
   D. Rectum
   E. Sacrum
2. A lead sheet is placed on the imaging table at the edge of the posterior collimation field.
3. A. Profile
   B. Femoral heads

4. A. Rectosigmoid region
   B. Midcoronal plane
   C. ASIS
5. Rectum, distal sigmoid, sacrum, and femoral heads
6. The patient's right side was rotated anteriorly.
7. The femoral heads are not superimposed; the right femoral head is rotated anterior to the left femoral head. Rotate the right side of the patient posteriorly until the posterior pelvic wings are superimposed and aligned perpendicular to the imaging table.
8. The femoral heads are not superimposed; the right femoral head is rotated posterior to the left femoral head. Rotate the right side of the patient anteriorly until the posterior pelvic wings are superimposed and aligned perpendicular to the imaging table.

Large Intestine: Lateral Decubitus Position (AP or PA Projection)

1. A. Descending colon
   B. Iliac ala
   C. Sigmoid
   D. Rectum
   E. Cecum
   F. Ascending colon
   G. Right colic flexure
   H. Transverse colon
   I. Left colic flexure
2. Attach a wedge-compensating filter to the x-ray collimator head with the thick end positioned toward the patient's "up" side (thinnest part of abdomen) and the thin end toward the patient's "down" side (thickest part of abdomen).
3. A. Vertebral bodies
   B. Spinous processes
   C. Iliac ala
4. Farther
5. Narrower
6. To prevent the lateral abdomen, adjacent to the cart or imaging table, from being clipped or covered with artifact lines
7. A. Fourth lumbar vertebra
   B. Midsagittal
   C. Iliac crest
8. A. Midsagittal
   B. Symphysis pubis
   C. ASIS
9. Entire large intestine, including the left colic (splenic) flexure and rectum
10. The patient was not elevated on a cardiac board or radiolucent sponge.
11. The patient's right side was positioned farther from the IR than the left side.
12. A decrease in density is present across the entire image, and grid artifact lines are demonstrated

longitudinally. Align the grid so it is perpendicular to the central ray.
13. This is an AP projection (the marker is correct). The distance from the right pedicles to the spinous processes is less than the distances from the left pedicles to the spinous processes, the left iliac ala is wider than the right, and the left colic (splenic) flexure demonstrates increased superimposition. Rotate the left side of the patient away from the IR until the shoulders and ASISs are at equal distances from the IR.
14. This is a PA projection (the marker is reversed). The distance from the right iliac ala is narrower than the left. Rotate the right side of the patient away from the IR until the shoulders and ASISs are at equal distances from the IR.

Large Intestine: PA Oblique Projection (RAO Positions)

1. A. Left colic flexure
   B. Right colic flexure
   C. Descending colon
   D. Ascending colon
   E. Sigmoid
2. A. Right colic (hepatic) flexure
   B. Left colic (splenic) flexure
   C. Right
3. A. 35 to 45
   B. Ascending
   C. Descending
   D. Rectum
4. A. Midabdomen
   B. Left
   C. Iliac crest
5. Entire large intestine
6. The patient was insufficiently rotated.

Large Intestine: PA Oblique Projection (LAO Position)

1. A. Left colic flexure
   B. Right colic flexure
   C. Transverse colon
   D. Descending colon
   E. Ascending colon
   F. Sigmoid
2. A. Left
   B. Left
3. A. 35 to 45
   B. Descending
   C. Ascending
4. A. Midabdomen
   B. Right
   C. Iliac crest
5. Entire large intestine

Large Intestine: PA Axial Oblique (RAO) or PA Axial Projections (Butterfly Positions)

1. A. Femoral head
   B. Inferior acetabulum
   C. Rectum
   D. Right superior acetabulum
   E. Sigmoid colon
   F. ASIS
2. A. Rectosigmoid segment
   B. Medial
   C. Left
3. A. Right
   B. Midcoronal
4. Symmetrical
5. A. Inferosuperior
   B. Distal rectum
   C. 30 to 40
   D. Caudally
6. A. Rectosigmoid segment
   B. ASIS
   C. ASIS
   D. Left
7. Rectum, sigmoid, and pelvic structures
8. The pelvis was rotated more than 45 degrees.
9. The central ray was insufficient.
10. The right SI joint is obscured, and the left obturator foramen is closed. The inferior aspect of the left acetabulum is demonstrated superior to the distal rectum. Decrease pelvic rotation until the midcoronal plane is at a 30- to 45-degree angle with the imaging table, and increase the degree of central ray angulation.
11. The right SI joint is obscured, and the left obturator foramen is closed. The inferior aspect of the left acetabulum is demonstrated inferior to the distal rectum. Decrease pelvic rotation until the midcoronal plane is at a 30- to 45-degree angle with the imaging table, and decrease the degree of central ray angulation.